The Central Nervous System in Pediatric Critical Illness and Injury

Derek S. Wheeler, Hector R. Wong, and Thomas P. Shanley (Eds.)

The Central Nervous System in Pediatric Critical Illness and Injury

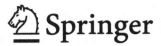 Springer

Editors

Derek S. Wheeler, MD
Assistant Professor of Clinical Pediatrics
University of Cincinnati College of Medicine
Division of Critical Care Medicine
Cincinnati Children's Hospital Medical Center
Cincinnati, OH, USA

Hector R. Wong, MD
Professor of Pediatrics
University of Cincinnati College of Medicine
Director, Division of Critical Care Medicine
Cincinnati Children's Hospital Medical Center
Cincinnati, OH, USA

Thomas P. Shanley, MD
Ferrantino Professor of Pediatrics and
   Communicable Diseases
University of Michigan Medical Center
Director, Division of Critical Care Medicine
C.S. Mott Children's Hospital
Ann Arbor, MI, USA

ISBN 978-1-84800-992-9   e-ISBN 978-1-84800-993-6
DOI 10.1007/978-1-84800-993-6

British Library Cataloguing in Publication Data
A catalogue record for this book is available from the British Library

Library of Congress Control Number: 2008940282

Springer Science+Business Media
springer.com

Preface

Neurologic emergencies are a common reason for admission to the pediatric intensive care unit (PICU). A thorough understanding of the diseases and disorders affecting the pediatric central nervous system is vital for any physician or healthcare provider working in the PICU. In the following pages, an international panel of experts provides an in-depth discussion on the resuscitation, stabilization, and ongoing care of the critically ill or injured child with central nervous system dysfunction. Once again, we would like to dedicate this textbook to our families and to the physicians and nurses who provide steadfast care every day in pediatric intensive care units across the globe.

Derek S. Wheeler
Hector R. Wong
Thomas P. Shanley

Preface to *Pediatric Critical Care Medicine: Basic Science and Clinical Evidence*

The field of critical care medicine is growing at a tremendous pace, and tremendous advances in the understanding of critical illness have been realized in the last decade. My family has directly benefited from some of the technological and scientific advances made in the care of critically ill children. My son Ryan was born during my third year of medical school. By some peculiar happenstance, I was nearing completion of a 4-week rotation in the newborn intensive care unit (NICU). The head of the pediatrics clerkship was kind enough to let me have a few days off around the time of the delivery—my wife, Cathy, was 2 weeks past her due date and had been scheduled for elective induction. Ryan was delivered through thick meconium-stained amniotic fluid and developed breathing difficulty shortly after delivery. His breathing worsened over the next few hours, so he was placed on the ventilator. I will never forget the feelings of utter helplessness my wife and I felt as the NICU transport team wheeled Ryan away in the transport isolette. The transport physician, one of my supervising third-year pediatrics residents during my rotation the past month, told me that Ryan was more than likely going to require extracorporeal membrane oxygenation (ECMO). I knew enough about ECMO at that time to know that I should be scared! The next 4 days were some of the most difficult moments I have ever experienced as a parent, watching the blood being pumped out of my tiny son's body through the membrane oxygenator and roller pump, slowly back into his body (Figures 1 and 2). I remember the fear of each day when we would be told of the results of his daily head ultrasound, looking for evidence of intracranial hemorrhage, and then the relief when we were told that there was no bleeding. I remember the hope and excitement on the day Ryan came off ECMO, as well as the concern when he had to be sent home on supplemental oxygen. Today,

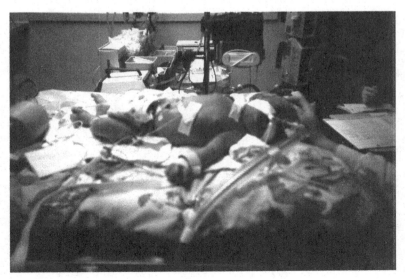

FIGURE 1

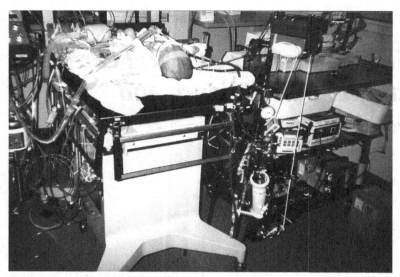

FIGURE 2

Ryan is happy, healthy, and strong. We are thankful to all the doctors, nurses, respiratory therapists, and ECMO specialists who cared for Ryan and made him well. We still keep in touch with many of them. Without the technological advances and medical breakthroughs made in the fields of neonatal intensive care and pediatric critical care medicine, things very well could have been much different. I made a promise to myself long ago that I would dedicate the rest of my professional career to advancing the field of pediatric critical care medicine as payment for the gifts with which we, my wife and I, have been truly blessed. It is my sincere hope that this textbook, which has truly been a labor of joy, will educate a whole new generation of critical care professionals and in so doing help make that first step toward keeping my promise.

Derek S. Wheeler

Contents

Contributors

Stephen Ashwal, MD
Professor of Pediatrics
Loma Linda University School of Medicine
Division of Child Neurology
Loma Linda University Children's Hospital
Loma Linda, CA, USA

Brenda L. Banwell, MD, FRPCP
Assistant Professor of Pediatrics
University of Toronto School of Medicine
Director, Pediatric Multiple Sclerosis Clinic
Associate Scientist, Research Institute
Division of Neurology
The Hospital for Sick Children
Toronto, Ontario, Canada

Raymond C. Barfield, MD, PhD
Division of Bone Marrow Transplantation
St. Jude Children's Research Hospital
Memphis, TN, USA

Michael J. Bell, MD
Associate Professor Pediatrics, Critical Care
  Medicine and Anesthesiology
Department of Critical Care Medicine
Investigator, Center for Neuroscience
  Research
Children's Research Institute
Children's National Medical Center
Washington, DC, USA

Taeun Chang, MD
Clinical Instructor
George Washington University Medical Center
Division of Neurology
Children's National Medical Center
Washington, DC, USA

Richard F.M. Chin, MRCPCH
Clinical Research Fellow in Paediatric
  Neuroscience
Institute of Child Health, University College
  London
London, UK

Dermot R. Doherty, MD, BCh, FCARCSI
Faculty of Medicine, University of Ottawa
Departments of Anaesthesia and
  Critical Care
Children's Hospital of Eastern Ontario
Ottawa, Ontario, Canada

Ann-Christine Duhaime, MD
Professor of Neurosurgery,
  Dartmouth Medical School
Program Director, Pediatric Neurosurgery
Children's Hospital at Dartmouth
Dartmouth-Hitchcock Medical Center
Lebanon, NH, USA

Amar Gajjar, MD
Director, Neuro-oncology
St. Jude Children's Research Hospital
Memphis, TN, USA

Cecil D. Hahn, MD, FRCPC
Fellow in Pediatric Neurocritical Care
  and Epilepsy
Department of Neurology
Harvard Medical School
Children's Hospital Boston
Boston, MA, USA

James S. Hutchison, MD, FRCPC
Director of Education
Department of Critical Care Medicine
Hospital for Sick Children
Hospital for Sick Children
  Research Institute
Toronto, Ontario, Canada

Steven G. Kernie, MD
Assistant Professor of Pediatrics and
  Developmental Biology
UT Southwestern Medical Center
Division of Pediatric Critical
  Care Medicine
Children's Medical Center
Dallas, TX, USA

Mark R. Lee, MD, PhD
Associate Professor of Neurosurgery
Medical College of Georgia
Allen Distinguished Chair in Neurosurgery
MCG Children's Medical Center
Augusta, GA, USA

Samuel M. Lehman, MD
UT Southwestern Medical Center
Division of Pediatric Critical
    Care Medicine
Children's Medical Center
Dallas, TX, USA

Eng H. Lo, PhD
Harvard Medical School
Neurosciences Center
Massachusetts General Hospital
    for Children
Boston, MA, USA

Darlene A. Lobel, MD
Department of Neurosurgery
Medical College of Georgia
Augusta, GA, USA

Josephine Lok, MD
Harvard Medical School
Pediatric Critical Care Medicine and
    Neurosciences Center
Massachusetts General Hospital
    for Children
Boston, MA, USA

Kathleen L. Meert, MD, FCCM
Professor of Pediatrics
Wayne State University School of Medicine
Division of Pediatric Critical
    Care Medicine
Children's Hospital of Michigan
Detroit, MI, USA

David J.J. Michelson, MD
Department of Pediatrics
Loma Linda University School of Medicine
Division of Child Neurology
Loma Linda University Children's Hospital
Loma Linda, CA, USA

Simon Nadel, MBBS, FRCP, MRCPCH
Consultant in Paediatric Intensive Care
St. Mary's Hospital
London, UK

Natan Noviski, MD
Harvard Medical School

Chief, Division of Critical Care Medicine
Massachusetts General Hospital for Children
Boston, MA, USA

Ashok P. Sarnaik, MD
Professor of Pediatrics
Wayne State University School of Medicine
Associate Pediatrician-in-Chief
Co-Chief, Division of Critical Care Medicine
Children's Hospital of Michigan
Detroit, MI, USA

Rod C. Scott, PhD, MRCPCH
Senior Lecturer in Paediatric Neuroscience
    and Honorary Consultant Paediatric
    Neurologist
Institute of Child Health
Great Ormond Street Hospital NHS Trust and
    The National Centre for Young People with
    Epilepsy (NCYPE)
London, UK

Robert Tamburro, MD
Associate Professor of Pediatrics
University of Tennessee Health Sciences
    Center–Memphis
Division of Critical Care Medicine
LeBonheur Children's Medical Center
St Jude Children's Research Hospital
Memphis, TN, USA

Robert C. Tasker, MD, FRCP
University Senior Lecturer in Pediatrics
School of Clinical Medicine
University of Cambridge
Addenbrooke NHS Trust
Cambridge, UK

Michael J. Whalen, MD
Assistant Professor of Paediatrics
Harvard Medical School
Pediatric Critical Care Medicine and
    Neurosciences Center
MassGeneral Hospital for Children
Boston, MA, USA

Phoebe Yager, MD
Assistant Professor of Pediatrics
Harvard Medical School
Pediatric Critical Care Medicine and
    Neurosciences Center
MassGeneral Hospital for Children
Boston, MA, USA

1

Central Nervous System Monitoring

Michael J. Bell and Taeun Chang

Introduction

The overall goal of monitoring the brains of critically ill children is to detect injurious processes at a time when they can be corrected. An ideal monitor of the central nervous system (CNS) function would have several properties. The theoretical monitor would be available at the bedside for minute-to-minute use. It would gather data through noninvasive means, posing no risk to the patient while deriving substantial benefits. The technology would be simple enough for widespread use, and it would be inexpensive. The data derived would have a high degree of reliability and would predict periods of injury in a timely manner so interventions could be implemented. Unfortunately, such a monitor does not exist at the present time. Instead, a number of monitoring systems can be used, and the most commonly used techniques are described below (Table 1.1).

Physical Examination

The most fundamental method to monitor the CNS of critically ill children is by consistent, repetitive physical examinations performed by caregivers. Observation of changes in cranial nerve function, muscular tone, strength, sensation, and levels of consciousness can be performed virtually continuously without undue harm to the child. Regular and frequent bedside assessment can definitively diagnose an evolving process (such as a new stroke or evolving encephalopathy) or can indicate the need for more definitive testing. Detection of new neurologic abnormalities is dependent on the experience of the examiner, the care in which the examination is performed, and the training of bedside caregivers.

A standardized tool to assess neurologic function in critically ill children is the Glasgow Coma Scale (GCS) score (Table 1.2) [1]. Initially developed to assess adults after traumatic brain injury,

this simple scale can provide a rapid, objective assessment of a child's level of consciousness (as measured by eye opening, verbal responses, and motor responses) that is reproducible between caregivers [2]. Modifications of the GCS for preverbal children have been proposed, but none has been rigorously validated. The GCS is an effective predictor of neurologic outcome of traumatically injured adults, but its predictive value in children has not been validated. This may be a result of poor reporting of the GCS by caregivers in children. In the stabilization of traumatically injured adults or children, the GCS can be used to track significant neurologic deterioration. As an example, a decrease of more than 3 points in the scale is indicative of a significant clinical change warranting further investigation according to published guidelines [3]. Its utility as a quantitative, repeatable assessment of mental status is clear and serves a valuable function as a neurologic screening tool.

Intracranial Pressure Monitoring

Measurement and management of abnormal increases in intracranial pressure (ICP) have been a mainstay of medical care of children and adults for decades [4]. Monitoring ICP after traumatic brain injury in adults became common practice decades ago and this technology was translated into childhood trauma as well as metabolic diseases, particularly Reye's syndrome [5–7]. The two scientific rationales for using this monitoring system are (1) prevention of cerebral herniation and (2) prevention of secondary injuries related to decreased brain perfusion. It is obvious to all that detecting an acute rise in ICP can presage a herniation event, leading to initiation of therapies to mitigate this process. It is also obvious that herniation must be prevented in order for neurologic recovery to occur. Prevention of secondary injuries caused by increased ICP is a more nebulous goal. Because up to 80% of autopsy specimens from patients with traumatic brain injury demonstrate significant ischemic lesions [8], it has been theorized that episodes of increased ICP represent periods of decreased brain perfusion. Early studies by Gopinath and colleagues demonstrated that episodes of ICP greater than 20 mm Hg correlated with poor neurologic outcome in adults after traumatic brain injury [9]. Currently, there is an ongoing debate regarding treatment of ICP versus maintenance of cerebral perfusion pressure (the difference between mean arterial pressure and ICP) [10].

D.S. Wheeler et al. (eds.), *The Central Nervous System in Pediatric Critical Illness and Injury*,
DOI 10.1007/978-1-84800-993-6_1, © Springer-Verlag London Limited 2009

TABLE 1.1. Comparisons of clinically available neuromonitors.

Monitor	Physiologic process measured	Sampling area	Advantages	Disadvantages
Intracranial pressure monitor	Intracerebral pressure	Global without localization	Bedside, reliable, therapeutic (intraventricular)	Invasive
Electroencephalogram	Cerebral activity and metabolism	Global with localization	Bedside, noninvasive, continuous data gathering available	Expertise required
Evoked potentials	Localized cerebral activity after applied stimuli	Global with localization	Bedside, noninvasive	Expertise required
Xenon techniques	Cerebral blood flow	Global with localization	Bedside (xenon-133 only), noninvasive, reliable	Patient transport required (xenon-CT), infrastructure costly, specialized instruments
Transcranial Doppler ultrasonography	Cerebral blood flow velocity of specified arteries	Regional	Bedside, noninvasive	Expertise required
Jugular venous oxygen saturation	Cerebral metabolism	Global without localization	Bedside, ideally reflects blood flow to metabolic demands	Invasive, thrombosis, infection, questionable reliability
Near-infrared spectroscopy	Cerebral oxygenation	Regional	Bedside, noninvasive, continuous data gathering	Reliability, standards unclear
Brain tissue oxygen tension	Cerebral oxygenation	Focal	Bedside, continuous data gathering	Invasive, threshold unclear
Cerebral microdialysis	Selected metabolites	Focal	Bedside, continuous data gathering, choice of metabolites for study	Invasive, thresholds unclear
Magnetic resonance spectroscopy	Cerebral metabolism	Focal with many areas available for sampling	Noninvasive, no radiation exposure	Patient transport required, limited number of samples to compare

Measuring ICP can be accomplished using monitors in a variety of locations [11]. Currently, ICP monitors are placed either in the brain parenchyma or in the ventricular space. Parenchymal monitors are easy to place (requiring only a reflection of the dura) and are believed to carry a decreased risk for infection. However, intraparenchymal monitors cannot be recalibrated, and first-generation intraparenchymal monitors were found to have significant drift [12]. Newer intraparenchymal monitors have corrected this problem. The advantages of intraventricular monitors are the ability to withdraw cerebrospinal fluid (CSF) as a therapy for increased ICP and the ease of recalibration, which can be accomplished using the same techniques as any intravascular catheter. Intraventricular monitors may be more technically challenging to place (especially when significant cerebral swelling has already occurred) and there have been anecdotal reports of an increased infection risk, although no systematic reviews of this complication are available at the time of the writing of this chapter. In selecting monitor location, we believe that intraventricular monitors should

be strongly considered when intracranial hypertension is likely to develop and when the procedure is technically feasible. Regardless, both locations accurately reflect ICP and can be used reliably to implement treatment strategies.

Electrophysiologic Monitoring

Electrophysiologic monitoring in the ICU has become more common over the last decade with portable digital systems. The various monitoring systems outlined below can serve any of four vital functions (detection of epileptiform activity; monitoring of cerebral metabolic rate as evidenced by depth of sedation or drug-induced coma; early detection of neurologic deterioration as in hypoxic–ischemic processes or herniation; prognostication of overall clinical outcome) in critically ill children. In general, electrophysiologic monitors have similar strengths and weaknesses. All of the monitors discussed below are noninvasive, can be used effectively at the patient's bedside, and can be used serially to follow interval changes in the child's condition. However, most of the monitors require relatively advanced training in interpretation (all except for the Bispectral index monitor) and can be adversely affected by the relatively hostile electrical environment within the ICU. Nevertheless, electrophysiologic monitoring is a mainstay in the care of children with critical neurologic disorders.

Bispectral Index Monitoring

Because most critically ill children require sedation for procedures (mechanical ventilation, in particular), an objective assessment of the depth of sedation is critical. Several physical examination scores (the COMFORT score, the Ramsey scale) have been used, but a more objective measure of sedation depth has been sought [13–15]. The bispectral (BIS) index is derived from two surface electroencephalographic (EEG) electrodes placed over the frontal cortex and generates numerical values that correlate with levels of

TABLE 1.2. The Glasgow Coma Scale.

Eye opening	4 = Spontaneously
	3 = To command
	2 = To painful stimuli
	1 = Closed
Verbal response	5 = Clear and appropriate words
	4 = Comprehensible words, but not appropriate to situation
	3 = Unintelligible words
	2 = Sounds in response to painful stimuli
	1 = No sounds
Motor response	6 = Obeys verbal commands
	5 = Localizes to a painful stimulus
	4 = Withdraws to pain but does not localize response
	3 = Abnormal flexion movements
	2 = Abnormal extension movements
	1 = No movements

sedation from a wide variety of anesthetics (0 = isoelectric, 100 = fully awake). The mathematical computations from the EEG signal used to generate the BIS index involve artifact filtering, suppression detection, fast Fourier transformation, and estimation of signal quality. Intraoperative studies have demonstrated that adequate anesthesia, as assessed by movement at incision, correlates well with BIS values <60 [16] and that BIS values of 40–60 are typical during maintenance of general anesthesia [17].

Most relevant to pediatric intensivists, studies suggest that amnesia reliably occurs at BIS values <64–80 [18]. Ideally, sedative medications could be administered to critically ill children and titrated to given BIS scores to maintain an adequate, but not overdose, of medication. At present, several small series have attempted to correlate BIS values with both clinical sedation scores and signs of drug withdrawal [13–15,19]. The correlations have been relatively weak, and, because of this, the BIS monitor has not yet become standard at this time. A final limitation of the BIS monitoring system is that the transformations of brain electrical activity assume the child has a relatively normal EEG. Therefore, its applicability in children with evolving or persistent brain injuries is questionable at this time.

Electroencephalography

Electroencephalograms are surface tracings of the brain's electrical activity. Traces are generated by measuring amplified electrical potential differences between two electrodes (represented as an EEG channel) placed in designated locations on the child's skull using the International 10–20 system (sometimes with modifications). Typically, 16 or 32 EEG channels are recorded in a variety of montages (which can be now be retrospectively montaged with digital machines). Rhythmicity, amplitude, and location of waveforms are determined and can be indicative of normal or abnormal function of the relevant brain regions. For instance, alpha waves of 8 to 13 Hz over the posterior portions of the head occur during wakefulness, whereas waves of frequencies over 13 Hz (designated as beta activity) can be seen with common intensive care unit (ICU) medications (i.e., benzodiazepines, phenytoin, and barbiturates). Young children have greater amounts of theta activity (frequencies of 4 to 7 Hz), but focal or lateralized theta activity is indicative of localizing CNS pathology. Overall, much can be gleaned from careful interpretation of EEG. However, more detailed examination of these waves is beyond the scope of this chapter.

Electroencephalograms can be performed as a single routine examination (rEEG) or as a continuous recording (cEEG). Provocative stimuli or commands (eye opening and closing, loud auditory stimuli, induced hyperventilation, photic stimuli) are routinely used in rEEG to elicit characteristic wave changes or epileptic events. With the advent of digital monitors to record and sometimes interpret data, cEEG has become more commonplace in neurologic intensive care [20]. The detection of status epilepticus is one of the most common indications for EEG monitoring in the PICU. Jordan applied continuous EEG to 124 consecutive neuro-ICU patients and recorded seizures in 35%, of which 76% were nonconvulsive epileptic seizures [21]. Continuous EEG is commonly used to monitor the depth of drug-induced coma in children because the duration of burst suppression is highly correlative with tissue concentrations of these agents. In adults, cEEG has also been used to detect impending cerebral ischemia caused by vasospasm after subarachnoid hemorrhage, a less common complication in children. Potential indications for continuous EEG monitoring include

severe head injury with GCS less than 13, elevated ICP, use of paralytic agents, early or partial seizures, use of hypothermia, treatment of refractory status epilepticus, coma of unknown etiology, and global brain ischemia [22–25].

Electroencephalographic monitoring is noninvasive and provides immediate bedside data. Limitations to EEG monitoring include the requirement for trained staff for lead placement, the necessity of frequent expert interpretation of waveforms, and the difficulties in obtaining clear signals in an artifact abundant environment. However, EEG monitoring is a mainstay of neurologic monitoring, and advances in technology will likely lead to an increased use of these monitors in the future.

Quantitative and Amplitude-Integrated EEG

Continuous trending of quantitative measures of EEG allows for compression of information, ability to trend data, and display long epochs of data. Three measures have been examined: total power trending, compressed spectral array (CSA), and amplitude-integrated EEG (aEEG). The compressed spectral array method displays a pseudo-three-dimensional image of the temporal evolution of the EEG frequency distribution and relative amplitude [26]. A fast Fourier transform analysis of the EEG generates a frequency spectrum for a given epoch of time. Serial epochs are then displayed behind each other, giving a three-dimensional appearance. The pattern of frequencies over time suggests different states (i.e., predominantly low frequencies suggesting sedation or coma and predominantly high frequencies suggesting seizures).

The first aEEG monitor was developed in the 1960s by Maynard and termed the *cerebral function monitor* (CFM) [26,27]. It allowed for the trending of EEG amplitude over extended time periods on a logarithmic scale. Patterns of amplitude changes were shown to correlate with cerebral states (burst suppression, seizures). The presence of only a single recording channel in CFM gives certain advantages over cEEG or CSA. It allows for greater ease of use in ICUs and less dependency on expert technical assistance for lead placement, a limitation for many ICUs in obtaining immediate EEG monitoring. Subsequent monitors have added a second recording channel to discern hemispheric differences. In conjunction, an rEEG is recommended for comprehensive and confirmatory study as artifacts can mimic real activity. Evolution of these technologies will allow expansion of the role of EEG in the evaluation of critically ill children.

Evoked Potentials

Evoked potentials are measurements of electrical activity of relevant brain regions after a peripheral stimulus has been applied. Stimuli are applied to sensory nerves (normally the median or posterior tibial nerve), visual fields, or auditory pathways, and the conduction of the impulses to the cortex is measured. Characteristic waves are generated, and amplitudes and latencies can implicate regions of damage to sensory nerves, pathways, or nuclei within the CNS.

Somatosensory (SSEP), brain stem (BAEP) and visual (VEP) evoked potentials serve predominantly as prognosticators of outcome in coma, spinal cord, and brain stem injury patients. After traumatic brain injury, absence of SSEP was associated with universally poor outcome in a relatively large series. Similarly, BAEP and VEP combined were prognostic of poor outcome in a series of children following hypoxic coma [23]. Abnormal SSEP latencies have been shown to correlate with encephalopathy secondary to sepsis in adults [28]. The main advantage of evoked potentials is that these waveforms are relatively unaffected by sedative medications. The tests are relatively labor intensive, require technical expertise, and can be performed only intermittently. These monitoring modalities are less frequently used than conventional EEG but are useful in select patient populations within the pediatric ICU.

Assessments of Blood Flow and/or Metabolism

Because of the brain's large requirement for oxygen and its dependence on aerobic respiration for optimal neuronal functioning, it has been widely accepted that measures of cerebral blood flow, metabolism, and oxygenation are useful indicators of local or global cerebral function. A variety of monitors have been developed to assess these parameters either locally or globally, and those that are in widespread use are summarized here. Some of the monitors directly measure one or more of these parameters, whereas others use inferences to derive data that can be used by clinicians. Monitoring techniques that are available at specialized centers for research purposes (such as positron emission tomography) are not discussed in this review.

Xenon Cerebral Blood Flow Determination

Xenon is an inert gas that is taken up by the brain but not metabolized. As such, it can be used in conjunction with a variety of detection devices to estimate both local and global cerebral blood flow by measuring its overall distribution and clearance [29]. Xenon can be administered via inhalation or intravenously. Intravenously-injected, radioactive xenon-133 can be detected within the cranial vault using multiple stationary scintillation detectors around the head. By this method, xenon-133 uptake and elimination can be measured, and global cerebral blood flow can be determined. This method is convenient, can be performed at bedside with minimal radiation exposure to patient or staff with serial use, and is effective at measuring hemispheric blood flow. However, focal areas of ischemia can be missed using this method because resolution is relatively poor. Alternatively, inhalation of xenon gas can be used to estimate blood flow using computed tomography (CT) imaging (Xe-CT). Using software and detection methods within the CT scanner, uptake of xenon within the brain can be measured, and a cerebral blood flow map can be generated. Cerebral blood flow of individual brain structures (white matter versus gray matter, structures within the deep brain structures, peritrauma areas, and others) can be quantified in milliliters per100g tissue per minute [29]. This technique has the disadvantage of requiring transportation to the imaging facility, a relatively high institutional cost for the technology, and the technical expertise required to interpret the test.

Xenon cerebral blood flow techniques have many clinical applications [30]. They can be used to detect focal areas of ischemia or hyperemia, providing clinical indications for lobectomy of unrecoverable injured brain. Adjusting pH or arterial blood pressure during sequential examinations can allow assessment of cerebral autoregulation in brain regions of interest. Confirmation of the clinical diagnosis of brain death can also be accomplished without the artifactual contribution from extracerebral blood sources that occurs with nuclear medicine techniques.

Transcranial Doppler Ultrasonography

Transcranial Doppler ultrasonography (TCD) is a noninvasive technique to determine the cerebral blood velocity in large intracranial vessels [31]. The handheld probe can be placed over the temporal bone window, foramen magnum window, and/or transorbital window, allowing evaluation of anterior cerebral circulation, vertebrobasilar circulation, and ophthalmic artery and carotid siphon circulation, respectively. Transcranial Doppler ultrasonography measures mean cerebral blood flow velocity (MCBFV) using the principles of ultrasound and spectral Doppler shift of blood cell flow through these large vessels and can (1) determine the presence or absence of flow; (2) calculate systolic, diastolic, and mean velocities; and (3) determine the direction of flow. With these determinations graphically represented, a pulsatility index (PI) can be calculated (PI = [Peak velocity – diastolic velocity]/ mean velocity) that represents downstream resistance to blood flow. The hemispheric index or Lindegaard's ratio of the mean velocity within the middle cerebral artery to that in the internal carotid artery (MCBFV$_{MCA}$/MCBFV$_{ICA}$) is indicative of cerebral vasospasm when >3 and of hyperemia (edema) <3.

The main clinical indications for TCD in children are determining vessel patency, detecting focal areas of vasospasm after intracerebral hemorrhage, and confirmation of the clinical diagnosis of brain death (criteria include severely diminished MCBFV$_{ICA}$, absent diastolic flow, reverberating flow, and severely elevated PI) [32]. Transcranial Doppler ultrasonography is readily available at the bedside but requires a relatively high level of technical expertise. Importantly, TCD measures cerebral blood flow velocity and not cerebral blood flow or cerebral blood volume. Because of this, extrapolations of TCD data to blood flow and volume may lack reliability. Furthermore, because vasospasm is uncommon in children, experience with TCD in children is limited.

Jugular Venous Oxygen Saturation

Measurement of the oxygen saturation in the blood leaving the brain (SjvO$_2$) is a global indirect measure of cerebral blood flow and metabolism. It identifies time periods in which cerebral blood flow is inadequate for metabolic demands. Under ideal conditions, blood returning to the body from the brain can be sampled for oxygen saturation. Suboptimal saturation (usually defined as <50% saturated), indicates cerebral blood flow and metabolism mismatch and potential time period of ongoing cerebral ischemia. Clinicians can then act to determine the cause of the abnormality, be it excessive hyperventilation, anemia, impaired oxygen content of arterial blood, or intracranial hypertension. Today, SjvO$_2$ monitoring is used in children after traumatic brain injury and during extracorporeal membrane oxygenation [33–35].

Despite the advantages of SjvO$_2$ monitoring (ease of placement and interpretation, relatively basic technology used, and real-time data generation), its use at the present time is limited by its questionable reliability and potential complications. Although commercially available monitors can accurately measure SjvO$_2$, the reliability of unilateral measurements to accurately sample *all of the blood leaving the brain* has been questioned. In a series of 32 adults in traumatic coma, both jugular vein saturations were measured simultaneously, and a difference of at least 15% between each monitor was noted in almost half of the patients during the study [36]. Rarely, catheter thrombosis and infection have been reported in adults and children may be a greater risk for these complications because of the smaller caliber of the jugular vein during development.

Near-Infrared Spectroscopy

Near-infrared spectroscopy (NIRS) uses the unique absorption characteristics of oxyhemoglobin, deoxyhemoglobin, and oxidized cytochrome aa$_3$ and the ability of light to pass through tissues (Lambert-Beer law) to estimate regional cerebral oxygenation. The NIRS probe contains a light source emitting a red (660 nm) and infrared (940 nm) light that penetrate into the superficial brain, and the state of oxygenation and oxidized state of cytochromes can be determined.

Near-infrared spectroscopy may be a better neuromonitor for children than adults because the quality of the signal will be affected by the density of the bones of the skull. It has been used in small studies to assess cerebral oxygenation in children with coma [37,38], during heart surgery [39], and in several other assorted conditions. In adults, the inability of the NIRS to detect occult ischemic events (infarctions in subcortical tissue directly under the probe) has been reported. Currently, NIRS is used as a bedside screening tool to rapidly diagnose accumulation of secondary hematomas after trauma (signal is lost as fluid accumulates) [40]. Because NIRS is noninvasive, it can be measured continuously, and both trends and absolute values of cerebral oxygenation can be followed. Near-infrared spectroscopy assumes that other forms of hemoglobin are not present within the blood at significant quantities and would be unreliable in these situations. Furthermore, the penetration of the light from NIRS is limited to several centimeters under normal conditions. Therefore, the calculated oxygenation index will not reflect the deeper structures of the brain in older children. Presently, NIRS is an intriguing clinical tool that needs to be fully evaluated.

Brain Oxygen Monitoring and Cerebral Microdialysis

Although SjvO$_2$ may detect global disturbances in cerebral blood flow and metabolism, monitors have emerged to assess the adequacy of some of these parameters in focal areas of the brain. Specifically, the partial pressure of oxygen of brain parenchyma (PbtO$_2$) and cerebral microdialysis can assess substrate delivery or metabolic conditions within the brain parenchyma. These devices require surgical implantation and can be performed concurrently to improve the information gathered from either device.

The PbtO$_2$ is measured using a small Clark electrode embedded at the end of a catheter. This electrode senses oxygen concentration, and the results are displayed on a screen in real time. Ideally, the sensor is placed in an area of brain at risk for cerebral injury. As with systemic measurements of PaO$_2$, normal values of PbtO$_2$ can vary over a wide physiologic range. Thresholds for periods of ischemia have been arbitrarily defined by individual investigators based on their experience. In general, PbtO$_2$ <10–15 mm Hg have been indicative of cerebral ischemia by most groups. More importantly, trends in PbtO$_2$ can be followed to determine the adequacy of oxygen delivered to the region immediately surrounding the electrode.

Experience with children is limited, but this monitoring technique is gaining acceptance for injured adults [41–44]. Monitoring PbtO$_2$ is invasive and gives information regarding a relatively small portion of brain parenchyma. Localized damage to tissue from electrode insertion is required, but extensive complications have not been reported. This monitoring technique is promising, but further studies regarding its use in children will aid in determining optimal usage.

Cerebral microdialysis has been performed the past two decades and serves to measure mediators of interest directly from the brain parenchyma. Microdialysis catheters are constructed with an inflow port, an outflow port, and a semipermeable membrane. Artificial CSF is perfused as a dialysate through the inflow port across the semipermeable membrane into the brain parenchyma. Solutes from the brain tissue can diffuse across the membrane and are recovered from the outflow port. The recovery of solutes is dependent on the dialysate flow rate, the membrane pore size, and solute concentrations within the brain. The relative change in dialysate concentration can reflect similar changes within the brain parenchyma. Samples are collected serially, and a wide variety of mediators can be measured from the dialysate (including glucose, pyruvate, lactate, glycerol, excitatory amino acids, purines, nitric oxide metabolites, and others).

Cerebral microdialysis has become more common over the past several years for a variety of disorders [45–53]. Microdialysis is a relatively invasive measure of local concentrations of metabolites within a small area of brain. For these reasons, extrapolations of this information to larger areas of brain are problematic. However, because serial measurements can be obtained, valuable information can be gleaned during the monitoring period regarding the state of the brain and the effect of various therapies.

Magnetic Resonance Spectroscopy

Nuclei of atoms, protons, or ^{31}P can be excited by a strong magnetic field. When the field is interrupted, the nuclei resonate in a frequency that can be detected and quantified. Using this method, metabolites of cellular metabolism can be detected with the spatial resolution of magnetic resonance images. Proton magnetic resonance spectroscopy (MRS) can detect N-acetyl compounds, primarily N-acetylaspartate, creatine (including phosphocreatine and its precursor, creatine) and choline-containing compounds (including free choline, phosphoryl, and glycerophosphoryl choline). N-acetylaspartate is a neuronal marker, whereas the choline compounds are released as glial membranes are damaged. Proton MRS can determine the concentration of lactate (accumulating from tissue damage) and various neurotransmitters (GABA and glutamate). Concentrations of adenosine triphosphate, phosphocreatine, and some of the other high-energy phosphates involved in cellular energetics can be assessed using ^{31}P-MRS. Spectra can be acquired within 1 hr, and changes in intracellular pH and metabolites can be studied.

Proton and ^{31}P-MRS has been used in the localization of epileptic foci, evaluation of the extent of post-traumatic lesions, classification of brain tumors, prediction of outcome after brain trauma, and diagnosis of the various mitochondrial disorders, leukodystrophies, and other demyelinating disorders [54,55]. The ability to noninvasively measure a host of metabolites within the brain is the unique function of MRS. However, scanning times are still prolonged and caution must be taken to ensure patient safety during the time the spectra are being generated. Furthermore, although studies can be repeated, each image reflects the brain milieu at a single time point.

Conclusion

Clinical neuromonitoring is a rapidly advancing field in pediatric critical care medicine, and the present chapter reviews the most commonly used modalities. Currently, no single monitor can effectively perform all of the functions demanded by clinicians caring for critically ill children. Developing the proper combination of techniques appropriate for each child is the challenge of the coming years to improve neurologic outcomes.

References

1. Lieberman JD, Pasquale MD, Garcia R, Cipolle MD, Mark Li P, Wasser TE. Use of admission Glasgow Coma Score, pupil size, and pupil reactivity to determine outcome for trauma patients. J Trauma 2003;55: 437–443.
2. Hooper SR, Alexander J, Moore D, Sasser HC, Laurent S, King J, Bartel S, Callahan B. Caregiver reports of common symptoms in children following a traumatic brain injury. NeuroRehabilitation 2004;19: 175–189.
3. Adelson PD, Bratton SL, Carney NA, Chesnut RM, du Coudray HE, Goldstein B, Kochanek PM, Miller HC, Partington MD, Selden NR, Warden CR, Wright DW. Guidelines for the acute medical management of severe traumatic brain injury in infants, children, and adolescents. Chapter 5. Indications for intracranial pressure monitoring in pediatric patients with severe traumatic brain injury. Pediatr Crit Care Med 2003;4:S19–S24.
4. Lundberg N, Troupp H, Lorin H. Continuous recording of the ventricular fluid pressure in patients with severe acute traumatic brain injury. J Neurosurg 1965;22:581–589.
5. Jenkins JG, Glasgow JF, Black GW, Fannin TF, Hicks EM, Keilty SR, Crean PM. Reye's syndrome: assessment of intracranial monitoring. BMJ (Clin Res Ed) 1987;294:337–338.
6. Alper G, Jarjour IT, Reyes JD, Towbin RB, Hirsch WL, Bergman I. Outcome of children with cerebral edema caused by fulminant hepatic failure. Pediatr Neurol 1998;18:299–304.
7. Luerssen TG. Intracranial pressure: current status in monitoring and management. Semin Pediatr Neurol 1997;4:146–155.
8. Graham D, Adams J, Doyle D. Ischemic brain damage in fatal, nonmissile head injuries. J Neurol Sci 1978;39:213–219.
9. Gopinath SP, Robertson CS, Contant CF, Hayes C, Feldman Z, Narayan RK, Grossman RG. Jugular venous desaturation and outcome after head injury. J Neurol Neurosurg Psychiatry 1994;57:717–723.
10. Robertson CS, Valadka AB, Hannay HJ, Contant CF, Gopinath SP, Cormio M, Uzura M, Grossman RG. Prevention of secondary ischemic insults after severe head injury. Crit Care Med 1999;27: 2086–2095.
11. North B, Reilly P. Comparison among three methods of intracranial pressure recording. Neurosurgery 1986;18:730–732.
12. Ghajar J. Intracranial pressure monitoring techniques. New Horiz 1995;3:395–399.
13. Courtman SP, Wardurgh A, Petros AJ. Comparison of the bispectral index monitor with the Comfort score in assessing level of sedation of critically ill children. Intensive Care Med 2003;29:2239–2246.
14. Crain N, Slonim A, Pollack MM. Assessing sedation in the pediatric intensive care unit by using BIS and the COMFORT scale. Pediatr Crit Care Med 2002;3:11–14.
15. Grindstaff RJ, Tobias JD. Applications of bispectral index monitoring in the pediatric intensive care unit. J Intensive Care Med 2004;19: 111–116.
16. Liu J, Singh H, White PF. Electroencephalographic bispectral index correlates with intraoperative recall and depth of propofol-induced sedation. Anesth Analg 1997;84:185–189.
17. Avramov MN, White PF. Methods for monitoring the level of sedation. Crit Care Clin 1995;11:803–826.
18. Simmons LE, Riker RR, Prato BS, Fraser GL. Assessing sedation during intensive care unit mechanical ventilation with the bispectral index and the Sedation-Agitation Scale. Crit Care Med 1995;27:1499–1504.
19. Tobias JD, Berkenbosch JW. Tolerance during sedation in a pediatric ICU patient: effects on the BIS monitor. J Clin Anesth 2001;13:122–124.
20. Procaccio F, Polo A, Lanteri L, Sala F. Electrophysiologic monitoring in neurointensive care. Curr Opin Crit Care 2001;7:74–80.
21. Jordan K. Continuous EEG and evoked potential monitoring in the neuroscience intensive care unit. J Clin Neurophysiol 1993;10:445–475.
22. Mandel R, Martinot A, Delepoulle F, Lamblin M, Laureau E, Vallee L, Leclerc F. Prediction of outcome after hypoxic–ischemic encephalopathy: a prospective clinical and electrophysiologic study. J Pediatr 2002;141:45–50.
23. Mewasingh L, Catherine Christophe C, Fonteyne C, Dachy B, Ziereisen F, Christiaens F, Deltenre P, De Maertelaer V, Dan B. Predictive value of electrophysiology in children with hypoxic coma. Pediatr Neurol 2003;28:178–183.
24. Hosaya M, Ushikua H, Arakawab H, Morikawa A. Low-voltage activity in EEG during acute phase of encephalitis predicts unfavorable neurological outcome. Brain Dev 2002;24:161–165.
25. Vespa P, Nenov V, Nuwer MR. Continuous EEG monitoring in the intensive care unit: early findings and clinical efficacy. J Clin Neurophysiol 1999;16:1–13.
26. Bickford R. The compressed spectral array. A pictorial EEG. Proc San Diego Biomed Symp 1972;11:365–370.
27. Prior P, DE M. Monitoring cerebral function: long-term monitoring of EEG and evoked potentials. Maynald DE Brit J Anesth 1986;57:63–81.
28. Zauner C, Gendo A, Kramer L, Funk G, Bauer E, Schenk P, Ratheiser K, Madl C. Impaired subcortical and cortical sensory evoked potential pathways in septic patients. Crit Care Med 2002;30:1136–1139.
29. Perez-Arjona E, Del Proposto Z, Sehgal V, Fessler R. New techniques in cerebral imaging. Neurol Res 2002;24:S17–S26.
30. Kilpatrick M, Yonas H, Goldstein S, Kassam A, Gebel J, •• JM, Wechsler L, Jungreis C, Fukui M. CT-based assessment of acute stroke: CT, CT angiography, and xenon-enhanced CT cerebral blood flow. Stroke 2001;32:2543–2549.
31. Manno E. Transcranial Doppler ultrasonography in the neurocritical care unit. Crit Care Clin 1997;13:79–104.
32. Hassler W, Steinmetz H, Gawlowski J. Transcranial Doppler ultrasonography in raised intracranial pressure and in intracranial circulatory arrest. J Neurosurg 1988;68:745–751.
33. Pettignano R, Labuz M, Gauthier TW, Huckaby J, Clark RH. The use of cephalad cannulae to monitor jugular venous oxygen content during extracorporeal membrane oxygenation. Crit Care (Lond) 1997;1: 95–99.
34. Perez A, Minces PG, Schnitzler EJ, Agosta GE, Medina SA, Ciraolo CA. Jugular venous oxygen saturation or arteriovenous difference of lactate content and outcome in children with severe traumatic brain injury. Pediatr Crit Care Med 2003;4:33–38.
35. Schneider GH, von Helden G, Lanksch WR, Unterberg A. Continuous monitoring of jugular bulb oxygen saturation in comatose patients-therapeutic implications. Acta Neurochir (Wien) 1995;134:71–75.
36. Stocchetti N, Paparella A, Bridelli F, Bacchi M, Piazza P, Zuccoli P. Cerebral venous oxygen saturation studied with bilateral samples in the internal jugular veins. Neurosurgery 1994;34:38–44.
37. Wagner BP, Pfenninger J. Dynamic cerebral autoregulatory response to blood pressure rise measured by near-infrared spectroscopy and intracranial pressure. Crit Care Med 2002;30:2014–2021.
38. Nagdyman N, Fleck T, Schubert S, Ewert P, Peters B, Lange PE, Abdul-Khaliq H. Comparison between cerebral tissue oxygenation index measured by near-infrared spectroscopy and venous jugular bulb saturation in children. Intensive Care Med 2005;31:846–850.
39. Hayashida M, Kin N, Tomioka T, Orii R, Sekiyama H, Usui H, Chinzei M, Hanaoka K. Cerebral ischaemia during cardiac surgery in children

detected by combined monitoring of BIS and near-infrared spectroscopy. Br J Anaesth 2004;92:662–669.

40. Gopinath S, Robertson C, Grossman R, Chance B. Near-infrared spectroscopic localization of intracranial hematomas. J Neurosurg 1993; 79:43–47.

41. Jodicke A, Hubner F, Boker DK. Monitoring of brain tissue oxygenation during aneurysm surgery: prediction of procedure-related ischemic events. J Neurosurg 2003;98:515–523.

42. Kett-White R, Hutchinson PJ, Al-Rawi PG, Czosnyka M, Gupta AK, Pickard JD, Kirkpatrick PJ. Cerebral oxygen and microdialysis monitoring during aneurysm surgery: effects of blood pressure, cerebrospinal fluid drainage, and temporary clipping on infarction. J Neurosurg 2002;96:1013–1019.

43. Sarrafzadeh AS, Kiening KL, Bardt TF, Schneider GH, Unterberg AW, Lanksch WR. Cerebral oxygenation in contusioned vs. nonlesioned brain tissue: monitoring of PtiO$_2$ with Licox and Paratrend. Acta Neurochir Suppl 1998;71:186–189.

44. Valadka AB, Gopinath SP, Contant CF, Uzura M, Robertson CS. Relationship of brain tissue PO$_2$ to outcome after severe head injury. Crit Care Med 1998;26:1576–1581.

45. Vespa P, Bergsneider M, Hattori N, Wu HM, Huang SC, Martin NA, Glenn TC, McArthur DL, Hovda DA. Metabolic crisis without brain ischemia is common after traumatic brain injury: a combined microdialysis and positron emission tomography study. J Cereb Blood Flow Metab 2005;25:763–774.

46. Parkin M, Hopwood S, Jones DA, Hashemi P, Landolt H, Fabricius M, Lauritzen M, Boutelle MG, Strong AJ. Dynamic changes in brain glucose and lactate in pericontusional areas of the human cerebral cortex, monitored with rapid sampling on-line microdialysis: relationship with depolarisation-like events. J Cereb Blood Flow Metab 2005; 25:402–413.

47. Johnston AJ, Steiner LA, Coles JP, Chatfield DA, Fryer TD, Smielewski P, Hutchinson PJ, O'Connell MT, Al-Rawi PG, Aigbirihio FI, Clark JC, Pickard JD, Gupta AK, Menon DK. Effect of cerebral perfusion pressure augmentation on regional oxygenation and metabolism after head injury. Crit Care Med 2005;33:189–195.

48. Nelson DW, Bellander BM, Maccallum RM, Axelsson J, Alm M, Wallin M, Weitzberg E, Rudehill A. Cerebral microdialysis of patients with severe traumatic brain injury exhibits highly individualistic patterns as visualized by cluster analysis with self-organizing maps. Crit Care Med 2004;32:2428–2436.

49. Bellander BM, Cantais E, Enblad P, Hutchinson P, Nordstrom CH, Robertson C, Sahuquillo J, Smith M, Stocchetti N, Ungerstedt U, Unterberg A, Olsen NV. Consensus meeting on microdialysis in neurointensive care. Intensive Care Med 2004;30:2166–2169.

50. Winter CD, Pringle AK, Clough GF, Church MK. Raised parenchymal interleukin-6 levels correlate with improved outcome after traumatic brain injury. Brain 2004;127:315–320.

51. Sarrafzadeh AS, Kiening KL, Callsen TA, Unterberg AW. Metabolic changes during impending and manifest cerebral hypoxia in traumatic brain injury. Br J Neurosurg 2003;17:340–346.

52. Vespa PM, McArthur D, O'Phelan K, Glenn T, Etchepare M, Kelly D, Bergsneider M, Martin NA, Hovda DA. Persistently low extracellular glucose correlates with poor outcome 6 months after human traumatic brain injury despite a lack of increased lactate: a microdialysis study. J Cereb Blood Flow Metab 2003;23:865–877.

53. Magnoni S, Ghisoni L, Locatelli M, Caimi M, Colombo A, Valeriani V, Stocchetti N. Lack of improvement in cerebral metabolism after hyperoxia in severe head injury: a microdialysis study. J Neurosurg 2003; 98:952–958.

54. Shutter L, Tong KA, Holshouser BA. Proton MRS in acute traumatic brain injury: role for glutamate/glutamine and choline for outcome prediction. J Neurotrauma 2004;21:1693–1705.

55. Brenner T, Freier M, Holshouser B, Burley T, Ashwal S. Predicting neuropsychologic outcome after traumatic brain injury in children. Pediatr Neurol 2003;28:104–114.

2

Molecular Biology of Brain Injury

Michael J. Whalen, Phoebe Yager, Eng H. Lo, Josephine Lok, and Natan Noviski

Neurotransmitters and Their Receptors

The concept that electrical activity between neurons is transmitted via chemical messengers was first demonstrated in 1921 by an Austrian physiologist, Otto Loewi. Using two frog hearts, he placed the first heart (still connected to its vagus nerve) into a saline-filled chamber. This chamber was connected to a second saline-filled chamber into which he placed the second heart. Electrical stimulation of the vagus nerve caused the first heart to slow. After a short delay, he noticed the second heart also slowed. From this experiment, he hypothesized that the electrical stimulation of the vagus nerve released a chemical into the first chamber that flowed into the second and caused the second heart to slow just as the first. He referred to the chemical as *Vagusstoff*. We now know this chemical to be acetylcholine, by far the best-studied neurotransmitter [1].

Neurotransmitters: Definition

Neurotransmitters are the chemical messengers synthesized and utilized by neurons to propagate electrical impulses from one neuron to the next. Neurotransmitters are produced and stored within presynaptic neurons, which when depolarized release neurotransmitters into the synaptic cleft. Neurotransmitters bind and activate specific membrane-bound receptors in the postsynaptic cell, leading to ion fluxes, such as inward sodium, calcium, or chloride currents, and to outward potassium efflux. Following their release, neurotransmitters are rapidly inactivated by reuptake and/ or degradation.

Neurotransmitters fall into two main categories: peptide neurotransmitters and small-molecule neurotransmitters, such as acetylcholine, biogenic amines, and amino acids. We focus primarily on the role of several major classes of neurotransmission in the normal brain and on the role of amino acid neurotransmitters in excitotoxicity, the process by which overstimulation of glutamate receptors induces cell death.

Neurotransmitter Receptors

There are over 100 putative neurotransmitters and a vast array of neurotransmitter receptors; the same neurotransmitter may be excitatory or inhibitory, depending on whether binding to a specific receptor results in depolarization versus hyperpolarization, respectively. In general, all neurotransmitter receptors function by opening or closing ion channels in the postsynaptic cell membrane. They can do this directly if the receptor functions as an ion channel or indirectly if the receptor lacking an ion channel activates a second messenger system. The former is referred to as an *ionotropic* or *ligand-gated receptor*, the latter as a *metabotropic receptor*.

Ionotropic receptors are generally composed of five membrane-spanning subunits that together form a central channel. The receptor is a multimer with several extracellular neurotransmitter binding sites, a number of transmembrane domains, and a single central ion channel connecting the extra- and intracellular compartments. In contrast, metabotropic receptors are monomeric, membrane-spanning proteins that stimulate intracellular G proteins that interact with separate membrane-spanning ion channels. When neurotransmitters bind the extracellular sites of metabotropic receptors, G proteins linked to the intracellular domain are activated, dissociate, and interact with ion channels or through intermediary proteins to alter conductance of neighboring ion channels. Metabotropic receptors generally modulate the function of ionotropic receptors and have longer lasting electrical effects as well as effects on gene expression and intracellular signaling important for synaptic plasticity, learning, and memory.

Acetylcholine

The two types of acetylcholine (ACh) receptors are nicotinic and muscarinic, named for synthetic chemicals that activate their respective extracellular binding sites on the ACh receptor. Nicotinic ACh (nACh) receptors are excitatory ligand-gated channels localized at the neuromuscular junction, as well as within the brain and autonomic nervous system. Although the role of ACh at the neuromuscular junction and autonomic ganglia is well understood, its role in the brain is less clear. Nicotinic ACh receptors, found throughout the cortex, induce arousal, euphoria, and relaxation. Nicotine and other nACh receptor agonists improve attention, enhance learning, and shorten reaction time. Muscarinic ACh receptors are metabotropic and are responsible for the majority of

D.S. Wheeler et al. (eds.), *The Central Nervous System in Pediatric Critical Illness and Injury*,
DOI 10.1007/978-1-84800-993-6_2, © Springer-Verlag London Limited 2009

acetylcholine effects in the brain. These receptors are found in abundance in the striatum and other forebrain regions in addition to postganglionic parasympathetic neurons.

Biogenic Amines

Biogenic amines are a group of small-molecule neurotransmitters and includes the three main catecholamines (dopamine, norepinephrine, and epinephrine) as well as serotonin and histamine. Together, the biogenic amines account for a complex array of brain function and clinical behavior.

Dopamine

Inhibitory dopaminergic neurons project from the substantia nigra to the corpus striatum, where they mediate control of motor activity. Disruption of dopaminergic neurons results in the abnormal shuffling gait and pill-rolling tremor described in patients suffering from Parkinson's disease. In addition, dopaminergic neurons arising from the ventral tegmental area and extending to the nucleus accumbens are believed to be involved in motivation, reward, and addictive behavior. Cocaine blocks norepinephrine, serotonin, and dopamine reuptake into presynaptic terminals by inhibiting the dopamine transporter, leading to an accumulation of dopamine in the synaptic cleft. This results in prolongation of dopaminergic effects in the limbic system, producing intense euphoria. Of note, dopamine receptors are exclusively metabotropic.

Norepinephrine

Norepinephrine is a key neurotransmitter of neurons in the locus coeruleus that project to the cerebral cortex, thalamus, and midbrain reticular activating system. Norepinephrine is an excitatory neurotransmitter that mediates sleep and wakefulness, attention, and feeding behavior. Norepinephrine is normally cleared from the synaptic cleft by the norepinephrine transporter (NET). As with cocaine, amphetamine blocks this reuptake mechanism. In addition, amphetamine inhibits monoamine oxidase (MAO) and catechol O-methyltransferase (COMT), the major enzymes that metabolize norepinephrine in neurons and glia. Disruption of norepinephrine metabolism increases synaptic norepinephrine, leading to insomnia, decreased appetite, and increased alertness.

Histamine

Histamine-containing neurons in the hypothalamus project to most regions of the brain and spinal cord, where they influence attention and arousal. Thus, drowsiness is caused by antihistaminic drugs that cross the blood–brain barrier, such as diphenhydramine. Neurons utilizing histamine as a neurotransmitter are also found in the vestibular system. This may explain why another antihistamine, meclizine, is effective as an antiemetic. All three known histamine receptors are metabotropic.

Serotonin

Serotonin, or 5-hydroxytryptamine (5-HT), is implicated in the pathophysiology of a number of psychiatric diseases, including depression, eating disorders, anxiety disorders, and obsessive-compulsive disorder. Serotonin-containing neurons predominate in the raphe region of the pons and upper brain stem and project into the forebrain. A wide variety of 5-HT receptors have been discovered, most of which are metabotropic. These receptors influence sleep and wakefulness, emotion, motor behaviors, and satiety. Once serotonin has been released into a synaptic cleft, its action is terminated by the serotonin reuptake transporter (SERT). The selective serotonin reuptake inhibitors (SSRIs) interfere with SERT and prolong the action of serotonin in the synaptic cleft.

Amino Acids

Four amino acids have been identified as neurotransmitters, including glutamate, aspartate, gamma-aminobutyric acid (GABA), and glycine. Most excitatory neurons in the brain utilize glutamate as a neurotransmitter and are referred to as *glutamatergic neurons*. The most important inhibitory neurotransmitters are GABA and glycine. Together, amino acid neurotransmitters are responsible for the majority of synaptic neurotransmission in the brain.

Gamma-Aminobutyric Acid and Glycine

The majority of inhibitory synapses in the brain utilize either GABA or glycine as neurotransmitters, which act on ionotropic and metabotropic receptors to decrease excitation by causing hyperpolarization of the postsynaptic membrane. In the normal brain, glucose is metabolized to glutamate via the tricarboxylic acid cycle. Glutamate is then converted to GABA by glutamic acid decarboxylase (GAD). Glutamic acid decarboxylase requires a cofactor, pyridoxal phosphate (derived from vitamin B_6), for normal function. Pyridoxine dependency is an autosomal recessive disorder manifest by intractable infantile seizures responsive to vitamin B_6 administration. The disorder is associated with high levels of glutamate in the cerebrospinal fluid and impaired GAD activity.

There are two types of GABA receptors: GABA-A and GABA-B. The GABA-A receptors are ligand gated and function by enhancing Cl^- conduction through the central pore, inducing hyperpolarization and reducing membrane excitability. Benzodiazepines and barbiturates induce sedation and anxiolysis and increase the seizure threshold by binding GABA-A receptors. The GABA-B receptors are metabotropic and inhibit depolarization via recruitment of a G-protein second messenger that blocks neighboring K^+ and Ca^{2+} channels.

Glutamate

Glutamate is a nonessential amino acid that does not cross the blood–brain barrier and therefore must be produced by neurons within the central nervous system in order to function as a neurotransmitter. Glutamine, the primary precursor to glutamate, is supplied by glial cells to neurons. Once within the presynaptic terminal of the neuron, glutaminase converts glutamine to glutamate. Glutamate is stored in vesicles until released by neuronal depolarization and is then transported back to glial cells, reconverted to glutamine via glutamine synthetase, and returned to the neuron.

Glutamate receptors are composed of five monomeric subunits that assemble in various combinations to form a variety of glutamate receptors, several of which may respond to glutamate simultaneously in a given postsynaptic neuron. Three ligand-gated (ionotropic) glutamate receptors have been described: N-methyl-D-aspartate (NMDA), α-amino-3-hydroxy-5-methyl-4-isoxazole propionate (AMPA), and kainite receptors. All three are excitatory. There are three specific properties that make NMDA receptors unique. First, their central pore conducts Na^+, K^+, and Ca^{2+}. Ca^{2+} influx serves as a second messenger to initiate intracellular signaling cascades and novel gene expression. Second, magnesium binds to glutamate receptors within the central pore, which inhibits channel function by maintaining hyperpolarization of the postsynaptic membrane. Magnesium is extruded from the pore during depolarization to allow free flow of other cations. This unique property adds voltage dependence to ionic flow across the pore and has been linked to brain functions such as learning and memory. Finally, a glycine binding site modulates channel opening in response to glutamate binding, and glycine is required for optimal NMDA receptor function.

Activation of NMDA receptors underlies the formation of novel memories by modulating the strength of the effect of a synapse on a postsynaptic cell [2]. For example, frequent and repetitive stimulation of a synapse containing NMDA receptors leads to augmentation of the postsynaptic response during future synaptic stimulation; this electrophysiologic phenomenon is known as *long-term potentiation* (LTP) and is mediated by calcium influx through the NMDA receptor. Conversely, a low frequency of synaptic stimulation, and failure to recruit firing from additional synapses, leads to long-term depression (LTD) and inhibitory effects on the postsynaptic cell. Long-term depression is also mediated by calcium currents in NMDA receptors. Long-term potentiation and LTD depression are ways in which synaptic strength is regulated, both acutely and on a long-term basis, and both are necessary for normal learning and memory. Both LTP and LTD are inhibited by NMDA receptor antagonists that impair memory function in rodents. Thus, NMDA receptors induce memory formation by calcium-dependent mechanisms that include LTP or LTD in hippocampal as well as cortical brain regions.

In addition to the ligand-gated glutamate receptors, three known metabotropic receptor subtypes modulate neurotransmission by altering postsynaptic Ca^{2+} and Na^+ channels and thereby modulating excitability of the postsynaptic neuron. Group I mGlu receptors coupled to phospholipase C modulate intracellular calcium signaling, whereas group II and group III receptors inhibit adenylyl cyclase. Metabotropic glutamate receptors also play important roles in synaptic plasticity by potentiating the effects of NMDA receptor activity in brain regions involved in learning and memory.

Excitotoxicity

Drs. Lucas and Newhouse first demonstrated the concept of excitotoxicity in 1957 by feeding glutamate to young mice and finding neuronal loss in the retina [3]. The relationship between increased extracellular glutamate concentrations and neuronal cell death was subsequently described in a number of acute brain injury models [4–8]. During acute insults to the brain, such as stroke, infection, trauma, seizures, hypoglycemia, or hemorrhage, glutamate is released by neurons and glia into the brain extracellular space [8]. High concentrations of glutamate overstimulate NMDA and calcium-permeable AMPA receptors and induce transient, massive influx of extracellular calcium. Calcium may also enter the neuron from voltage-gated calcium channels, sodium/calcium transporters, and from intracellular stores. Intracellular calcium activates proteolytic enzymes that cleave substrates essential for cellular survival, such as cytoskeletal proteins, DNA repair enzymes, and other key cellular constituents. In addition, increased intracellular calcium induces mitochondrial electron transport chain dysfunction and subsequent generation of oxygen free radicals that, in concert with activation of proteases and other "death effectors," leads to necrotic or apoptotic cell death [9]. Recent studies have shown that calpains and caspases (two classes of death proteases activated by increased intracellular calcium) contribute to prolonged increases of intracellular calcium following excitotoxic stimuli by cleaving and inactivating membrane calcium pumps [10,11]. Thus, following an initial (sublethal) calcium increase, defective cellular calcium clearance magnifies the initial insult by prolonging the duration of increased intracellular calcium. Cell injury and death that occur as a result of overactivity of glutamatergic neurotransmission is referred to as *excitotoxicity*.

Despite a wealth of preclinical data implicating excitotoxicity in the pathogenesis of central nervous system injury, efforts to interrupt excitotoxicity using glutamate receptor antagonists are only effective if given before or shortly after the time of ischemic or traumatic injury in experimental animals [12–15]. In human trials, administration of NMDA receptor antagonists up to several hours after stroke and traumatic brain injury was not effective and actually increased mortality and morbidity in some patients [6,16–20]. One explanation for these negative results is that, following traumatic brain injury, NMDA receptor deactivation occurs between 15 min and 1 hr in regions of injured cortex and hippocampus; NMDA receptors remain deactivated for at least 7 days; and NMDA receptor deactivation correlates with deficits in a working memory task at 2 weeks after injury [21]. Interestingly, administration of NMDA reversed the cognitive deficits associated with NMDA receptor deactivation after acute traumatic brain injury [21]. Taken together with other studies implicating acute central nervous system inflammation as one cause of NMDA receptor deactivation [22], the data suggest that long-term memory deficits induced by acute central nervous system injury may be initiated by an acute neuroinflammatory response that inhibits NMDA receptor function in cortical and hippocampal brain regions critical for learning and memory. This hypothesis, testable in the laboratory, may elucidate relationships between acute brain injury, the associated inflammatory response, and lasting learning and memory dysfunction in experimental animals and patients with acute brain injury.

Cell Death After Acute Brain Injury

A number of insults to the central nervous system may initiate complex cascades of intracellular biochemical events that lead to delayed neuronal death, as well as death of other vulnerable cell types remote from the injury center [9,23–29]. Because cell death may occur hours to weeks after central nervous system injury, it is hoped that a better mechanistic understanding will result in novel treatments to preserve tissue and neurologic function. The last 30 years has witnessed impressive advances in understanding basic mechanisms of how cells die after acute brain injury. Excitotoxicity, oxidative stress, and programmed cell death are major pathways that are central to the pathogenesis of ischemic and traumatic brain cell death [30]. Understanding how injured brain cells die is difficult because numerous interrelated, complex mechanisms contribute to the execution phases, and little is known about the mechanisms that initiate death programs after acute brain injury [29,31,32]. This section presents an overview of three modes of cell death, the major pro-cell death pathways, and initiating mechanisms involved in acute brain cell death. Figure 2.1 summarizes some of the pathways involved.

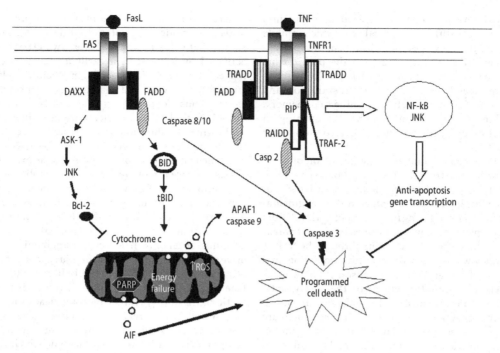

FIGURE 2.1. Cell death pathways and acute brain injury. Fas and tumor necrosis factor receptor 1 (TNFR1) are prototypical death receptors that signal apoptosis through Fas-associated protein with a death domain (FADD), by activating initiator caspases such as caspases (Casp) 8, 10, and 2. Mitochondria release cytochrome c and other apoptogenic factors (e.g., apoptosis-inducing factor[AIF]), leading to programmed cell death. In addition, TNFR and Bid activation can also induce necrosis through oxidative stress and mechanisms that remain to be clarified. APAF1, apoptotic protease activating factor 1; FasL, Fas ligand; TRADD, TNFR-associated protein with a death domain; RIP, receptor interacting protein; RAIDD, RIP-associated ICH-1 homologous protein with a death domain; TRAF-2, TNF receptor-associated factor-2 ; JNK, jun N–kinase; NFκB, nuclear factor-kappa B; ASK-1, apoptosis signal-regulating kinase 1; Bcl-2, B-cell lymphoma-2; DAXX, death associated protein 6; PARP, poly-ADP(ribose)polymerase; ROS, reactive oxygen species.

Necrosis

Severe ischemic, infectious, epileptogenic, or traumatic insults to the brain induce early cell death that is characterized by cell membrane permeability, organelle swelling, cellular and nuclear shrinkage, metabolic failure and depletion of cellular energy reserves, loss of ion pump function, and cell death that induces a marked local inflammatory response that propagates tissue injury. This mode of neuronal cell death is referred to as *necrosis* [33]. Necrosis is traditionally viewed as resulting from physical cellular disruption, as in severe traumatic brain injury, or from severe ischemic/metabolic insults that induce profound energy failure and cell death, such as severe ischemia or prolonged seizures. The exact biochemical mechanisms that mediate necrosis are relatively unknown but include activation of calpains and other proteolytic enzymes, oxidant injury resulting from generation of toxic oxygen species in the setting of mitochondrial dysfunction, and energy failure resulting from collapse of the mitochondrial transmembrane potential and rapid depletion of intracellular adenosine triphosphate stores [32]. However, recent studies suggest that necrosis can also occur as a form of programmed cell death initiated by activation of tumor necrosis family receptor members [34], and it is likely that necrotic cell death programs will be discovered that contribute to acute brain injury.

Excitotoxic death can be necrotic in the context of extreme insults, whereas milder forms of excitotoxic injury may trigger delayed programmed cell death, commonly referred to as *apoptosis*. Whether necrosis or apoptosis results from excitotoxic insults likely depends on the resulting magnitude and duration of increased intracellular calcium as well as on other factors such as depletion of cellular energy stores. Therapeutic attempts to inhibit necrotic cell death will likely require intervention early after brain injury, as necrosis occurs rapidly after acute central nervous system insults but may also be delayed and progressive.

Programmed Cell Death

Programmed cell death (apoptosis) is an evolutionarily conserved, genetically programmed cell suicide process that is mediated by new protein synthesis and activation of death-inducing proteases [35–37]. Caspase-dependent programmed cell death is mediated by a family of cysteine proteases known as *caspases*, a family of at least 14 known cysteine proteases that promote apoptosis by cleaving substrates at specific tetrapeptide amino acid sequences [33,38]. Caspases exist as proforms that when cleaved at specific aspartate residues form tetrameric active complexes that cleave and inactivate diverse cellular substrates, such as cytoskeletal proteins, inhibitors of DNA endonucleases, and cellular enzymes required for survival. Activity of effector caspases results in classic apoptotic cellular morphology and cell death. Initiator caspases, such as caspases 2, 8, and 9, cleave and activate effector caspases 3, 6, and 7. Other caspases are involved in inflammatory responses and do not directly mediate cell death.

Activated caspases are found in ischemic and traumatic brain tissue and cerebrospinal fluid of humans [29,32]. Genetic or pharmacologic inhibition of caspases reduces tissue damage in experimental stroke and traumatic brain injury but does not always improve functional outcome [39].

Apoptosis is characterized by morphologic and biochemical features distinct from necrosis. Caspase-dependent apoptosis, for example, is characterized by cell shrinkage, chromatin condensation, internucleosomal DNA fragmentation in multiples of 280 bp (known as *DNA laddering* because of the classic pattern produced by DNA gel electrophoresis), formation of nuclear apoptotic bodies, and engulfment of dying cells by phagocytes or neighboring cells in the absence of a local inflammatory response [40]. At the molecular level, activated caspases and proteolytic products of their substrates are detectable, as well as externalization of membrane phosphatidylcholine (which signals phagocytosis) and internucleosomal DNA fragmentation that reacts with terminal transferase in the TUNEL assay, a commonly used in situ marker for apoptosis.

Caspase-independent programmed cell death is mediated by apoptosis-inducing factors released from mitochondria, without concomitant activation of caspases [41–44]. One such factor, named *apoptosis-inducing factor* (AIF), is a phylogenetically ancient flavoprotein encoded by a gene on the X chromosome and expressed in most tissues (45). Apoptosis-inducing factor functions as an electron acceptor/donor and has a second apoptogenic function as well. Precursor AIF is synthesized in the cytosol and imported into the intermembrane space of mitochondria. Following acute cellular injury, AIF translocates through the outer mitochondrial membrane into the cytosol and to the nucleus, where it induces nuclear chromatin condensation and large-scale (approximately 50 kb) DNA fragmentation. This mode of cell death produces margination of nuclear chromatin and cellular morphology distinct from that of caspase-dependent apoptosis. It is likely that other mitochondrial and cytosolic apoptotic proteins also contribute to caspase-independent cell death following acute central nervous system injury.

Intrinsic Pathway of Apoptotic Cell Death

The *intrinsic pathway* is a major apoptotic pathway that involves release of proapoptotic factors from injured mitochondria. Proteins involved in the intrinsic cell death pathway include the Bcl-2 family of proapoptotic proteins (i.e., Bax and Bad), mitochondrial oxidoreductases such as cytochrome c and AIF, some caspases, and DNA fragmentation factors such as caspase-activated DNAse and endonuclease G. Following acute brain injury, apoptosis may be triggered by a number of pathologic mechanisms, including ischemia, trauma, excitotoxicity, oxidative stress, energy failure, and others [24,32]. These pathologic events can lead to depolarization of the mitochondrial inner membrane and release of cytochrome c (or other apoptogenic factors such as AIF in caspase-independent death). Cytochrome c interacts with an adapter protein *apoptotic protease activating factor* (Apaf-1), adenosine triphosphate, and procaspase-9 in the cytosol to form an *apoptosome*, where caspase-9 is autoactivated by self-oligomerization. Caspase-9 cleaves and activates caspase-3, leading to caspase-dependent apoptosis.

Other mechanisms of mitochondrial-mediated cell death include generation of reactive oxygen species in response to excitotoxic and other stimuli and energy failure through overactivation of the DNA repair enzyme poly(ADP)-ribose polymerase (PARP, discussed later). Thus, the mitochondrion not only controls cellular respiration but is a rheostat for cellular damage and a central mediator of cell death after acute central nervous system injury.

The Extrinsic Pathway of Apoptotic Cell Death

Another route to programmed cell death (and even necrosis) involves activation of membrane bound *death receptors* of the tumor necrosis factor receptor (TNFR) superfamily, such as Fas and TNFR1 [46–49]. Ligand binding induces activation of death receptors, which then recruit cytosolic adapter proteins such as Fas-associated protein with a death domain (FADD) and TNFR-associated protein with a death domain (TRADD). Binding between death receptors and their adapter proteins occurs via homotypic interactions between evolutionarily conserved death domain sequences. Activated adapter proteins bind initiator procaspases, such as procaspases 2, 8, and 10, through death effector domain (DED) sequences present in adapter proteins and procaspases. The resulting complex formed by a death receptor, adapter protein(s), and procaspase is a death-inducing signaling complex (DISC). Self-aggregation of initiator procaspases at the DISC induces their autoactivation, and activated initiator caspases process and activate procaspases 3, 6, and 7, which mediate cell death. Alternatively, activated caspase-8 can cleave and activate cytosolic Bid, a proapoptotic Bcl-2 family member that induces release of cytochrome c from mitochondria [50,51]. Of note, mice deficient in Bid have reduced infarct volume and caspase-3 activation after experimental cerebral ischemic injury [52], and Bid can also induce necrotic cell death [53]. Thus, activation of Bid links the extrinsic death pathway, initiated by death receptor activation, to mitochondrial (intrinsic) pathways that may culminate in apoptosis or necrosis.

In addition to cell death pathways, activated TNFRs may induce intracellular signaling pathways and novel gene expression that favor cell survival. For example, activation of nuclear factor-κB (NFκB) is antiapoptotic in the setting of central nervous system injury, whereas activation of jun N-kinase (JNK) by death receptors is proapoptotic in ischemic brain. In neuronal cells, JNK activation is involved in apoptosis in response to stress or withdrawal of survival signals, whereas NFκB protects against TNF- and Fas-induced apoptosis by promoting transcription of antioxidant and antiapoptotic genes, including Bcl-2 family members that inhibit cytochrome c translocation and other apoptotic and necrotic death pathways [54–57]. Thus, TNFR family members may activate multiple intracellular signaling pathways that initiate complex, redundant, and often opposing responses, the net effect of which determines cell survival, death, or even proliferation.

Our group and others have studied death receptor signaling in acute brain injury. In experimental cerebral ischemia, inhibition of TNF-α and Fas ligand together reduces infarction volume by as much as 80% [58]. Following cerebral contusion in mice and humans, a Fas-FADD-procaspase-8 DISC assembles in brain early after trauma and is associated with activation of caspases and ongoing cell death [59]. Because death receptor signaling is highly redundant, it is not surprising that genetic inhibition of Fas alone fails to reduce lesion volume or acute cell death after experimental cerebral contusion [60], although Fas inhibition does reduce cerebral ischemic infarction volume [61] and sequelae of traumatic spinal cord injury [62–64]. We have found that genetic or genetic/pharmacologic inhibition of TNF-α and Fas receptor together reduces post-traumatic brain lesion volume, and, more importantly, seems to improve neurologic function after controlled cortical impact in adult and immature mice [60]. Based on these preliminary findings, we believe that TNFRs, and their downstream adapter proteins, are attractive therapeutic targets to ameliorate tissue damage and functional neurologic deficits after ischemic, traumatic, and other forms of central nervous system injury and degenerative central nervous system diseases.

The Poly(ADP-Ribose) Polymerase Suicide Hypothesis

Poly(ADP-ribose) polymerase-1 (PARP-1) is an abundant nuclear DNA repair enzyme that stabilizes damaged DNA for subsequent repair. Upon activation by severe DNA damage, PARP-1 hydrolyzes NAD(+) to nicotinamide and transfers adenosine diphosphate ribose units to histones and other nuclear proteins, including PARP-1 itself. Adenosine diphosphate ribosylation inhibits protein function and facilitates DNA repair, but overactivation of PARP-1 can deplete cellular stores of NAD(+) and adenosine triphosphate, resulting in energy failure and cell death. DNA damage by oxygen radicals, or excitotoxicity injury, induces PARP-1 activation during acute ischemic and traumatic brain injury. Lesion size after experimental stroke is dramatically reduced in PARP-1 knockout mice. Following traumatic brain injury, PARP-1 knockout mice had similar lesion size but improved neurologic function than wild type [65]. Excessive PARP-1 activation is also implicated in models of Parkinson's disease and traumatic spinal cord injury [66–68]. In addition to necrosis via depleted energy reserves, PARP-1 can also induce release of AIF from mitochondria and induce caspase-independent programmed cell death [69]. Finally, PARP-1 is a transcription factor that modulates expression of genes involved in cell death and survival. Recent studies using specific PARP-1 inhibitors show that partial inhibition of PARP-1 preserves brain NAD(+) stores and improves functional outcome after traumatic brain injury in mice, whereas more complete pharmacologic PARP-1 inhibition impairs spatial learning in naïve as well as injured mice [70]. These studies highlight the multiple roles of PARP-1 in traumatic and ischemic brain injury and underscore the difficulties involved in development of therapies targeting proteins with complex and multiple diverse functions in the brain.

Studies in experimental traumatic brain injury often demonstrate very little correlation between cell death and functional outcome, and interventions that inhibit cell death may or may not influence motor and memory function. Thus, it is not yet clear that inhibiting apoptotic cell death will prove beneficial to patients with head injury [32]. The most effective therapeutic strategies will probably target multiple mechanisms in addition to cell death, such as derangements in cerebral blood flow and energy metabolism, or neurotransmitters and their receptors that are involved in the motor and cognitive functions adversely affected by acute brain injury (discussed below).

The Mitochondrial Permeability Transition Pore

The mitochondrial permeability transition (MPT) pore is a voltage-gated channel that, when open, allows molecules and ions with a mass <1,500 Daltons to pass through the inner mitochondrial membrane to the intermembrane space. Oxidative stress, or rapid and extreme increases in intracellular calcium associated with excitotoxicity, triggers the assembly of an MPT pore, which consists of cyclophilin D binding to an adenine nucleotide translocator [71]. Opening of the MPT pore releases stored calcium into the cytosol, and dissipation of the mitochondrial inner transmembrane potential uncouples the electron transport system from adenosine triphosphate hydrolysis. These events lead to energy failure, enhanced production of reactive oxygen species, a secondary increase in intracellular calcium, release of apoptogenic factors from the mitochondria, and cell death [72]. Compounds that block the MPT pore, such as cyclosporine A and its derivatives, are protective in experimental stroke and traumatic brain injury models, suggesting that the MPT pore is a key regulator of cell death mechanisms, both necrotic and apoptotic [71].

Oxidative Damage in Acute Brain Injury

Under normal conditions, a critical balance exists between the production of oxidant free radicals and the antioxidant defense that protects cells in vivo. Free radicals are defined as molecular species that contain one or more unpaired electrons. During normal metabolism, they are involved in enzymatic reactions, mitochondrial electron transport, signal transduction, activation of nuclear transcription factors, gene expression, and the antimicrobial action of neutrophils and macrophages [73]. The balance between oxidants and antioxidants in injured brain may be disturbed by increased production of free radicals because antioxidant defenses in brain (such as superoxide dismutase, catalase, glutathione, ascorbate, and α-tocopherol) are not adequate to completely neutralize the increase of oxidant species present after trauma or ischemia–reperfusion [74]. The severity of oxidant–antioxidant imbalance determines the magnitude of injury to the cell.

Free radicals can react with almost every molecule found in living cells, including DNA, membrane lipids, proteins, and carbohydrates. A major consequence of oxidative stress is damage to cellular macromolecules. During lipid peroxidation, peroxyl or hydroxyl groups may be added to unsaturated fatty acids, or fatty acid carbon chains may be cleaved during reaction with unpaired electrons to generate aldehydes. Free radical damage to proteins may cause cross-linking, carbonyl formation, and protein denaturation. DNA bases may also be modified by oxidation, resulting in single- and double-strand breaks or mispairing of purine and pyrimidine during DNA replication.

The brain has a number of characteristics that make it especially susceptible to free radical–mediated damage. Brain lipids are highly enriched in polyunsaturated fatty acids, and brain regions such as substantia nigra and striatum have high concentrations of iron, which catalyzes production of free radicals. Both of these factors increase the susceptibility of brain cell membranes to lipid peroxidation. Because the brain is critically dependent on aerobic metabolism, mitochondrial respiratory activity is higher than in many other tissues, increasing the risk of free radical *leak* from mitochondria; conversely, free radical damage to mitochondria in brain may be tolerated relatively poorly because of this dependence on aerobic metabolism.

Free radicals have been implicated in the pathogenesis of central nervous system injury, including traumatic brain injury, spinal cord injury, cerebral ischemia, and neurodegenerative diseases [28,73,75–78]. Reactive oxygen species may modify excitotoxicity by downregulating ion flux through NMDA receptors; however, exposure to oxidative stress can also enhance NMDA receptor-mediated neurotoxicity, particularly when antioxidant defenses are depleted. Free radicals contribute to cell death at several points in the apoptotic cascade, serving as initiators, early signals, and possibly late effectors of apoptotic neuronal death. As previously mentioned, oxidative stress can also contribute to cell death by facilitating mitochondria transition pore formation [74]. Proof that excessive oxygen radical generation is fundamental to the pathogenesis of acute brain injury derives from studies in which superoxide dismutase (SOD) knockout mice had increased damage, and SOD overexpressors had reduced brain damage and improved functional neurologic outcome after experimental stroke and traumatic brain injury [79–82].

Reactive Oxygen Species

Reactive oxygen species formation during ischemia–reperfusion may originate from several sources (Figure 2.2), including nitric oxide synthase (NOS) activity, mitochondrial electron transport, multiple steps in the metabolism of arachidonic acid, and, in some species (e.g., rodents), xanthine oxidase, which is produced by hydrolysis of xanthine dehydrogenase. Oxygen (O_2) qualifies as a radical because it has two unpaired electrons, each located in a different orbital, both *spinning* in the same direction. This parallel spin is one reason for poor reactivity of O_2 with cellular constituents, despite its potential as an oxidizing agent. Acceptance of a single electron by an O_2 molecule forms the superoxide radical, O_2^-, which has one unpaired electron. Superoxide itself has limited reactivity and is capable of inactivating only a few enzymes directly. The NADH dehydrogenase complex of the mitochondrial electron transport chain is one of the enzymes shown to be a direct target for superoxide attack [83].

Excess superoxide is removed by converting it to H_2O_2, a reaction that is catalyzed by SOD. This reaction is an important defense mechanism in aerobic organisms [83]. Overall, both O_2^- and H_2O_2 have limited chemical reactivity, but they can generate highly reactive hydroxyl radicals (OH·) by reacting with transition metals such as iron and copper. After closed head injury in rats, peak hydroxyl radical formation occurred by 40 min, and hydroxyl radicals are increased for several hours after experimental acute subdural hematoma [84–86]. Increased hydroxyl radical production also occurs in brain after focal cerebral ischemic injury in rodents [87]. Superoxide production has been detected after experimental spinal

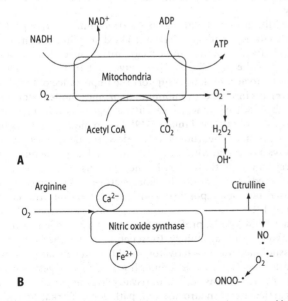

A

B

Figure 2.2. Oxidative stress pathways. **(A)** Reactive oxygen species generated by mitochondrial electron transport and **(B)** reactive nitrogen species generated by nitric oxide synthase. Peroxynitrite (ONOO-) is a highly toxic species that signals apoptosis and necrosis after acute brain injury. Other oxidants are generated in damaged mitochondria by the electron transport chain and molecular oxygen. NO, nitric oxide; $O_2^{·-}$, singlet oxygen; H_2O_2, hydrogen peroxide; OH·, hydroxyl radical. ADP, adenosine diphosphate; ATP, adenosine triphosphate; NAD+, oxidized form of nicotinamide adenine dinucleotide; NADH, reduced form of nicotinamide adenine dinucleotide.

cord injury [88], central nervous system inflammation and ischemia–reperfusion [89], and fluid percussion traumatic brain injury [90]. Superoxide radical is believed to be the principal mediator of microvascular damage after traumatic brain injury, and SOD attenuates brain microvascular damage after traumatic brain injury [91,92].

Reactive Nitrogen Species

Nitric oxide synthase has been identified as another source of reactive oxygen and reactive nitrogen species with special relevance to pathologic conditions (see Figure 2.2). Nitric oxide synthase is homologous to P-450 cytochrome c reductase; cofactors in the reaction-mediated by NOS are flavin mononucleotide, flavin adenine dinucleotide, tetrahydrobiopterin, and nicotinamide adenine dinucleotide phosphate. Three types of NOS have been identified: Ca^{2+}/calmodulin-activated neuronal NOS (nNOS), endothelial NOS (eNOS), and inducible NOS (iNOS). Nitric oxide synthase normally converts arginine and molecular oxygen to citrulline and nitric oxide (NO), a free radical gas. Nitric oxide is lipid soluble, readily crosses cell membranes, and functions in control of cerebral blood flow (NO mediates vasodilatation), neuronal communication, synaptic plasticity and memory formation, intracellular signal transmission, and release of neurotransmitters [93]. Nitric oxide may exist as nitrosonium (NO+), NO·, and nitroxyl anion (NO-). NO+ is thought to contribute to NMDA toxicity, whereas NO- is thought to be neuroprotective by downregulating the NMDA receptor and inhibiting glutamate release presynaptically, through activation of guanylate cyclase. Nitric oxide, which has limited radical reactivity, can combine readily with O_2 and possibly H_2O_2 to produce peroxynitrite (ONOO-), a highly oxidizing, nonradical compound that oxidizes lipids, proteins, and DNA. Nitric oxide-mediated peroxynitrite contributes to acute brain injury in part by inducing DNA damage and activating PARP, as well as directly by oxidizing key cellular constituents. On the other hand, NO can inhibit excitotoxicity by downregulating NMDA receptor function via S-nitrosylation; NO may inhibit caspase activity in a similar manner. Thus, reactive nitrogen species may have both beneficial and detrimental effects in acute brain injury.

Inhibition of the early peak of NO in brain following traumatic brain injury, which is likely mediated by nNOS, improves neurologic outcome after experimental traumatic brain injury [93]. However, later after injury there is a relative NO deficiency associated with cerebral hypoperfusion; augmentation of NO during this time, by administering L-arginine, improves cerebral blood flow and outcome in several models [93]. A delayed increase in NO after traumatic injury, mediated by iNOS, is also observed in experimental traumatic brain injury; experimental studies suggest both deleterious and protective effects of iNOS in rodent traumatic brain injury models. Formation of peroxynitrite by iNOS early after injury is detrimental, and iNOS inhibition may therefore be protective [94]. In contrast, iNOS knockout mice have impaired long-term spatial memory acquisition after experimental traumatic brain injury, suggesting that iNOS is critical for recovery mechanisms [95]. Recent studies support a beneficial role for iNOS in traumatic brain injury by maintaining endogenous antioxidant reserves [94]. Thus, NO can exert beneficial and detrimental effects in the injured brain, depending on the magnitude of its production, temporal distribution after injury, and other factors.

In the first comprehensive clinical study of oxidative injury in children with traumatic brain injury, Bayir and colleagues found progressive depletion of antioxidant reserves and evidence for free radical–mediated lipid peroxidation in cerebrospinal fluid samples [96]. These investigators later reported increased S-nitrosothiols (transfer of NO groups to cysteine sulfhydryls on proteins) in cerebrospinal fluid of children with severe traumatic brain injury and increased intracranial pressure and postulated that S-nitrosothiols could be neuroprotective after traumatic brain injury by virtue of nitrosylation and inhibition of NMDA receptors and caspases [97]. In adult patients, lipid peroxidation was noted early after severe traumatic brain injury and was more prominent in males than in females, suggesting that females have less oxidative damage than males during acute brain injury and enhanced neuroprotection mediated by female gonadal hormones [98]. In that study, therapeutic hypothermia tended to decrease lipid peroxidation in males but not females. These data suggest that differences in susceptibility to oxidative injury may explain, at least in part, gender-specific differences in pathophysiology and outcome observed after acute and neurodegenerative brain injury [99].

Oxidative Stress and Neuroinflammation: Mediators of Neurologic Dysfunction After Brain Injury?

Does the brain's endogenous inflammatory response to acute injury influence subsequent neurologic dysfunction observed in patients with traumatic brain injury, meningitis, and other forms of acute central nervous system injury? Our preliminary data suggest that this may indeed be the case, as immature mice lacking TNF-α and Fas receptor had decreased neurologic dysfunction compared with wild-type mice or mice deficient in TNF or Fas alone [60]. Recent studies provide one possible explanation linking neuroinflammation, NMDA receptor deactivation, and motor and cognitive deficits in experimental meningitis and traumatic brain injury [21,22]. In mice subjected to closed head injury, an initial increase in NMDA receptor activation, consistent with acute excitotoxicity, is observed in brain regions proximal to the injury site. From 1 hr to 1 week later, however, pronounced NMDA receptor deactivation is observed in cortex and hippocampal regions involved in learning and memory and is associated with motor and cognitive dysfunction after traumatic brain injury [21]. Downregulation of NMDA receptor function is also observed after injection of lipopolysaccharide into rat brain and is prevented by treatment with an antioxidant [22]. The above observations suggest a link between acute brain injury, neuroinflammation, oxidant stress, and postinjury neurologic dysfunction. Furthermore, desensitization of NMDA receptors after stroke and traumatic brain injury may in part account for the failure of clinical trials using NMDA receptor antagonists to improve outcome in patients with stroke and traumatic brain injury [21].

Extracellular Matrix Proteases

In addition to intracellular proteases, extracellular proteases may also play important roles in brain injury. Data emerging in the past 6 years implicate proteases from the matrix metalloproteinase (MMP) family of genes as well as serine proteases from the plasminogen axis [100]. These proteases play major roles during brain development by altering extracellular matrix and allowing cellular migration and neurite and axonal extension [101]. Dysregulation of MMPs after brain injury leads to aberrant proteolysis of the neurovascular matrix, resulting in blood–brain barrier (BBB) damage and cell death.

In experimental models of cerebral ischemia, many MMPs are significantly increased at the levels of expression and activity [102–105]. Overall data point to a deleterious role for MMPs, at least acutely. Matrix metalloproteinase injection into brain is neurotoxic [106]. Treatment with inhibitors or MMP-neutralizing antibodies reduce edema and infarction in rat and mouse models of cerebral ischemia [103,107–109]. Recently, it was demonstrated that MMP-9 knockout mice had significantly smaller lesion volumes than wild-type mice after focal cerebral ischemia and traumatic brain injury, emphasizing the central role of this protease, at least in murine systems [102,103,110]. A similar finding was obtained after transient global cerebral ischemia, with hippocampal neuron death being significantly ameliorated in MMP-9 knockout mice [111].

After neurovascular injury, MMPs may degrade basal lamina, weaken vessels, and predispose vessels to leakage and rupture. In experimental studies, activation of MMP-9 and degradation of critical protein components of cerebral blood vessels have been correlated with the development of hemorrhage and edema [112,113]. In a recent study, pharmacologic inhibition of MMPs significantly decreased the incidence of hemorrhage in a rabbit model of embolic stroke [102], and matrix degradation and subsequent BBB leakage was reduced after cerebral ischemia in MMP-9 knockout mice [102]. Matrix metalloproteinase activation and BBB disruption is associated with the generation of reactive oxygen radicals [114]; thus interactions between oxidative stress and the proteolytic cascade may ultimately mediate the progression of edema and infarction. Within the context of early neurovascular inflammation, cytokines and vascular adhesion molecules may further amplify MMPs in activated endothelium [115–117]. Cell adhesion molecules themselves may also be substrates for MMPs, thus comprising a complex interactive system of response to brain injury.

In addition to vascular leakage, extracellular matrix proteases may also directly induce cell death. The disruption of homeostatic signals between cells and matrix can initiate specialized modes of apoptosis called *anoikis* [118]. In vivo and in vitro evidence is beginning to accumulate to support the importance of these novel mechanisms in stroke. In a nonhuman primate model of focal cerebral ischemia, areas in which vascular antigens were lost correlated with regions of neuronal injury [119]. Loss of neuron–matrix interactions promotes neurotoxicity by downregulating cell survival pathways associated with integrin signaling [120]. The importance and relevance of these matrix mechanisms has recently been underscored by the finding that fibronectin knockout mice suffered increased neuronal apoptosis and brain infarction after cerebral ischemia [121].

Apart from MMPs, proteases from the plasminogen system are also involved in brain injury. In ischemic stroke, the primary role for tissue plasminogen activator would be beneficial lysis of the offending clot. However, accumulating data now suggest that pleiotropic and deleterious actions of tissue plasminogen activator may also participate in neurovascular pathology. Tsirka, Strickland, Lipton, and colleagues first demonstrated that tissue plasminogen activator knockout mice were protected against excitotoxic hippocampal injury and focal cerebral ischemia [122,123]. Tissue plasminogen activator knockout mice suffered significantly less brain damage after trauma than did wild-type mice [124]. Tissue plasminogen activator may interact with the NR1 subunit of the NMDA receptor complex and amplify damaging calcium currents during excitotoxicity [125]. Tissue plasminogen activator (and plasmin) may also target nonfibrin substrates in brain extracellular matrix, leading to augmented excitotoxic neuronal death in the hippocampus via degradation of interneuronal laminin and disruption of prosurvival cell-matrix signaling (126). Although the main effect of tissue plasminogen activator administration in stroke certainly occurs within the targeted vessel, these findings suggest that extravascular actions of tissue plasminogen activator may complicate its intended role in clot lysis.

Most brain injury research has been focused on intracellular mechanisms of cell death. However, accumulating data now suggest that extracellular proteases can also play key roles by degrading neurovascular matrix and inducing both BBB disruption and cell death. Hence, targeting both intra- and extracellular proteases may offer more effective approaches for treating stroke and brain trauma in the future.

Cortical Spreading Depression

During acute brain injury such as stroke or trauma, neurons and glia may undergo spontaneous depolarizations that spread in waves to distant regions of uninjured brain. These waves, known as *cortical spreading depression* (CSD), propagate at 2–4 mm/min over cerebral cortex and are associated with marked increases in extracellular K^+ and glutamate and intracellular Na^+ and Ca^{2+} [127]. Although neuronal firing may initially increase, it is subsequently depressed, and the electroencephalographic silence outlasts the period of tissue depolarization by several minutes [127]. Cortical spreading depression causes a large transient cerebral blood flow increase, followed by delayed, prolonged cerebral blood flow decrease [128]. In experimental animal models, NMDA receptor inhibitors (e.g., ketamine) and Ca^{2+} channel antagonists block CSD [129]. The factors that mediate cerebral blood flow changes during CSD remain unknown, although K^+, H^+, prostanoids, nitric oxide (NO), and calcitonin gene-related peptide have been implicated [130–133].

Following experimental cerebral ischemia, repetitive spontaneous waves of spreading depolarizations resembling CSD originate from focal ischemic cortex [134]. Like CSD, these periinfarct spreading depressions cause massive K^+, Na^+, and Ca^{2+} shifts, reduce intracellular adenosine triphosphate, and cause tissue acidosis. Periinfarct spreading depressions decrease cerebral blood flow and worsen hypoperfusion under ischemic conditions and enlarge cerebral infarcts presumably by exacerbating the energy deficit in ischemic neurons [135–137]. More work needs to be done to understand the contribution of CSD to acute brain injury in humans and to determine whether targeting CSD in the postinjury period is a useful therapeutic strategy [138].

References

1. Purves DAG, Fitzpatrick D, Hall W, LaMantia A, McNamara J, Williams S. Neuroscience. Sunderland, MA: Sinauer Associates;2004: 773.
2. Stevens CF. Spatial learning and memory: the beginning of a dream. Cell 1996;87:1147–1148.
3. Lucas DR, Newhouse JP. The toxic effect of sodium L-glutamate on the inner layers of the retina. AMA Arch Ophthalmol 1957;58:193–201.
4. Arundine M, Tymianski M. Molecular mechanisms of glutamate-dependent neurodegeneration in ischemia and traumatic brain injury. Cell Mol Life Sci 2004;61:657–668.
5. Choi DW. Excitotoxic cell death. J Neurobiol 1992;23:1261–1276.
6. Choi D. Antagonizing excitotoxicity: a therapeutic strategy for stroke? Mt Sinai J Med 1998;65:133–138.
7. Duhaime AC. Exciting your neurons to death: can we prevent cell loss after brain injury? Pediatr Neurosurg 1994;21:117–123.
8. Hillered L, Vespa PM, Hovda DA. Translational neurochemical research in acute human brain injury: the current status and potential future for cerebral microdialysis. J Neurotrauma 2005;22:3–41.
9. Chan PH. Mitochondria and neuronal death/survival signaling pathways in cerebral ischemia. Neurochem Res 2004;29:1943–1949.
10. Schwab BL, Guerini D, Didszun C, et al. Cleavage of plasma membrane calcium pumps by caspases: a link between apoptosis and necrosis. Cell Death Differ 2002;9:818–831.
11. Bano D, Young KW, Guerin CJ, et al. Cleavage of the plasma membrane Na^+/Ca^{2+} exchanger in excitotoxicity. Cell 2005;120:275–285.
12. Kroppenstedt SN, Schneider GH, Thomale UW, Unterberg AW. Protective effects of aptiganel HCl (Cerestat) following controlled cortical impact injury in the rat. J Neurotrauma 1998;15:191–197.
13. Chen M, Bullock R, Graham DI, Frey P, Lowe D, McCulloch J. Evaluation of a competitive NMDA antagonist (D-CPPene) in feline focal cerebral ischemia. Ann Neurol 1991;30:62–70.
14. Rod MR, Auer RN. Pre- and post-ischemic administration of dizocilpine (MK-801) reduces cerebral necrosis in the rat. Can J Neurol Sci 1989;16:340–344.
15. Shapira Y, Yadid G, Cotev S, Niska A, Shohami E. Protective effect of MK801 in experimental brain injury. J Neurotrauma 1990;7:131–139.
16. Fisher M. The travails of neuroprotective drug development for acute ischemic stroke. Eur Neurol 1998;40:65–66.
17. Maas AI, Steyerberg EW, Murray GD, et al. Why have recent trials of neuroprotective agents in head injury failed to show convincing efficacy? A pragmatic analysis and theoretical considerations. Neurosurgery 1999;44:1286–1298.
18. Narayan RK, Michel ME, Ansell B, et al. Clinical trials in head injury. J Neurotrauma 2002;19:503–557.
19. Ikonomidou C, Turski L. Why did NMDA receptor antagonists fail clinical trials for stroke and traumatic brain injury? Lancet Neurol 2002;1:383–386.
20. Hoyte L, Barber PA, Buchan AM, Hill MD. The rise and fall of NMDA antagonists for ischemic stroke. Curr Mol Med 2004;4:131–136.
21. Biegon A, Fry PA, Paden CM, Alexandrovich A, Tsenter J, Shohami E. Dynamic changes in N-methyl-D-aspartate receptors after closed head injury in mice: implications for treatment of neurological and cognitive deficits. Proc Natl Acad Sci USA 2004;101:5117–5122.
22. Biegon A, Alvarado M, Budinger TF, et al. Region-selective effects of neuroinflammation and antioxidant treatment on peripheral benzodiazepine receptors and NMDA receptors in the rat brain. J Neurochem 2002;82:924–934.
23. Bittigau P, Sifringer M, Felderhoff-Mueser U, Ikonomidou C. Apoptotic neurodegeneration in the context of traumatic injury to the developing brain. Exp Toxicol Pathol 2004;56:83–89.
24. Zhang F, Yin W, Chen J. Apoptosis in cerebral ischemia: executional and regulatory signaling mechanisms. Neurol Res 2004;26:835–845.
25. Tolias CM, Bullock MR. Critical appraisal of neuroprotection trials in head injury: what have we learned? Neurorx 2004;1:71–79.
26. Mergenthaler P, Dirnagl U, Meisel A. Pathophysiology of stroke: lessons from animal models. Metab Brain Dis 2004;19:151–167.
27. Charriaut-Marlangue C. Apoptosis: a target for neuroprotection. Therapie 2004;59:185–190.
28. Starkov AA, Chinopoulos C, Fiskum G. Mitochondrial calcium and oxidative stress as mediators of ischemic brain injury. Cell Calcium 2004;36:257–264.
29. Raghupathi R. Cell death mechanisms following traumatic brain injury. Brain Pathol 2004;14:215–222.
30. Lo EH, Moskowitz MA, Jacobs TP. Exciting, radical, suicidal: how brain cells die after stroke. Stroke 2005;36:189–192.
31. Kochanek PM, Clark RS, Ruppel RA, et al. Biochemical, cellular, and molecular mechanisms in the evolution of secondary damage after

severe traumatic brain injury in infants and children: lessons learned from the bedside. Pediatr Crit Care Med 2000;1:4–19.

32. Zhang X, Chen Y, Jenkins LW, Kochanek PM, Clark RS. Bench-to-bedside review: apoptosis/programmed cell death triggered by traumatic brain injury. Crit Care 2005;9:66–75.

33. Yuan J, Lipinski M, Degterev A. Diversity in the mechanisms of neuronal cell death. Neuron 2003;40:401–413.

34. Vanden Berghe T, van Loo G, Saelens X, et al. Differential signaling to apoptotic and necrotic cell death by Fas-associated death domain protein FADD. J Biol Chem 2004;279:7925–7933.

35. Lockshin RA. Programmed cell death. Activation of lysis by a mechanism involving the synthesis of protein. J Insect Physiol 1969;15:1505–1516.

36. Webster DA, Gross J. Studies on possible mechanisms of programmed cell death in the chick embryo. Dev Biol 1970;22:157–184.

37. Marovitz WF, Shugar JM, Khan KM. The role of cellular degeneration in the normal development of (rat) otocyst. Laryngoscope 1976;86:1413–1425.

38. Thornberry NA. Caspases: key mediators of apoptosis. Chem Biol 1998;5:R97–R103.

39. Clark RS, Kochanek PM, Watkins SC, et al. Caspase-3 mediated neuronal death after traumatic brain injury in rats. J Neurochem 2000;74:740–753.

40. Kerr JF. A histochemical study of hypertrophy and ischaemic injury of rat liver with special reference to changes in lysosomes. J Pathol Bacteriol 1965;90:419–435.

41. Susin SA, Lorenzo HK, Zamzami N, et al. Molecular characterization of mitochondrial apoptosis-inducing factor. Nature 1999;397:441–446.

42. Lorenzo HK, Susin SA, Penninger J, Kroemer G. Apoptosis inducing factor (AIF): a phylogenetically old, caspase-independent effector of cell death. Cell Death Differ 1999;6:516–524.

43. Joza N, Susin SA, Daugas E, et al. Essential role of the mitochondrial apoptosis-inducing factor in programmed cell death. Nature 2001;410:549–554.

44. Cande C, Cohen I, Daugas E, et al. Apoptosis-inducing factor (AIF): a novel caspase-independent death effector released from mitochondria. Biochimie 2002;84:215–222.

45. Daugas E, Nochy D, Ravagnan L, et al. Apoptosis-inducing factor (AIF): a ubiquitous mitochondrial oxidoreductase involved in apoptosis. FEBS Lett 2000;476:118–123.

46. Choi C, Benveniste EN. Fas ligand/Fas system in the brain: regulator of immune and apoptotic responses. Brain Res Brain Res Rev 2004;44:65–81.

47. Thorburn A. Death receptor-induced cell killing. Cell Signal 2004;16:139–144.

48. Wallach D, Boldin M, Varfolomeev E, Beyaert R, Vandenabeele P, Fiers W. Cell death induction by receptors of the TNF family: towards a molecular understanding. FEBS Lett 1997;410:96–106.

49. Nagata S. Apoptosis by death factor. Cell 1997;88:355–365.

50. Wei MC, Lindsten T, Mootha VK, et al. tBID, a membrane-targeted death ligand, oligomerizes BAK to release cytochrome c. Genes Dev 2000;14:2060–2071.

51. Leonard JR, D'Sa C, Cahn BR, Korsmeyer SJ, Roth KA. Bid regulation of neuronal apoptosis. Brain Res Dev Brain Res 2001;128:187–190.

52. Plesnila N, Zinkel S, Le DA, et al. BID mediates neuronal cell death after oxygen/ glucose deprivation and focal cerebral ischemia. Proc Natl Acad Sci USA 2001;98:15318–15323.

53. Wang X, Ryter SW, Dai C, et al. Necrotic cell death in response to oxidant stress involves the activation of the apoptogenic caspase-8/bid pathway. J Biol Chem 2003;278:29184–29191.

54. Mattson MP, Goodman Y, Luo H, Fu W, Furukawa K. Activation of NF-kappaB protects hippocampal neurons against oxidative stress-induced apoptosis: evidence for induction of manganese superoxide dismutase and suppression of peroxynitrite production and protein tyrosine nitration. J Neurosci Res 1997;49:681–697.

55. Ashkenazi A, Dixit VM. Death receptors: signaling and modulation. Science 1998;281:1305–1308.

56. Le-Niculescu H, Bonfoco E, Kasuya Y, Claret FX, Green DR, Karin M. Withdrawal of survival factors results in activation of the JNK pathway in neuronal cells leading to Fas ligand induction and cell death. Mol Cell Biol 1999;19:751–763.

57. Cassarino DS, Halvorsen EM, Swerdlow RH, et al. Interaction among mitochondria, mitogen-activated protein kinases, and nuclear factor-kappaB in cellular models of Parkinson's disease. J Neurochem 2000;74:1384–1392.

58. Martin-Villalba A, Hahne M, Kleber S, et al. Therapeutic neutralization of CD95-ligand and TNF attenuates brain damage in stroke. Cell Death Differ 2001;8:679–686.

59. Qiu J, Whalen MJ, Lowenstein P, et al. Upregulation of the Fas receptor death-inducing signaling complex after traumatic brain injury in mice and humans. J Neurosci 2002;22:3504–3511.

60. Bermpohl D YZ, Lai C, Moskowitz MA, Whalen MJ. Cell death and neurologic dysfunction after controlled cortical impact in immature mice deficient in TNF alpha and Fas genes. J Neurotrauma 2004;21:1332.

61. Martin-Villalba A, Herr I, Jeremias I, et al. CD95 ligand (Fas-L/APO-1L) and tumor necrosis factor–related apoptosis-inducing ligand mediate ischemia-induced apoptosis in neurons. J Neurosci 1999;19:3809–3817.

62. Yoshino O, Matsuno H, Nakamura H, et al. The role of Fas-mediated apoptosis after traumatic spinal cord injury. Spine 2004;29:1394–1404.

63. Beattie MS. Inflammation and apoptosis: linked therapeutic targets in spinal cord injury. Trends Mol Med 2004;10:580–583.

64. Demjen D, Klussmann S, Kleber S, et al. Neutralization of CD95 ligand promotes regeneration and functional recovery after spinal cord injury. Nat Med 2004;10:389–395.

65. Whalen MJ, Clark RS, Dixon CE, et al. Reduction of cognitive and motor deficits after traumatic brain injury in mice deficient in poly(ADP-ribose) polymerase. J Cereb Blood Flow Metab 1999;19:835–842.

66. Casey PJ, Black JH, Szabo C, et al. Poly(adenosine diphosphate ribose) polymerase inhibition modulates spinal cord dysfunction after thoracoabdominal aortic ischemia-reperfusion. J Vasc Surg 2005;41:99–107.

67. Genovese T, Mazzon E, Muia C, et al. Inhibitors of poly(ADP-ribose) polymerase modulate signal transduction pathways and secondary damage in experimental spinal cord trauma. J Pharmacol Exp Ther 2005;312:449–457.

68. Skaper SD. Poly(ADP-ribosyl)ation enzyme-1 as a target for neuroprotection in acute central nervous system injury. Curr Drug Targets CNS Neurol Disord 2003;2:279–291.

69. Yu SW, Wang H, Poitras MF, et al. Mediation of poly(ADP-ribose) polymerase-1-dependent cell death by apoptosis-inducing factor. Science 2002;297:259–263.

70. Satchell MA, Zhang X, Kochanek PM, et al. A dual role for poly-ADP-ribosylation in spatial memory acquisition after traumatic brain injury in mice involving NAD+ depletion and ribosylation of 14-3-3gamma. J Neurochem 2003;85:697–708.

71. Sullivan PG, Rabchevsky AG, Waldmeier PC, Springer JE. Mitochondrial permeability transition in CNS trauma: cause or effect of neuronal cell death? J Neurosci Res 2005;79:231–239.

72. Siesjo BK, Elmer E, Janelidze S, et al. Role and mechanisms of secondary mitochondrial failure. Acta Neurochir Suppl 1999;73:7–13.

73. Warner DS, Sheng H, Batinic-Haberle I. Oxidants, antioxidants and the ischemic brain. J Exp Biol 2004;207:3221–3231.

74. Lo EH, Dalkara T, Moskowitz MA. Mechanisms, challenges and opportunities in stroke. Nat Rev Neurosci 2003;4:399–415.

75. Dawson VL. Nitric oxide: role in neurotoxicity. Clin Exp Pharmacol Physiol 1995;22:305–308.

76. Beckman JS. Peroxynitrite versus hydroxyl radical: the role of nitric oxide in superoxide-dependent cerebral injury. Ann NY Acad Sci 1994;738:69–75.

77. Buonocore G, Perrone S, Bracci R. Free radicals and brain damage in the newborn. Biol Neonate 2001;79:180–186.

78. Chan PH. Reactive oxygen radicals in signaling and damage in the ischemic brain. J Cereb Blood Flow Metab 2001;21:2–14.

79. Kinouchi H, Epstein CJ, Mizui T, Carlson E, Chen SF, Chan PH. Attenuation of focal cerebral ischemic injury in transgenic mice overexpressing CuZn superoxide dismutase. Proc Natl Acad Sci USA 1991; 88:11158–11162.

80. Kondo T, Reaume AG, Huang TT, et al. Reduction of CuZn-superoxide dismutase activity exacerbates neuronal cell injury and edema formation after transient focal cerebral ischemia. J Neurosci 1997;17:4180–4189.

81. Pineda JA, Aono M, Sheng H, et al. Extracellular superoxide dismutase overexpression improves behavioral outcome from closed head injury in the mouse. J Neurotrauma 2001;18:625–634.

82. Mikawa S, Kinouchi H, Kamii H, et al. Attenuation of acute and chronic damage following traumatic brain injury in copper, zinc-superoxide dismutase transgenic mice. J Neurosurg 1996;85:885–891.

83. Zhang Y, Marcillat O, Giulivi C, Ernster L, Davies KJ. The oxidative inactivation of mitochondrial electron transport chain components and ATPase. J Biol Chem 1990;265:16330–16336.

84. Sen S, Goldman H, Morehead M, Murphy S, Phillis JW. alpha-Phenyl-tert-butyl-nitrone inhibits free radical release in brain concussion. Free Radic Biol Med 1994;16:685–691.

85. Smith SL, Andrus PK, Zhang JR, Hall ED. Direct measurement of hydroxyl radicals, lipid peroxidation, and blood-brain barrier disruption following unilateral cortical impact head injury in the rat. J Neurotrauma 1994;11:393–404.

86. Doppenberg EM, Rice MR, Di X, Young HF, Woodward JJ, Bullock R. Increased free radical production due to subdural hematoma in the rat: effect of increased inspired oxygen fraction. J Neurotrauma 1998; 15:337–347.

87. Ste-Marie L, Vachon P, Vachon L, Bemeur C, Guertin MC, Montgomery J. Hydroxyl radical production in the cortex and striatum in a rat model of focal cerebral ischemia. Can J Neurol Sci 2000;27:152–159.

88. Liu D, Sybert TE, Qian H, Liu J. Superoxide production after spinal injury detected by microperfusion of cytochrome c. Free Radic Biol Med 1998;25:298–304.

89. Kontos CD, Wei EP, Williams JI, Kontos HA, Povlishock JT. Cytochemical detection of superoxide in cerebral inflammation and ischemia in vivo. Am J Physiol 1992;263:H1234–H1242.

90. Kontos HA, Wei EP. Superoxide production in experimental brain injury. J Neurosurg 1986;64:803–807.

91. Kukreja RC, Kontos HA, Hess ML, Ellis EF. PGH synthase and lipoxygenase generate superoxide in the presence of NADH or NADPH. Circ Res 1986;59:612–619.

92. Wei EP, Kontos HA, Dietrich WD, Povlishock JT, Ellis EF. Inhibition by free radical scavengers and by cyclooxygenase inhibitors of pial arteriolar abnormalities from concussive brain injury in cats. Circ Res 1981;48:95–103.

93. Cherian L, Hlatky R, Robertson CS. Nitric oxide in traumatic brain injury. Brain Pathol 2004;14:195–201.

94. Bayir H, Kagan VE, Borisenko GG, et al. Enhanced oxidative stress in iNOS-deficient mice after traumatic brain injury: support for a neuroprotective role of iNOS. J Cereb Blood Flow Metab 2005;25:673–684.

95. Sinz EH, Kochanek PM, Dixon CE, et al. Inducible nitric oxide synthase is an endogenous neuroprotectant after traumatic brain injury in rats and mice. J Clin Invest 1999;104:647–656.

96. Bayir H, Kagan VE, Tyurina YY, et al. Assessment of antioxidant reserves and oxidative stress in cerebrospinal fluid after severe traumatic brain injury in infants and children. Pediatr Res 2002;51:571–578.

97. Bayir H, Kochanek PM, Liu SX, et al. Increased S-nitrosothiols and S-nitrosoalbumin in cerebrospinal fluid after severe traumatic brain injury in infants and children: indirect association with intracranial pressure. J Cereb Blood Flow Metab 2003;23:51–61.

98. Bayir H, Marion DW, Puccio AM, et al. Marked gender effect on lipid peroxidation after severe traumatic brain injury in adult patients. J Neurotrauma 2004;21:1–8.

99. Czlonkowska A, Ciesielska A, Gromadzka G, Kurkowska-Jastrzebska I. Estrogen and cytokines production—the possible cause of gender differences in neurological diseases. Curr Pharm Des 2005;11:1017–1030.

100. Lo EH, Wang X, Cuzner ML. Extracellular proteolysis in brain injury and inflammation: role for plasminogen activators and matrix metalloproteinases. J Neurosci Res 2002;69:1–9.

101. Levicar N, Nuttall RK, Lah TT. Proteases in brain tumour progression. Acta Neurochir (Wien) 2003;145:825–838.

102. Asahi M, Wang X, Mori T, et al. Effects of matrix metalloproteinase-9 gene knock-out on the proteolysis of blood-brain barrier and white matter components after cerebral ischemia. J Neurosci 2001;21:7724–7732.

103. Asahi M, Asahi K, Jung JC, del Zoppo GJ, Fini ME, Lo EH. Role for matrix metalloproteinase 9 after focal cerebral ischemia: effects of gene knockout and enzyme inhibition with BB-94. J Cereb Blood Flow Metab 2000;20:1681–1689.

104. Fujimura M, Gasche Y, Morita-Fujimura Y, Massengale J, Kawase M, Chan PH. Early appearance of activated matrix metalloproteinase-9 and blood–brain barrier disruption in mice after focal cerebral ischemia and reperfusion. Brain Res 1999;842:92–100.

105. Mun-Bryce S, Rosenberg GA. Matrix metalloproteinases in cerebrovascular disease. J Cereb Blood Flow Metab 1998;18:1163–1172.

106. Anthony DC, Miller KM, Fearn S, et al. Matrix metalloproteinase expression in an experimentally-induced DTH model of multiple sclerosis in the rat CNS. J Neuroimmunol 1998;87:62–72.

107. Rosenberg GA, Estrada EY, Dencoff JE. Matrix metalloproteinases and TIMPs are associated with blood–brain barrier opening after reperfusion in rat brain. Stroke 1998;29:2189–2195.

108. Jiang X, Namura S, Nagata I. Matrix metalloproteinase inhibitor KB-R7785 attenuates brain damage resulting from permanent focal cerebral ischemia in mice. Neurosci Lett 2001;305:41–44.

109. Romanic AM, White RF, Arleth AJ, Ohlstein EH, Barone FC. Matrix metalloproteinase expression increases after cerebral focal ischemia in rats: inhibition of matrix metalloproteinase-9 reduces infarct size. Stroke 1998;29:1020–1030.

110. Wang X, Jung J, Asahi M, et al. Effects of matrix metalloproteinase-9 gene knock-out on morphological and motor outcomes after traumatic brain injury. J Neurosci 2000;20:7037–7042.

111. Lee SR, Tsuji K, Lo EH. Role of matrix metalloproteinases in delayed neuronal damage after transient global cerebral ischemia. J Neurosci 2004;24:671–678.

112. Hamann GF, Okada Y, del Zoppo GJ. Hemorrhagic transformation and microvascular integrity during focal cerebral ischemia/reperfusion. J Cereb Blood Flow Metab 1996;16:1373–1378.

113. Heo JH, Lucero J, Abumiya T, Koziol JA, Copeland BR, del Zoppo GJ. Matrix metalloproteinases increase very early during experimental focal cerebral ischemia. J Cereb Blood Flow Metab 1999;19:624–633.

114. Gasche Y, Fujimura M, Morita-Fujimura Y, et al. Early appearance of activated matrix metalloproteinase-9 after focal cerebral ischemia in mice: a possible role in blood-brain barrier dysfunction. J Cereb Blood Flow Metab 1999;19:1020–1028.

115. Rosenberg GA, Estrada EY, Dencoff JE, Stetler-Stevenson WG. Tumor necrosis factor-alpha–induced gelatinase B causes delayed opening of the blood–brain barrier: an expanded therapeutic window. Brain Res 1995;703:151–155.

116. Aoudjit F, Potworowski EF, St-Pierre Y. Bi-directional induction of matrix metalloproteinase-9 and tissue inhibitor of matrix metalloproteinase-1 during T lymphoma/endothelial cell contact: implication of ICAM-1. J Immunol 1998;160:2967–2973.

117. May AE, Kalsch T, Massberg S, Herouy Y, Schmidt R, Gawaz M. Engagement of glycoprotein IIb/IIIa (alpha(IIb)beta3) on platelets upregulates CD40L and triggers CD40L-dependent matrix degradation by endothelial cells. Circulation 2002;106:2111–2117.

118. Michel JB. Anoikis in the cardiovascular system: known and unknown extracellular mediators. Arterioscler Thromb Vasc Biol 2003;23:2146–2154.

119. Tagaya M, Haring HP, Stuiver I, et al. Rapid loss of microvascular integrin expression during focal brain ischemia reflects neuron injury. J Cereb Blood Flow Metab 2001;21:835–846.

120. Gary DS, Milhavet O, Camandola S, Mattson MP. Essential role for integrin linked kinase in Akt-mediated integrin survival signaling in hippocampal neurons. J Neurochem 2003;84:878–890.

121. Sakai T, Johnson KJ, Murozono M, et al. Plasma fibronectin supports neuronal survival and reduces brain injury following transient focal cerebral ischemia but is not essential for skin-wound healing and hemostasis. Nat Med 2001;7:324–330.

122. Indyk JA, Chen ZL, Tsirka SE, Strickland S. Laminin chain expression suggests that laminin-10 is a major isoform in the mouse hippocampus and is degraded by the tissue plasminogen activator/plasmin protease cascade during excitotoxic injury. Neuroscience 2003;116:359–371.

123. Junge CE, Sugawara T, Mannaioni G, et al. The contribution of protease-activated receptor 1 to neuronal damage caused by transient focal cerebral ischemia. Proc Natl Acad Sci USA 2003;100:13019–13024.

124. Mori T, Wang X, Kline AE, et al. Reduced cortical injury and edema in tissue plasminogen activator knockout mice after brain trauma. Neuroreport 2001;12:4117–4120.

125. Nicole O, Docagne F, Ali C, et al. The proteolytic activity of tissue-plasminogen activator enhances NMDA receptor-mediated signaling. Nat Med 2001;7:59–64.

126. Hacke W, Brott T, Caplan L, et al. Thrombolysis in acute ischemic stroke: controlled trials and clinical experience. Neurology 1999;53:S3–S14.

127. Somjen GG. Mechanisms of spreading depression and hypoxic spreading depression-like depolarization. Physiol Rev 2001;81:1065–1096.

128. Zhang ZG, Chopp M, Maynard KI, Moskowitz MA. Cerebral blood flow changes during cortical spreading depression are not altered by inhibition of nitric oxide synthesis. J Cereb Blood Flow Metab 1994;14:939–943.

129. Kunkler PE, Kraig RP. P/Q Ca^{2+} channel blockade stops spreading depression and related pyramidal neuronal Ca^{2+} rise in hippocampal organ culture. Hippocampus 2004;14:356–367.

130. Colonna DM, Meng W, Deal DD, Busija DW. Calcitonin gene-related peptide promotes cerebrovascular dilation during cortical spreading depression in rabbits. Am J Physiol 1994;266:H1095–H1102.

131. Colonna DM, Meng W, Deal DD, Gowda M, Busija DW. Neuronal NO promotes cerebral cortical hyperemia during cortical spreading depression in rabbits. Am J Physiol 1997;272:H1315–H1322.

132. Meng W, Colonna DM, Tobin JR, Busija DW. Nitric oxide and prostaglandins interact to mediate arteriolar dilation during cortical spreading depression. Am J Physiol 1995;269:H176–H181.

133. Kraig RP, Cooper AJ. Bicarbonate and ammonia changes in brain during spreading depression. Can J Physiol Pharmacol 1987;65:1099–1104.

134. Hossmann KA. Periinfarct depolarizations. Cerebrovasc Brain Metab Rev 1996;8:195–208.

135. Selman WR, Lust WD, Pundik S, Zhou Y, Ratcheson RA. Compromised metabolic recovery following spontaneous spreading depression in the penumbra. Brain Res 2004;999:167–174.

136. Sonn J, Mayevsky A. Effects of brain oxygenation on metabolic, hemodynamic, ionic and electrical responses to spreading depression in the rat. Brain Res 2000;882:212–216.

137. Hopwood SE, Parkin MC, Bezzina EL, Boutelle MG, Strong AJ. Transient changes in cortical glucose and lactate levels associated with peri-infarct depolarisations, studied with rapid-sampling microdialysis. J Cereb Blood Flow Metab 2005;25:391–401.

138. Strong AJ, Fabricius M, Boutelle MG, et al. Spreading and synchronous depressions of cortical activity in acutely injured human brain. Stroke 2002;33:2738–2743.

3

Pediatric Intensive Care Unit Management of Neurosurgical Diseases

Darlene A. Lobel, Mark R. Lee, and Ann-Christine Duhaime

Introduction

Care of the pediatric neurosurgical patient in the postoperative setting requires a generalized knowledge of pediatric intensive care unit (PICU) management as well as specialized knowledge of disease specific concerns in the neurosurgical population. Although postoperative care for each distinct neurosurgical procedure will necessarily vary, several common threads of care must be observed in all of these patients. Specific emphasis for all postoperative neurosurgical patients must be placed on performing a detailed neurologic examination, recognizing signs of elevated intracranial pressure (ICP), and stringent management of fluids and electrolytes [1]. Each of these topics is discussed in detail; is followed by a discussion of specific issues that arise after several common neurosurgical procedures requiring postoperative PICU care.

General Concerns

The Neurologic Examination

A detailed neurologic examination should be performed hourly following admission to the PICU. The child's history and preoperative physical examination findings should be reviewed in order to ascertain any changes in the examination that may occur during the perioperative period. An assessment of the child's mental status is perhaps the most important component of the postoperative neurosurgical examination. Children are commonly less responsive during the first 1–2 hr following craniotomy compared with their baseline because of the lingering effects of general anesthesia. However, after this time period has passed, these children should be oriented to person and time and at a minimum should be able to recognize family members. Speech fluency and patterns should be assessed for any new deficits. Finally, these children should be assessed for the ability to follow both simple and complex commands, as well as their ability to symmetrically move their upper and lower extremities.

Cranial nerves (CNs) II–XII should be evaluated (Table 3.1). First and foremost, it is critical to perform a baseline pupillary examination. Changes in pupillary diameter or pupils that have a sluggish response to light often may precede other changes in the neurologic examination and indicate an early elevation in ICP. However, certain medications may also alter pupil size and reactivity to light. For example, narcotics may cause pupillary constriction, whereas sympathomimetics may cause a symmetric pupillary dilation. Regardless, unequal pupil size in a postoperative neurosurgical patient always warrants further investigation. Of note, papilledema in children is present in chronically elevated ICP, and so the presence of papilledema may not be a reliable indicator of acute intracranial hypertension [2]. Extraocular movements should be assessed to evaluate the function of CNs III (oculomotor nerve), IV (trochlear nerve), and VI (abducens nerve). Occasionally, the first sign of elevated ICP will be a bilateral CN VI palsy. Extraocular muscle palsies are often associated with brain-stem lesions or acute elevations in ICP, although they also may be indicative of meningitis. Infants will often have a physiologic dysconjugate gaze [2]. Parinaud's syndrome, caused by pressure on the tectal plate, causes a characteristic *setting sun sign* in which the upward gaze is impaired and the eyelids are lowered. This sign is readily apparent even in infants and may suggest hydrocephalus. The lower cranial nerves VII–XII should be assessed, as well. Deficits here are noted most commonly after surgical resection of brain stem tumors.

A thorough motor examination should be completed as soon as possible after arrival to the PICU. Even if the child is initially not alert, he should be able to localize to stimuli in all extremities. Once the child is alert, a more detailed motor examination should be performed, including strength testing of the upper and lower extremities. Testing for pronator drift can be a useful adjunct to the formal motor examination, and evidence of a drift is often a more sensitive sign of paresis. Any changes in the child's motor examination from the baseline preoperative examination should be further assessed with an urgent computed tomography (CT) scan. Abnormalities in the sensory examination and the reflex examination may result from effects of a mass lesion, although these findings are often subtle and are difficult to assess in young children.

The Glasgow Coma Scale (GCS) is a useful tool to assess all postoperative neurosurgical patients. As in cases of neurotrauma, all children with a GCS score <8 should be invasively monitored with either a parenchymal ICP monitor or an external ventricular drain

D.S. Wheeler et al. (eds.), *The Central Nervous System in Pediatric Critical Illness and Injury*,
DOI 10.1007/978-1-84800-993-6_3, © Springer-Verlag London Limited 2009

TABLE 3.1. The cranial nerves.

Cranial nerve	Function	Deficit
I Ophthalmic	Smell	Loss of smell—noticeable only if bilateral injury
II Optic	Vision; pupillary response	Nonreactive pupils or blindness
III Oculomotor	Eye movements; pupillary constriction	Large pupil, eye deviated "down and out"; diplopia
IV Trochlear	Eye movements	Diplopia with downgaze
V Trigeminal	Facial sensation; corneal reflex; jaw muscles	Decreased facial sensation; absent corneal reflex
VI Abducens	Eye movements	Diplopia, eye deviated inward
VII Facial	Facial muscles	Unilateral facial droop
VIII Vestibulocochlear	Hearing; balance; doll's eyes response	Decreased hearing; ataxia
IX Glossopharyngeal	Palatal elevation; gag reflex	Poor gag reflex
X Vagus	Pharyngeal muscles	Difficulty swallowing
XI Spinal accessory	Sternocleidomastoid	Head deviation
XII Hypoglossal	Tongue movement	Ipsilateral tongue deviation

(EVD). Typically an EVD is placed in addition to an ICP monitor to allow for both treatment of elevated ICP as well as minute-to-minute monitoring of ICP [3].

Cerebral Edema

Cerebral edema is defined as an absolute increase in the water content of the brain and can arise from a variety of different insults. Cerebral edema is classically divided into three subtypes: (1) vasogenic edema, (2) cytotoxic edema, and (3) interstitial edema. Vasogenic edema is characterized by disruption of the blood-brain barrier (BBB), which leads to the accumulation of fluid in the extracellular space. The inflammatory response to ischemic or traumatic injury results in recruitment and activation of leukocytes, generation of proinflammatory mediators (cytokines, eicosanoids, etc.), release of oxygen radicals, and production of nitric oxide. Vasogenic edema therefore commonly occurs in inflammatory disease processes such as head trauma, meningoencephalitis, and intracranial hemorrhage. It also occurs in areas surrounding tumors and brain abscesses. Vasogenic edema typically responds to osmotic agents such as mannitol and hypertonic saline, as well as to corticosteroids.

Cytotoxic edema results from failure of the brain cells (neuronal cells, glial cells) to maintain their transmembrane ionic gradients. As sodium accumulates in the intracellular space, water follows passively, resulting in intracellular edema. Cytotoxic edema results

from severe cellular dysfunction and cell death and therefore is not readily responsive to therapy with either osmotic agents or corticosteroids. Cytotoxic edema is characteristic of hypoxic-ischemic brain injury. Interstitial edema results from increased cerebrospinal fluid hydrostatic pressure (imbalance in Starling forces across the BBB, which is intact) and typically occurs in periventricular regions of the brain. Interstitial edema is also commonly called *hydrostatic edema* (Table 3.2) [4,5].

Intracranial Hypertension

Most pediatric neurosurgical procedures will not require placement of an ICP monitor or an EVD for postoperative monitoring, with the notable exceptions of placement of subdural grids or postcraniotomy following trauma. Thus, close observation for early signs of elevated ICP is imperative, particularly in the immediate perioperative period. Changes in the neurologic examination, as mentioned above, often indicate early signs of elevations in ICP. Continuous monitoring of vital signs is essential, as bradycardia, hypertension, and irregular respiratory pattern (Cushing's triad) indicate intracranial hypertension. An emergent CT scan should be obtained for any suspicion of intracranial hypertension. If hemorrhage is present, the neurosurgeon must be contacted immediately to assess the need for repeat craniotomy. For cases of stroke, or focal or global cerebral edema, the management becomes more complex and varies based on the pathologic lesion that was originally treated. However, in general, placement of an ICP monitor and/or EVD should be considered for all postoperative patients with a GCS score <8 [1,3,4,6,7].

In general, children should be placed in bed with the head of the bed elevated to 30° following admission to the PICU. Fever should be aggressively treated when present. Treatment measures for acute episodes of intracranial hypertension include administration of sedation and neuromuscular blockade (if the child is tracheally intubated), drainage of cerebrospinal fluid via an indwelling EVD, if available, administration of hypertonic fluids such as 3% normal saline and mannitol, optimization of cerebral perfusion pressure (CPP), and, in severe cases, the use of pentobarbital, hyperventilation, and even decompressive surgical measures [1,4,7–9]. Collaboration between the PICU and neurosurgical faculty is essential when establishing treatment plans.

Cerebral perfusion pressure is a critical indicator of brain oxygenation and is a better predictor of long-term outcome than ICP. Cerebral perfusion pressure is calculated by subtracting the ICP from the mean arterial pressure. Cerebral perfusion pressure should be at least 70 mm Hg to ensure adequate perfusion of the adult brain [10]. If the ICP is below 15 mm Hg, monitoring CPP

TABLE 3.2. Classification of cerebral edema.

Type	Location	Site	Blood–brain barrier integrity	Mechanism	Example
Vasogenic	Extracellular	White matter	Disrupted	Increased vascular permeability	Tumor Trauma Meningitis Abscess Intracerebral hemorrhage
Cytotoxic	Intracellular	Predominantly gray matter	Intact	Na+/K+ pump failure	Anoxia Ischemia
Interstitial	Extracellular	White matter	Intact	Periventricular extravasation	Hydrocephalus

becomes less critical as cerebral autoregulation should provide adequate brain perfusion. If the ICP rises above 15 mm Hg, then pharmacologic agents should be used to maintain the CPP above 60 mm Hg [1,3,4,7,8,11,12]. Management of intracranial hypertension is discussed in further detail in a subsequent chapter.

Fluid and Electrolyte Management

Electrolyte abnormalities are common following craniotomy. Isotonic fluids (e.g., 0.9% saline) administered at maintenance are generally recommended for the first 24 hr following craniotomy. Additionally, blood chemistry levels should be obtained upon arrival to the PICU and periodically during the first 24 hr after surgery. Any abnormalities should be corrected in an expeditious manner. Hyponatremia is commonly observed in the postoperative period and most likely occurs secondary to the syndrome of inappropriate antidiuretic hormone secretion (SIADH). SIADH is best treated by volume restriction.

In certain cases, particularly after head trauma, hyponatremia may be caused by the cerebral salt wasting syndrome, which is best treated with sodium and volume replacement. Blood chemistries are similar in both of these disorders; therefore, the best way to differentiate between these two causes of hyponatremia is to assess the intravascular volume status with a central venous pressure (CVP) monitor. A high CVP is indicative of fluid overload and usually suggests SIADH rather than cerebral salt wasting. Conversely, a low or normal CVP is more suggestive of cerebral salt wasting as the etiology of hyponatremia.

Additionally, some children, particularly after craniotomy for head trauma or for suprasellar or intrasellar tumors, will develop diabetes insipidus (DI). It is therefore critical to monitor urine output closely. Urine output greater than 4 mL/kg/hr for 2 consecutive hours warrants evaluation for DI. Diagnostic criteria for DI include a urine specific gravity of <1.005 and a serum Na^+ level >145 [1,13]. In these cases, lost volume is replaced milliliter for milliliter with normal saline, and a vasopressin infusion should be started and titrated to a normal urine output. It is imperative to check serum sodium levels every 4 hours and continue to monitor urine output to ensure that treatment is adequate.

Hemodynamic Monitoring

It is critical to monitor the child's hemodynamic status after all neurosurgical procedures. Typically an arterial line is placed intraoperatively and is maintained in place while the child is monitored in the PICU. It is imperative that blood pressure be maintained in a normal physiologic range in the immediate postoperative period. Uncontrolled hypertension increases the risk of postoperative hemorrhage, whereas hypotension increases the risk of inadequate cerebral perfusion. The child's hemoglobin level and coagulation factors must be evaluated and corrected to normal levels. Generally, transfusion with packed red blood cells should be considered for a hemoglobin value less than 8.0 g/dL, and fresh-frozen plasma, cryoprecipitate, or vitamin K should be administered to normalize the international normalized ratio (INR) to ≤1.4. Typically laboratory values are assessed in the immediate postoperative period and again the day following surgery. Some children require chronic anticoagulation therapy for co-morbid conditions, although anticoagulation should be withheld in most cases for at least 72 hr after neurosurgical procedures [1].

Management Strategies for Specific Neurosurgical Diseases

Brain Tumors

Brain tumors are the second most common tumor in children, with an incidence of 2.5 cases per 100,000 in children under the age of 15 years [14,15]. Neonates most commonly present with supratentorial neuroectodermal tumors, such as teratomas. Conversely, children over 2 years of age most commonly present with tumors located in the posterior fossa, including medulloblastomas, cerebellar astrocytomas, ependymomas, and brain stem gliomas [16]. Unfortunately, many tumors remain undiagnosed for long periods of time, especially in infants and young children because of the delayed closure of the fontanelles, requiring tumors to reach a large volume before symptoms develop. Most tumors are treated with an attempt at gross total resection, which may be followed by radiation therapy and/or chemotherapy. Prognosis after brain tumor resection varies, ranging from 30% survival at 5 years for the most malignant tumors up to 100% survival for benign tumors [16]. Tumors of the central nervous system are discussed in further detail in a subsequent chapter.

In general, it is not unusual for a child to have transient hemiparesis or even aphasia following resection of a brain tumor, depending on the location of the tumor; this is often due to necessary brain retraction during the surgery, which may cause an increase in edema of the surrounding parenchyma. Corticosteroids are frequently administered in the operating room and continued postoperatively for several days in these patients specifically to address cerebral edema caused by surgical manipulation or by the cytotoxic effects of the tumor itself. Of note, because the brain continues to grow and develop postnatally, children, particularly under the age of 10 years, will often exhibit remarkable recovery after sustaining a neurologic injury.

Other postoperative complications vary based on the location and type of the tumor. Magnetic resonance imaging (MRI) or CT of the head is generally performed within 48 hr following surgical resection of a brain tumor. Delaying imaging beyond this point frequently leads to confounding results with contrast enhancement because of a reactive gliosis, making it difficult to assess for residual tumor. Gliosis is a hypertrophic and hyperplastic response to many types of central nervous system injury, including trauma, stroke, seizure, and neurosurgery, which may obscure the radiographic appearance of any residual tumor during the immediate postoperative period [17–19].

Medulloblastoma

Medulloblastoma is classified as one of the primitive neuroectodermal tumors (PNETs) and is the most common pediatric brain tumor [20]. These tumors are typically located in the midline of the cerebellum, and as a result affected children frequently present with ataxia. Because of the mass effect on the fourth ventricle, these tumors typically cause obstructive hydrocephalus as well. Rarely, children also may present with torticollis. Medulloblastoma may exhibit leptomeningeal dissemination and metastasis to the spinal nerve roots. Cerebrospinal fluid is typically obtained preoperatively to assess for leptomeningeal dissemination, as false-positive CSF is commonly observed in the postoperative period. Recommended treatment of medulloblastoma includes surgical resection followed by chemotherapy and focal radiation treatment. Five-year survival rates vary between 60% and 80% [20,21]. However, even with gross total resection of the tumor, recurrence is common within a 2-year period.

Hydrocephalus is the most common complication associated with medulloblastoma resection. Therefore, an EVD is typically placed preoperatively or intraoperatively in children with suspected medulloblastoma. This drain is typically clamped approximately 3 days after tumor resection. Less than 50% of children will require a long-term ventricular shunt, and, in some patients, hydrocephalus may be treated with a third ventriculostomy.

Resection of posterior fossa tumors often results in transient cerebellar dysfunction. Most commonly, ataxia and nystagmus may worsen in the immediate postoperative period. Occasionally, a constellation of symptoms collectively termed the *posterior fossa syndrome* is observed [22,23]. Irritation or damage to the deep cerebellar nuclei leads to mutism, swallowing apraxia, ataxia, and emotional lability in these children. Fortunately, this syndrome is transient and self-limiting, resolving within a few weeks. Aseptic meningitis occurs occasionally after surgical resection of posterior fossa tumors. Children develop severe headaches and meningismus, but, upon sampling, the cerebrospinal fluid is sterile. These symptoms associated with aseptic meningitis typically respond well to a short course of corticosteroids.

The most concerning complication following surgical resection of a medulloblastoma is development of a hematoma in the posterior fossa. Posterior fossa hematomas are a neurosurgical emergency. Intracranial pressure monitoring may not reveal any abnormalities in the ICP in the posterior fossa, so clinical examination as discussed in the preceding paragraphs is paramount. Altered mental status, slurred speech, respiratory difficulty, and confusion should not be simply attributed to the prolonged effects of anesthesia. Rather, an immediate noncontrast head CT should be obtained. These children frequently require emergent craniotomy. Some neurosurgeons will even forego CT and proceed directly to the operating room in this clinical scenario, as time is of the essence to relieve compression on the brain stem.

Ependymoma

An ependymoma is composed of glial cells that have differentiated along ependymal lines. These tumors occur most commonly in the ependymal lining of the ventricles but may also arise in the filum terminale and in the central spinal canal. The most common location for ependymomas is in the fourth ventricle. Affected children typically present with nausea, vomiting, ataxia, and occasionally cranial nerve palsies. These children will sometimes present with hydrocephalus, although this presentation is less commonly observed than medulloblastomas. Occasionally an EVD will be placed intraoperatively and left in situ for a few days after surgery to treat potential hydrocephalus. Treatment of ependymoma involves surgical resection followed by radiation therapy and/or chemotherapy. Five-year survival rates frequently surpass 85%, particularly in older children [24–26]. As with medulloblastoma, posterior fossa syndrome may occur following surgical resection of ependymoma. As with all surgical procedures in the posterior fossa, careful attention to assessment of the child's neurologic status postoperatively is paramount, as development of a posterior fossa hematoma can be devastating if not treated emergently.

Pilocytic Astrocytoma

Juvenile pilocytic astrocytomas (JPAs) are the most common astrocytic tumor in children. These tumors typically arise in the cerebellum or brain stem, but they can occur anywhere along the cranial–spinal axis. Children initially present with symptoms of elevated intracranial pressure. Depending on the location in the brain, these tumors may also present with hydrocephalus and may require an EVD or a definitive shunt. Gross total surgical resection of JPAs is associated with a nearly 100% 10-year survival rate [27]. Again, these children have the potential to develop posterior fossa syndrome during the immediate postoperative period. Resection of JPAs located in the brain stem carry the additional risk of injury to cranial nerve nuclei.

Nontraumatic Intracerebral Hemorrhage

Nontraumatic intracerebral hemorrhage (ICH) is rare in the pediatric population. Etiology is dependent on the age of the child. Premature infants are at risk for developing intraventricular hemorrhage (IVH) (Table 3.3). This disorder is believed to be caused by the relative immaturity of the germinal matrix in premature infants [28]. Management of IVH typically requires placement of a ventriculoperitoneal shunt only in severe cases. Birth trauma may also lead to ICH in neonates. Older children present with ICH because of a number of factors, including a ruptured arteriovenous malformation, cavernous malformation, tumor, hemorrhagic conversion of an ischemic stroke, venous thrombosis, arterial hypertension, or a ruptured aneurysm [29–31]. Prognosis after nontraumatic ICH varies based on the etiology of the hemorrhage and on the child's GCS at presentation, with a GCS of 3 or 4 portending a dismal prognosis.

Coagulopathies, such as disseminated intravascular coagulation, although common in the PICU, remain an infrequent cause of nontraumatic ICH. Numerous clotting factor deficiencies, such as factor VII deficiency, have been associated with spontaneous intraparenchymal, subdural, or subarachnoid hemorrhages, although ICH in these patients has been most often in the setting of a traumatic injury. Pharmacologic use of anticoagulants such as heparin and warfarin is associated with the feared complication of spontaneous ICH, although this too remains infrequent outside of the setting of full anticoagulation associated with extracorporeal support (e.g., extracorporeal membrane oxygenation). Finally, severe thrombocytopenia (platelet count <10,000) carries the potential risk of nontraumatic ICH particularly in the setting of chemotherapeutic-induced marrow suppression. Thus, a common goal in this setting is to maintain platelet counts >20,000 via transfusion. Idiopathic thrombocytopenic purpura, which is the most common cause of severe thrombocytopenia in childhood, remains a risk factor of ICH. However, a large recent epidemiologic study from the Intercontinental Childhood ITP Study showed that

TABLE 3.3. Classification of head ultrasound findings for intraventricular hemorrhage in the preterm infant.

Classification	Findings
Grade 1	Germinal matrix hemorrhage
Grade 2	Blood within the ventricular system but not distending it
Grade 3	Intraventricular hemorrhage with ventricular dilatation
Grade 4	Parenchymal involvement

only 3 of 1,742 patients suffered an ICH (http://www.itppeople.com/kids.htm).

In children without a history of trauma, further investigation as to the cause of the hemorrhage is essential. Typically this will consist of an MRI with and without contrast and a magnetic resonance angiogram (MRA) to evaluate for structural causes of the hemorrhage. If the results of the MRI/MRA are equivocal, a cerebral angiogram may be indicated to evaluate for aneurysm or arteriovenous malformation. Central nervous system vascular malformations, of a variety of histologic types—venous, arteriovenous, cavernous, capillary telangiectasia—are estimated to be present in up to 4% of the population. Certain diseases, such as Rendu-Osler-Weber syndrome, can be associated with an increased presence of intracranial lesions. Although the data on children are scarce, natural history studies in adults suggests a spontaneous hemorrhage rate between 0.1% and 1.3% per year for cavernous malformations [32], whereas arteriovenous malformations, which account for a large percentage of nontraumatic ICH in children, carry a rebleeding risk of 1.4%–7% per year and a mortality rate of 1% per year for adults [33,34].

In general, most pediatric intracranial hemorrhages that are not caused by structural lesions are treated with medical management for elevated ICP. Surgical evacuation of the hematoma becomes necessary only when there is a rapid decline the child's mental status or in the presence of a progressive neurologic deficit, such as a hemiparesis. In these cases, rapid surgical evacuation of an expanding hematoma can improve outcome in young patients [35].

As a general rule, children with a nontraumatic ICH should undergo a baseline CT scan and a repeated scan at 24 hr. If this scan is stable, repeated CT scanning should be performed if there is a change in the child's neurologic status, or several days after the original scan, to evaluate hematoma resolution. Treatment of venous sinus thrombosis, which requires anticoagulation therapy, will require more frequent CT scans, however. In these cases, CT scans should be attained daily while the child is under anticoagulation therapy, as a rapid expansion in the size of the hematoma may require surgical decompression even in the absence of a change in the child's neurologic examination.

Hematoma caused by an arteriovenous malformation or tumor will be managed medically during the initial hospital stay, unless the child shows signs of progressive rise in ICP. Ruptured aneurysms, however, are treated with surgical clipping or coiling as soon as possible after presentation because of the high risk of rerupture of aneurysms in the first 14 days after hemorrhage. Treatment of ruptured cerebral aneurysms postoperatively requires specialized management to avoid the common complication of cerebral vasospasm, which can lead to stroke.

Traumatic Head Injury

Head injury is most common in infants less than 1 year of age and in children older than 15 years. Many infants are injured during falls or as a result of nonaccidental trauma. Trauma is the most common cause of skull fractures and ICH (e.g., epidural hematomas and subdural hematomas) beyond the newborn period. In practice, most clinical head injuries include a combination of two types of forces, which result in a spectrum of different types of hemorrhages. Contact forces are those that occur when the head is struck or strikes an object. These result in scalp lacerations or contusions, skull fractures, epidural hematomas, and brain surface contusions. Inertial forces are those that occur from movement of the brain within the cranium and generally occur as a result of deceleration of the head. These forces cause concussion (i.e., brief loss of consciousness or alteration in consciousness with amnesia for the event), subdural hematomas, deeper subcortical or brain stem hemorrhages, and diffuse axonal injury. The specific injuries incurred depend on both the type of force and its magnitude, with the latter being dependent of the velocity and/or degree of deceleration, although many patients have a combination of these types of forces and findings.

Epidural Hematomas

Epidural hematoma (Figure 3.1) occurs when a skull fracture or surface contact force traverses an epidural vessel with sufficient force to rupture the vessel. These injuries can occur from low-height falls, especially in infants and young children whose skulls are thin and malleable. Because an arterial epidural hematoma can expand rapidly, a potentially life-threatening injury can occur from *household* falls and should be kept in mind when this mechanism is reported. Affected children may cry initially after the injury and appear well but then may suddenly deteriorate as the clot expands and present in a delayed fashion up to 12 hr after the initial injury [36]. The interval period is frequently referred to as the *lucid interval*. Therefore, children with a significant mechanism of injury should be followed with frequent neurologic examinations and should undergo an early repeated head CT to assess for delayed development of epidural hematoma. Two-thirds of epidural hematomas result from a tear of the middle meningeal artery, and thus cannot be managed without surgical evacuation and cauterization of this vessel. Epidural hematoma, when treated with immediate surgical evacuation, carries a relatively good prognosis, with <10% mortality rate [37].

Venous epidural hematomas may also occur, most often in association with skull fractures. In this instance, the bleeding source is the interdiploic space of the bone itself. These collections usually are small and enlarge gradually. Most of these are managed nonoperatively, but an enlarging clot as determined by serial CT

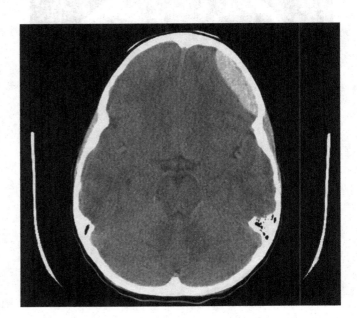

Figure 3.1. Computed tomography appearance of an epidural hematoma.

scanning and/or one that is symptomatic may warrant surgical evacuation. Venous epidural hemorrhages may also occur from tears of the venous dural sinuses. The posterior fossa is a common location for clots of this type, which may be associated with falls onto the back of the head or fractures that traverse the transverse sinus. Children may present with persistent vomiting or worsening mental status in a late fashion, sometimes several days after injury. Clots associated with significant mass effect are evacuated surgically.

Subdural Hematomas

Subdural hematomas (Figure 3.2) usually occur from traumatic events with significant force, most often involving motor vehicles. Acute subdural hematomas are generally evacuated emergently but, because of the large forces involved, are often associated with significant underlying primary brain injury and carry a much worse prognosis than epidural clots [38]. In infants, the most common etiology for acute subdural hematoma is nonaccidental injury. In this setting, the volume of hemorrhage is usually small and can often be managed nonoperatively [39]. When the impact resulting in subdural hematoma is substantial, deep intraparenchymal hemorrhages can occur most often associated with diffuse axonal injury. In these cases, hemorrhages with mass effect warranting surgery are uncommon. Intraventricular hemorrhage may also occur in this setting and may be managed with ventriculostomy drainage.

General Management Approach

Antiepileptic drug therapy is always instituted when children present with seizures after head injury. Typically, 7 days of antiepileptic therapy is recommended for cases of traumatic head injury, even when no seizures were witnessed, because of the high risk of associated seizures [4,6,7,2,39]. Coagulopathy is common in

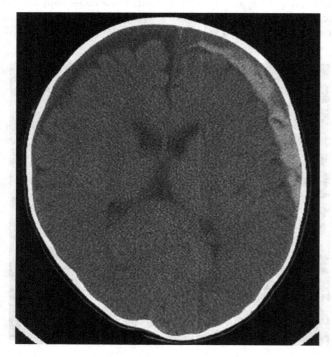

FIGURE 3.2. Computed tomography appearance of a subdural hematoma.

children who sustain head injury because of the release of brain tissue thromboplastin [41]. Therefore, it is integral to monitor coagulation factors and correct them to normal levels. As with the adult population, clinical presentation correlates with long-term outcome in children who suffer head injuries. In general, children who present with a CGS <5 have a dismal prognosis with or without surgical intervention.

Skull fractures often do not require surgical intervention, with a few notable exceptions. Open, depressed skull fractures are often treated with immediate surgical debridement and fracture repair to lessen the risk of developing meningitis, cerebrospinal fluid leak, or seizures. However, some neurosurgeons may choose to defer surgery until the swelling has lessened if there is no obvious cerebrospinal fluid leak at the time of injury. In these cases, children are treated with local wound washout at the bedside with primary closure of the skin and treatment with several days of antibiotics, such as cefazolin. Skull fractures that are associated with underlying brain injury, such as an epidural hematoma, require immediate evacuation and surgical repair in the vast majority of cases.

Occasionally, small epidural hematomas (less than 3 mm in greatest diameter) may be followed clinically, if the child presents with a stable neurologic examination. However, it is essential to obtain frequent CT scans in the first 24 hr after injury to assess for hematoma expansion. In these cases, intravenous isotonic fluid therapy should be used judiciously, as high intravenous volume may worsen cerebral edema and increase the risk of intracranial hypertension. However, intravenous fluids should not be withheld when there is evidence of hemodynamic instability, as hypotension significantly worsens outcome following closed head injury. If there is a change in neurologic status or pupillary size during this observation period, it is critical to obtain a repeated CT scan of the head to be followed by surgical evacuation of the expanding hematoma, if indicated.

Subdural hematomas may be managed either medically or surgically in children. Generally, subdural hematomas >5 mm should be treated with surgical evacuation, as they can precipitate cerebral edema, leading to a significant mass effect and shift, which may progress to subfalcine and uncal herniation and eventually death. As with medical management of epidermal hematomas, subdural hematomas should be followed with frequent CT scans in the first 24 hr after injury.

After surgical evacuation of either a subdural or an epidural hematoma, the child's neurologic examination should be monitored closely. There is a moderate incidence of recurrence of subdural and epidural hematomas after craniotomy for trauma. A CT scan is typically obtained at 24 hr after surgery or sooner if there is a change in the neurologic examination. Repeated craniotomy is occasionally required for recurrent hematomas. The management of children with head trauma frequently becomes complicated by management of concomitant injuries. Not only do children present with multisystem trauma, but also traumatic brain injury itself can precipitate pulmonary edema, acute respiratory distress syndrome, and other systemic complications (so-called *neurogenic pulmonary edema*). Therefore, collaboration between the PICU team, the neurosurgeon, and the pediatric trauma team is essential to provide optimal care to these children.

Finally, presentation of a child with a subdural or epidural hematoma or a skull fracture without appropriate history of trauma must be considered nonaccidental trauma. In these cases, a full skeletal survey, ophthalmologic assessment for retinal hemorrhages, and social services evaluation must be pursued.

Spinal Cord Injury

Approximately 20% of all spinal cord injuries occur in children under the age of 20 years [42]. Because of the relative cephalocervical disproportion in younger children as well as ligamentous laxity in the developing spine, children often present with different mechanisms of spinal cord injury from adults [43]. Often, there is no evidence of fracture or dislocation on plain radiographs and CT scans, and injuries are identified only after obtaining an MRI [44]. Hemodynamic instability often accompanies acute spinal cord injury. Neurogenic shock, which results in hypotension and bradycardia, is a result of decreased sympathetic tone. Neurogenic shock most commonly presents within the first few hours after spinal cord injury and is treated with the use of vasopressors and sympathomimetics. Hypotension typically resolves spontaneously after 2–3 days. Autonomic dysreflexia (AD), caused by a supranormal response of the sympathetic nervous system, is a common, often life-threatening, complication of high thoracic and cervical cord injuries. Often precipitated by bladder and bowel distention, AD may also occur after urinary tract infections, deep venous thromboses, or any surgical procedure. Classic symptoms of AD include hypertension, tachycardia, and cardiac arrhythmias. Treatment is focused on removal of the inciting stimulus.

Significant controversy exists over the use of intravenous corticosteroids for the treatment of acute spinal cord injury. Preclinical data and the results from the landmark studies in the 1980s [45–47] suggest that treatment with high-dose intravenous methylprednisolone may improve neurologic function after spinal cord injury. According to the National Acute Spinal Cord Injury Study protocol, any patient who presents within 3 hr of injury of injury should receive a 30 mg/kg bolus of intravenous methylprednisolone over 15 min, followed by a continuous infusion of 5.4 mg/kg/hr for 23 hr. If the patient presents within 3 to 8 hr of injury, the hourly dosage is continued for a total of 48 hr. Results from these studies suggest that treatment with intravenous methylprednisolone may result in recovery of one to two levels of function above the level of injury. Importantly, however, these studies included no pediatric patients, and, to date, no randomized trials have been conducted to assess the benefit of corticosteroid use in acute spinal cord injury in children. Furthermore, recent publications have called into question the results of the original studies and point to serious potential side effects from this treatment [48–51].

Timing of surgery to decompress and stabilize the spine after spinal cord injury is somewhat controversial [52–54]. Some neurosurgeons advocate early surgery, even in cases of complete spinal cord injury, whereas others recommend delaying surgery until the patient is more stable. Incomplete spinal cord injury due to a lesion causing mass effect, such as a traumatic disc herniation or an epidural hematoma, should always be treated early in order to allow for maximal recovery potential [55]. Optimal timing of surgery should be decided upon by both the neurosurgeons and pediatric intensivists to allow maximum recovery and address medical issues.

Intracranial Abscess

Brain abscess is a rare but serious condition in children (Figure 3.3). The peak age for children to develop brain abscesses is between 4 and 7 years [56]. Abscesses often occur secondary to direct contiguous spread from ear, sinus, or dental infections, but may also arise because of hematogenous seeding in children with

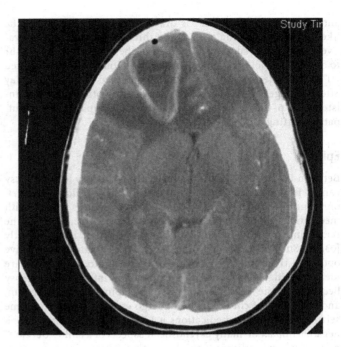

FIGURE 3.3. Computed tomography appearance of a brain abscess.

cyanotic congenital heart disease [55]. With an increase in the number of pediatric immunizations and better treatment of systemic infections in recent years, the incidence of brain abscesses in children has diminished significantly. The classic triad for symptomatic presentation of brain abscess is headache, focal neurologic deficit, and fever. However, this triad is found in <30% of children with brain abscess [49], so, even in absence of these symptoms, a high index of suspicion must be maintained. Additionally, lack of fever should not rule out brain abscess, as low-grade fever is observed in 50% of children with this condition. Contrasted CT of the head and MRI of the brain with gadolinium are the imaging modalities of choice to diagnose brain abscess.

Most brain abscesses are caused by streptococci; however, *Staphylococcus* species and occasionally enteric bacteria may be isolated from cultures as well [58]. Sterile cultures are found in a significant number of abscesses, so generally antibiotic treatment should be tailored toward Gram-positive and Gram-negative bacteria, as well as anaerobes, unless a specific bacteria is isolated from cultures. We generally avoid intravenous corticosteroid therapy with brain abscess, as this can decrease the ability of the antibiotics to penetrate the abscess cavity; however, occasionally abscesses may cause malignant cerebral edema, and patients will require short-term intravenous dexamethasone administration. Brain abscesses carry a high risk of seizure; therefore, we recommend short-term treatment with antiepileptic agents, such as phenytoin, for these children.

Small abscesses, less than 2.5 cm, or those in eloquent areas of the brain, such as the brain stem, may be treated medically with intravenous antibiotic therapy. In these cases, frequent CT scans will need to be obtained to assess for an enlarging abscess. Larger abscesses should be drained either stereotactically or through craniotomy [59]. It is important to tailor therapy to prevent intraventricular rupture of the abscess, as the mortality rate increases from 15% to 80% with this complication [60]. If surgical intervention is deemed necessary, generally we do not administer intravenous antibiotics until the abscess is drained, in order to increase the likelihood of obtaining a diagnosis through cultures. Postoperatively, children need to be monitored in the PICU for at least 24 hr to observe for potential postoperative hematoma. A noncontrasted CT scan of the head will typically be obtained the following day after drainage of the abscess. Intravenous antibiotics will be administered for 6–8 weeks after surgical drainage, typically in an outpatient setting [61].

Epilepsy

Between 1% and 2% of children suffer from epilepsy [62]. Epilepsy cannot be controlled medically in 20% of these children. In fact, only one third of patients with intractable seizures treated with medications alone eventually become seizure free, and, of the remaining two thirds, one half cannot function independently [63,64]. Surgical treatment of epilepsy offers a safe and effective option to treat epilepsy in many of these children. Children are ideal candidates for surgical treatment of intractable epilepsy because of the plasticity of the developing nervous system, and 60%–80% of children who undergo epilepsy surgery become seizure free, without medications [63,65]. Chronic seizures have a negative impact on many psychosocial aspects of a child's development; thus, the earlier in a child's life that surgical intervention is pursued, the better the prognosis. Major surgical complications are rare, ranging from 2% to 4% [61], and these risks are lower with modern surgical techniques, such as image guidance and brain mapping.

Prior to resective surgery, children undergo Phase I monitoring, which involves placement of surface electrodes to identify seizure foci. This is followed by Phase II monitoring, which involves craniotomy with placement of subdural electrodes and possibly depth electrodes. Typically, only children under 2 years of age are monitored in the PICU during Phase II monitoring. Computed tomography scan is difficult to interpret in these children because of the significant artifact from the grids and thus is not routinely performed postoperatively. When postoperative CT is obtained, it is common to see a small epidural hematoma in these patients; however, it is rarely clinically significant. Infection is also rare, occurring in less than 5% of these patients. The most common complication after subdural grid placement is the development of cerebral edema. Therefore, we typically place an ICP monitor in these children. We find that ICP >20 mm Hg in these children typically responds to treatment with intravenous dexamethasone and mannitol. Only very rarely do we find that removal of grids is necessary to control ICP in these children [63].

Several surgical procedures are performed to treat epileptogenic foci. The most common procedure is extratemporal lobectomy, performed in about 50% of patients, followed by temporal lobectomy, comprising about 25% of cases. Lobectomy involves removal of a seizure focus, demonstrated by preoperative and intraoperative electroencephalography. Functional hemispherectomy and hemispherotomy account for 15% of cases, and, finally, corpus callosotomy comprises about 10% of cases. Postoperatively, children are transported to the PICU and monitored overnight. Postoperative CT of the head is obtained only when indicated by deterioration in the neurologic examination. Of note, seizures may actually become more frequent in the immediate postoperative period because of local edema near the resection site. Thus, the patient is typically kept on preoperative doses of antiepileptic drugs for several weeks after surgery.

Complications of resective surgery typically are related to the location of the resection. The most common postoperative finding is cerebral edema that may result in a temporary hemiparesis, which typically resolves in a few days. Patients are therefore maintained on intravenous corticosteroids for about 2 weeks after surgery. Stroke is a rare complication, occurring in only a small percentage of these children, and is more common in reoperations. Disconnection syndrome, which is characterized by mutism, apraxia, and inattention, is common after corpus callosotomy. Often, younger children and those whose resection is limited to the anterior two thirds of the corpus callosum are spared from this complication. Split brain syndrome, which results in nondominant hand apraxia and sensory disconnection, occurs rarely after complete sectioning of the corpus callosum.

Children often require only 1–2 days' stay in the PICU after these procedures. As with all neurosurgical procedures, careful monitoring of electrolytes and neurologic examination is critical in the first 24 hr after epilepsy surgery. In general, imaging is not indicated in the immediate postoperative period, unless there is a change in the neurologic examination from baseline. Outcome is quite good in these patients, resulting in 65%–75% of children being seizure free children at 1-year follow up [66–68].

References

1. Hammer GB, Krane EJ. Perioperative care of the child with acute neurological disease. In: Andrews BT, Hammer GB, eds. Pediatric Neurosurgical Intensive Care. Park Ridge, IL: AANS; 1997:25–36.
2. Andrews BT, Hammer GB. The neurological examination and neurological monitoring in pediatric intensive care. In: Andrews BT, Hammer GB, eds. Pediatric Neurosurgical Intensive Care. Park Ridge, IL: AANS; 1997:1–11.
3. Narayan RK, Kishore PR, Becker DP, et al. Intracranial pressure: to monitor or not to monitor? A review of our experience with acute head injury. J Neurosurg 1982;56:650–659.
4. Luerssen TG, Wolfla CE. Pathophysiology and management of increased intracranial pressure in children. In: Andrews BT, Hammer GB, eds. Pediatric Neurosurgical Intensive Care. Park Ridge, IL: AANS; 1997: 37–57.
5. Gomes JA, Stevens RD, Lewin JJ III, Mirski MA, Bhardwaj A. Glucocorticoid therapy in neurologic critical care. Crit Care Med 2005;33: 1214–1224.
6. Dutton RP, McCunn M. Traumatic brain injury. Curr Opin Crit Care 2003;9:503–509.
7. Vincent JL, Berre J. Primer on medical management of severe brain injury. Crit Care Med 2005;33:1392–1399.
8. Adelson PD, Bratton SL, Carney NA, et al. Guidelines for the acute medical management of severe traumatic brain injury in infants, children, and adolescents: critical pathway for the treatment of established intracranial hypertension in pediatric traumatic brain injury. Pediatr Crit Care Med 2003;4:S65–S67.
9. Bracken MB, Collins WF. Randomized clinical trials of spinal cord injury treatment. In: Becker DP, Polishock JT eds. Central Nervous System Trauma Status Report. Washington, DC: National Institute of Neurological Disorders and Stroke; 1985.
10. Bullock R, Chesnut R, Clifton G, et al. Severe Head Injury Guidelines. New York: Brain Trauma Foundation; 1995.
11. Elf K, Nilsson P, Enblad P. Outcome after traumatic brain injury improved by an organized secondary insult program and standardized neurointensive care. Crit Care Med 2002; 30:2129–2134.
12. Hackbarth RM, Rzeszutko KM, Sturm G, et al. Survival and functional outcome in pediatric traumatic brain injury: a retrospective review and analysis of predictive factors. Crit Care Med 2002; 30:1630–1635.

13. Wise-Faberowski L, Soriano SG, Ferrari L, et al. Perioperative management of diabetes insipidus in children. J Neurosurg Anesth 2004; 16:220–225.

14. Vernon-Levett P, Geller M. Posterior fossa tumors in children: a case study. AACN Clin Issue 1997;8:214–226.

15. Warnick RE, Edwards MSB. Pediatric brain tumors. Curr Probl Pediatr 1991;21:129–173.

16. Pollack IF. Brain tumors in children. N Engl J Med 1994;331:1500–1507.

17. Norton WT, Aquino DA, Hozumi I, Chiu FC, Brosnan CF. Quantitative aspects of reactive gliosis: a review. Neurochem Res 1992;17:877–885.

18. McGraw J, Hiebert GW, Steeves JD. Modulating astrogliosis after neurotrauma. J Neurosci Res 2001;63:109–115.

19. Pekny M, Nilsson M. Astrocyte activation and reactive gliosis. Glia 2005;50:427–434.

20. Stavrou T, Bromley CM, Nicholson HS, et al. Prognostic factors and secondary malignancies in childhood medulloblastoma. J Pediatr Hematol Oncol 2001;23:431–436.

21. Paulino AC, Wen BC, Mayr NA, et al. Protracted radiotherapy treatment duration in medulloblastoma. Am J Clin Oncol 2003;26: 55–59.

22. Ersahin Y, Mutluer S, Cagli S, et al. Cerebellar mutism: report of seven cases and review of the literature. Neurosurgery 1996;38:60–66.

23. Ildan F, Tuna M, Erman T, et al. The evaluation and comparison of cerebellar mutism in children and adults after posterior fossa surgery: report of two adult cases and review of the literature. Acta Neurochir 2002;144:463–473.

24. Horn B, Heideman R, Geyer R, et al. A multi-institutional retrospective study of intracranial ependymoma in children: identification of risk factors. J Pediatr Hematol Oncol 1999;21:203–211.

25. Merchant T. Current management of childhood ependymoma. Oncology 2002;16:629–644.

26. Paulino AC, Wen BC, Buatti JM, et al. Intracranial ependymomas: an analysis of prognostic factors and patterns of failure. Am J Clin Oncol 2002;25:117–222.

27. Morantz RA. Low grade astrocytomas. In: Kaye AH and Laws ER, eds. Brain Tumors: An Encyclopedic Approach, 2nd ed. London, England: Harcourt Publishers; 2001:467–491.

28. Volpe JJ. Intracranial hemorrhage: germinal matrix hemorrhage of the premature infant. In: Volpe JJ ed. Neurology of the Newborn. Philadelphia: WB Saunders; 1995:403–463.

29. Ciricillo SF, Cogen PH, Edwards MSB. Pediatric cryptic vascular malformations: presentation, diagnosis, and treatment. Pediatr Neurosurg 1994;20:137–147.

30. Obana WG, Andrews BT. The intensive care management of nontraumatic intracerebral hemorrhage. In: Andrews BT, ed. Neurosurgical Intensive Care. New York: McGraw-Hill; 1993:311–327.

31. Ruiz-Sandoval JL, Cantu C, Barinagarrementeria F. Intracerebral hemorrhage in young people: analysis of risk factors, location, causes, and prognosis. Stroke 1999;30:537–541.

32. Kondziolka D, Lunsford LD, Kestle JR. The natural history of cerebral cavernous malformations. J Neurosurg 1995; 83:820–824.

33. Halim AX, Johnston SC, Singh V, McCulloch CE, Bennett JP, Achrol AS, Sidney S, Young WL. Longitudinal risk of intracranial hemorrhage in patients with arteriovenous malformation of the brain within a defined population. Stroke 2004;35:1697–1702.

34. Stapf C, Labovitz DL, Sciacca RR, Mast H, Mohr JP, Sacco RL. Incidence of adult brain arteriovenous malformation hemorrhage in a prospective population-based stroke survey. Cerebrovasc Dis 2002;3:43–46.

35. Auer L, Deinsberger W, Niederkorn K, et al. Endoscopic surgery versus medical treatment for spontaneous intracerebral hematoma: a randomized study. J Neurosurg 1989;70:530–535.

36. Mandavia DP, Villagomez J. The importance of serial neurologic examination and repeat cranial tomography in acute evolving epidural hematoma. Pediatr Emerg Care 2001;17:193–195.

37. Shutzman SA, Barnes PD, Mantello M, et al. Epidural hematomas in children. Ann Emerg Med 1993;22:535–541.

38. Wilberger JE, Harris M, Diamond DL. Acute subdural hematoma: morbidity, mortality, and operative timing. J Neurosurg 1991;74:212–218.

39. Duhaime AC, Christian CW, Rorke LB, Zimmerman RA. Nonaccidental head injury in infants—the "shaken baby syndrome." N Engl J Med 1998;338:1822–1829.

40. Chang BS, Lowenstein DH. Antiepileptic drug prophylaxis in severe traumatic brain injury: report of the Quality Standards Subcommittee of the American Academy of Neurology. Neurology 2003;60:10–16.

41. Utter GH, Owings JT, Jacoby RC, et al. Injury induces increased monocyte expression of tissue factor: factors associated with head injury attenuate the injury-related monocyte expression of tissue factor. J Trauma 2002;52:1071–1077.

42. Vogel LC, Hickey KJ, Klaas SJ, et al. Unique issues in pediatric spinal cord injury. Orthop Nurs 2004;23:300–308.

43. Di Martino A, Madigan L, Silber JS, et al. Pediatric spinal cord injury. Neurosurg Q 2004;14:184–197.

44. Proctor MR. Spinal cord injury. Crit Care Med 2002;30:S489–S499.

45. Bracken MB. Methylprednisolone and acute spinal cord injury: an update of the randomized evidence. Spine 2001;26:S47–S54.

46. Bracken MB, Collins WF, Freeman DF, et al. Efficacy of methylprednisolone in acute spinal cord injury. JAMA 1984;251:45–52.

47. Bracken MB, Shepard MJ, Hellenbrand KG, et al. Methylprednisolone and neurological function one year after spinal cord injury. J Neurosurg 1985;63:704–713.

48. Nesathurai S. Steroids and spinal cord injury: revisiting the NASCIS 2 and NASCIS 3 trials. J Trauma 1998;45:1088–1093.

49. Coleman WP, Benzel E, Cahill DW, et al. A critical appraisal of the reporting of the National Acute Spinal Cord Injury Studies (II and III) of methylprednisolone in acute spinal cord injury. J Spinal Disord 2000;13:185–199.

50. Hurlbert RJ. Methylprednisolone for acute spinal cord injury: an inappropriate standard of care. J Neurosurg (Spine) 2000;93:1–7.

51. Hurlbert RJ. The role of steroids in acute spinal cord injury: an evidence-based analysis. Spine 2001;26:S39–S46.

52. Kishan S, Vives MJ, Reiter MF. Timing of surgery following spinal cord injury. J Spinal Cord Med 2005;28:11–19.

53. Tator CH, Fehlings MG, Thorpe K, et al. Current use and timing of spinal surgery for management of acute spinal surgery for management of acute spinal cord injury in North America: results of a retrospective multicenter study. J Neurosurg 1999;91:12–18.

54. Vaccaro AR, Daugherty RJ, Sheehan TP, et al. Neurologic outcome of early versus late surgery for cervical spinal cord injury. Spine 1997;22: 2609–2613.

55. Fehlings MG, Sekhon LH, Tator C. The role and timing of decompression in acute spinal cord injury: What do we know? What should we do? Spine 2001;26:S101–S110.

56. Yogev R, Bar-Meir M. Management of brain abscesses in children. Pediatr Infect Dis J 2004;23:157–159.

57. Takeshita M, Kagawa M, Yato S, et al. Current treatment of brain abscess in patients with congenital cyanotic heart disease. Neurosurgery 1997;41:1270–1279.

58. Mampalam TJ, Rosenblum ML. Trends in the management of bacterial brain abscesses: a review of 102 cases over 17 years. Neurosurgery 1988;23:451–458.

59. Mamelak AN, Mampalam TJ, Obana WG, et al. Improved management of multiple brain abscesses: a combined surgical and medical approach. Neurosurgery 1995;36:76–86.

60. Zeidman SM, Geisler FH, Olivi A. Intraventricular rupture of a purulent brain abscess: case report. Neurosurgery 1995;36:189–193.

61. Cowan LD, Bodensteiner JB, Leviton A, et al. Prevalence of the epilepsies in children and adolescents. Epilepsia 1989;30:94–106.

62. Lindsey J, Ounsted C, Richards P. Long-term outcome in children with temporal lobe seizures: social outcome and childhood factors. Dev Med Child Neurol 1979;21:630–636.

63. Lobel DA, Park YP, Lee MR. Surgical treatment of epilepsy in children. Contemp Neurosurg 2004;26:1–8.

64. Morrison G, Duchowny M, Resnick T, et al. Epilepsy surgery in childhood. Pediatr Neurosurg 1992;18:291–297.

65. Pilcher WH, Ojemann GA. Presurgical evaluation and epilepsy surgery. In: Apuzzo ML, ed. Brain Surgery: Complication Avoidance and Management. New York: Churchill Livingstone; 1993:1525–1555.

66. Dlugos DJ. The early identification of candidates for epilepsy surgery. Arch Neurol 2001;58:1543–1546.

67. Engel J Jr. Current concepts: surgery for seizures. N Engl J Med 1996;334:647–652.

68. Davidson S, Falconer MA. Outcome of surgery in 40 children with temporal lobe epilepsy. Lancet 1973;1:1260–1263.

4

Tumors of the Central Nervous System

Robert Tamburro, Raymond C. Barfield, and Amar Gajjar

Introduction

Primary malignancies of the central nervous system are the second most common type of malignancy during childhood, second only to the leukemias. Although this chapter focuses primarily on central nervous system tumors and their treatment, it is important to realize that neurologic symptoms in the pediatric oncology patient may result from a variety of conditions. These conditions may, or may not, be related to their cancer and its treatment. Table 4.1 illustrates a broad differential diagnosis of an altered mental status in the pediatric cancer patient.

Brain Tumors

Incidence

Approximately 2,200 children under the age of 20 years are diagnosed with a brain tumor each year in the United States [1,2]. Primary brain tumors are the most common solid tumor in the pediatric population, comprising 20%–25% of all childhood cancers, and are the second most common childhood malignancy overall [2–4]. Although significant progress has been made in the diagnosis and treatment of childhood brain tumors, they are still responsible for the majority of cancer-related deaths in children [3,5,6]. Table 4.2 depicts the most common brain tumors in children by histology [7]. Table 4.3 depicts the most common pediatric brain tumors by location, an important consideration, as symptoms of brain tumors are frequently related to the location of the tumor [4]. Children with brain tumors frequently require critical care services for management of increased intracranial pressure (ICP), postoperative care, and treatment of other tumor or treatment-related morbidity.

Presenting Signs and Symptoms

The presenting signs and symptoms of pediatric brain tumors vary by the age of the child and by the location of the primary tumor.

Tumors that present in infancy tend to be more insidious because of the nonspecific nature of the clinical symptoms, including vomiting, irritability, lethargy, macrocephaly, failure to thrive, and loss of, or delay in, attaining developmental milestones [4,6]. Older children may better communicate specific neurologic deficits. Additionally, signs and symptoms related to increased ICP, including headache, nausea, and vomiting (particularly upon awakening in the morning), frequently occur in this age group as well [4,6].

Supratentorial tumors produce signs and symptoms according to the area of the brain that is affected [4,6]. For example, cerebral hemispheric lesions may present with focal neurologic findings or seizures, whereas tumors proximal to the optic chiasm and hypothalamus may produce vision loss, visual field defects, or endocrine abnormalities [6]. Cerebellar tumors, on the other hand, frequently result in ataxia, gait disturbances, and signs of increased ICP secondary to obstruction of the fourth ventricle [4,6]. Brain stem tumors present with cranial nerve abnormalities and/or upper motor neuron signs [4,6]. Signs and symptoms associated with specific tumor types are discussed in more detail in the following sections.

Gliomas

Tumors of glial origin constitute approximately 50% of all primary brain tumors in children and are grouped based on histopathologic appearance into low-grade and high-grade gliomas [4,6,8,9]. These tumors are found throughout the central nervous system, and location is an important prognostic factor [3,10]. Low-grade gliomas are a heterogeneous group of tumors with an overall 10-year survival rate of greater than 80% with appropriate treatment [3,11]. The most frequent low-grade gliomas are posterior fossa and cerebral hemisphere astrocytomas. Most low-grade gliomas are classified into two histopathologic types: pilocytic astrocytomas (World Health Organization, WHO grade I) and diffuse or fibrillary astrocytomas (WHO grade II) [3].

Pilocytic astrocytomas occur primarily in young children with a median age of 4 years [3]. These tumors can occur at all levels of the neuroaxis but occur most frequently in the cerebellum and the optic pathways [12]. On radiographic imaging, nearly all are brightly enhancing, well-circumscribed tumors that are clearly demarcated from surrounding brain tissue and have little surrounding edema; about half of them are cystic [3,12]. In contrast,

D.S. Wheeler et al. (eds.), *The Central Nervous System in Pediatric Critical Illness and Injury*,
DOI 10.1007/978-1-84800-993-6_4, © Springer-Verlag London Limited 2009

TABLE 4.1. Etiology of acute alterations in consciousness in children with cancer.

Tumor
- Primary central nervous system tumor
- Metastatic tumor
- Leukemic meningitis
- Hyperleukocytosis

Infection
- Meningitis: bacterial, fungi
- Viral encephalitis
- Brain abscess
- Septic shock

Cerebrovascular accident
Seizure/postictal state
Disseminated intravascular coagulation
Treatment
- Cytotoxic chemotherapy
  - Methotrexate
  - Cytosine arabinoside
  - Corticosteroids
  - Ifosfamide
  - 5-Fluorouracil

- Supportive care
  - Opioids
  - Benzodiazepines
  - Antihistamines
  - Anticonvulsants
  - Tricyclic antidepressants

Leukoencephalopathy
Metabolic abnormality
- Hyponatremia (syndrome of inappropriate secretion of antidiuretic hormone)
- Hypoglycemia/hyperglycemia
- Hypomagnesemia
- Uremia

Postradiation somnolence syndrome
Hypotension/hypertension
Dehydration
Hypoxia
Anemia
Liver failure
Depression

Source: Adapted from Rheingold SR, Lange BJ. Oncologic emergencies. In: Pizzo PA, Poplack DG, eds. Principles and Practice of Pediatric Oncology, 4th ed. Philadelphia: Lippincott, Williams & Wilkins; 2002:1189.

grade II astrocytomas occur at a median age of 10 years, infiltrate into the surrounding normal brain, do not enhance with contrast on diagnostic imaging, and mostly occur as cerebral hemisphere and intrinsic pontine tumors [3].

Pediatric high-grade gliomas are also a diverse group of tumors with different sites of origin and histologic features that affect children of different ages [13]. They account for approximately 14% of all childhood central nervous system tumors and consist of WHO grade III anaplastic astrocytomas and grade IV glioblastoma multiforme [3]. The overall incidence of high-grade gliomas in children less than 19 years of age is 0.63 per 100,000 person-years, with a roughly equal distribution across age groups and gender [13]. These tumors can arise from any location in the central nervous system but are most common in the supratentorial region and the brain stem. They rarely originate from the spinal cord or the cerebellum [13]. Regardless of location, these poorly circumscribed, highly infiltrative tumors are difficult to treat effectively, with long-term survival rates ranging from less than 10% to 30% for most supratentorial tumors and less than 10% for diffuse brain stem gliomas [3,13]. The prognosis seems to be better for patients with anaplastic astrocytomas than for those with glioblastoma multiforme, although the degree of surgical resection is the most important clinical prognostic factor for children with supratentorial high-grade astrocytomas [3,13–18].

TABLE 4.2. Selected childhood primary (malignant and nonmalignant) brain and central nervous system tumor age-specific incidence rates* (ages 0–19), by age at diagnosis, CBTRUS 1997–2001.[†]

Histology	Age at Diagnosis											
	0–4		5–9		10–14		15–19		0–19		0–14	
	NO.	Rate	NO.	Rate	NO.	Rate	NO.	Rate	NO.	Rate	NO.	Rate
Tumors of Neuroepithelial tissue	1,225	4.02	1,099	3.45	867	2.75	701	2.26	3,892	3.12	3,191	3.40
Pilocytic astrocytoma	260	0.85	316	0.99	242	0.77	181	0.58	999	0.80	818	0.87
Anaplastic astrocytoma	18	0.06	31	0.10	23	0.07	33	0.11	105	0.08	72	0.08
Astrocytoma, NOS	76	0.25	79	0.25	75	0.24	63	0.20	293	0.23	230	0.25
Glioblastoma	31	0.10	38	0.12	51	0.16	44	0.14	164	0.13	120	0.13
Ependymoma/anaplastic ependymoma	134	0.44	69	0.22	48	0.15	35	0.11	286	0.23	251	0.27
Glioma malignant, NOS	168	0.55	158	0.50	100	0.32	58	0.19	484	0.39	426	0.45
Benign and malignant neuronal/ glial, neuronal and mixed	104	0.34	52	0.16	79	0.25	79	0.25	314	0.25	235	0.25
Embryonal/primitive/ medulloblastoma	296	0.97	253	0.79	133	0.42	78	0.25	760	0.61	682	0.73
Tumors of cranial and spinal nerves	10	0.03	24	0.08	32	0.10	67	0.22	133	0.11	66	0.07
Tumors of meninges	38	0.12	28	0.09	44	0.14	97	0.31	207	0.17	110	0.12
Lymphomas and hemopoietic neoplasms	6	—	—	—	12	0.04	8	—	30	0.02	22	0.02
Germ cell tumors	33	0.11	39	0.12	75	0.24	76	0.24	223	0.18	147	0.16
Tumors of sellar region	24	0.08	55	0.17	60	0.19	139	0.45	278	0.22	139	0.15
Craniopharyngioma	24	0.08	51	0.16	40	0.13	32	0.10	147	0.12	115	0.12
Local extensions from regional tumors	—	—	—	—	—	—	7	—	17	0.01	10	0.01
Unclassified tumors	77	0.25	45	0.14	68	0.22	58	0.19	248	0.20	190	0.20
TOTAL[§]	1,414	4.63	1,298	4.08	1,163	3.69	1,153	3.71	5,028	4.02	3,875	4.13

*Rates are per 100,000 person-years.

[†]Includes data from 15 of 17 registries; North Dakota and Rhode Island are excluded.

[‡]Counts are not presented when fewer than 6 cases were reported for the specific histology category, and rates are not presented when fewer than 10 cases were reported for the specific histology category. The suppressed cases are included in the counts and rates for totals.

[§]Refers to all childhood brain tumors, including histologies not presented in this table.

Source: Central Brain Tumor Registry of the United States. Statistical Report: Primary Brain Tumors in the United States, 1997–2001. Hillsdale, IL: CBTRUS; 2004:40, Table 15.

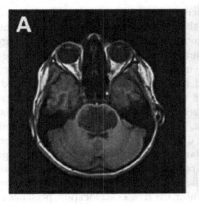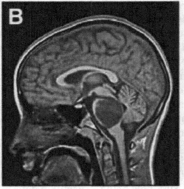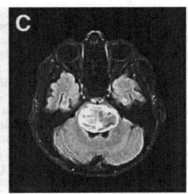

FIGURE 4.1. Typical appearance of magnetic resonance imaging scans of a patient with diffuse brain stem glioma. **(A,B)** T1-weighted axial and sagittal images without contrast. **(C)** Axial fluid-attenuated inversion recovery (FLAIR) image (Data from Broniscer and Gajjar [13].)

Supratentorial high-grade astrocytomas make up one third of all pediatric high-grade gliomas and more commonly affect children during late adolescence (ages 15–19 years) [13]. These astrocytomas constitute 6%–12% of all primary pediatric brain tumors [19]. Children with supratentorial high-grade astrocytomas present with signs and symptoms attributable to the specific area of involved brain, as well as signs and symptoms of increased ICP and seizures [13].

Diffuse brain stem gliomas occur with an incidence of 0.18 per 100,000 person-years and constitute 3%–10% of all primary pediatric brain tumors [4,13,20]. Children with diffuse brain stem high-grade gliomas classically present between 5 and 10 years of age with a brief history (<2–6 months) of pyramidal tract signs, cranial nerve deficits, and cerebellar signs and symptoms [13,21]. This clinical picture differs from that of most pediatric posterior fossa tumors in which signs and symptoms of increased ICP dominate, and focal deficits assume a secondary place [22]. Moreover, this clinical picture, in conjunction with typical magnetic resonance imaging findings of an intrinsic, pontine-based infiltrative lesion that exerts significant mass effect on adjacent structures, including the basilar artery and the fourth ventricle, is highly specific for a diffuse brain stem glioma, precluding the need for histologic confirmation (Figure 4.1) [13,21]. The time between the onset of symptoms and diagnosis, as well as the degree of neurologic deficits, are important prognostic factors [19]. Although outcomes are generally poor (as described above), patients with diffuse brain stem gliomas in association with neurofibromatosis type 1 tend to have better outcomes than anticipated [23,24].

Medulloblastomas

Medulloblastoma is the most common malignant central nervous system tumor in children and the second most common pediatric brain neoplasm, accounting for 12%–25% of all central nervous system tumors in children [3,25,26]. More than 90% of medulloblastomas occur in the cerebellum, and medulloblastomas account for nearly 40% of all pediatric posterior fossa tumors, the most common pediatric posterior fossa tumor overall (Table 4.3) [25,27]. Among children, the mean age at presentation is approximately 7 years, and there is a slight male predilection [25,27]. Clinical symptoms are usually brief (<3 months), reflecting the aggressive nature of the tumor, and commonly include headache and persistent vomiting [3,25,28,29]. Because more than three fourths of medulloblas-

tomas arise from the midline cerebellar vermis and involve the fourth ventricle, it is not uncommon for patients to present with obstructive hydrocephalus, at times requiring emergent placement of an external ventricular drain [3,25,27]. Macrocephaly, lethargy, and cerebellar signs such as ataxia and dysmetria may also be reported [3]. Truncal ataxia is the most common objective clinical sign and is frequently accompanied by spasticity [25,28,29]. Other clinical signs may include papilledema, nystagmus, and positive Babinski and Hoffmann signs [25,28,29]. Limb ataxia and dysdiadokokinesis suggest a laterally located mass within the cerebellar hemisphere [25,28,29]. Abducens nerve palsy results from compression of the nucleus of the sixth cranial nerve and suggests extraventricular tumor extension [25,29].

Although histologically similar, gene expression analyses show that medulloblastoma is a tumor type distinct from supratentorial primitive neuroectodermal tumors [3,30]. The classic CT appearance of a medulloblastoma is a hyperattenuated, well-defined vermian cerebellar mass with surrounding vasogenic edema, evidence of hydrocephalus, and homogeneous enhancement on contrasted studies in a child less than 10 years of age [25]. Magnetic resonance imaging generally reveals a brightly enhancing posterior fossa mass with low T1 signal and intermediate T2 and FLAIR signals [3].

Surgical resection to maximally reduce tumor burden and to relieve obstructive hydrocephalus is the initial intervention. A gross total resection of the tumor has been documented to offer

TABLE 4.3. Relative incidence of common brain tumors in children by location.

Supratentorial tumors (45%–50%)		Infratentorial tumors (50%–55%)	
Astrocytoma	23%	Medulloblastoma	20%
Malignant gliomas	6%	Astrocytoma	15%
Craniopharyngioma	6%	Brain stem glioma	10%
Embryonal tumors (PNET and others)	4%	Ependymoma	6%
Pineal region/intracranial germ cell tumors	4%		
Ependymoma	3%		
Other	4%		

Note: PNET, primitive neuroectodermal tumor.
Adapted from Kline and Sevier [4] and from Halperin E, Constine L, Tarbell N, Kun L. *Pediatric Radiation Oncology.* New York: Lippincott, Williams & Wilkins, 1999;38.

patients long-term survival advantage [3]. Postoperative mutism is not an uncommon complication of posterior fossa resections in children [3,32]. In one large series, 8.5% of infratentorial tumor resections resulted in postoperative mutism. In each case, the tumor (medulloblastomas, N = 7; astrocytomas, N = 3; and ependymomas, N = 2) involved the vermis. The incidence among children with vermian neoplasms was 13% [32]. Other postoperative complications may include ataxia, hemiparesis, hydrocephalus, hematoma, aseptic meningitis, gastrointestinal hemorrhage, cervical instability, and sixth cranial nerve palsy [3,31]. Surgery is followed by adjuvant radiation, and, perhaps, chemotherapy based on the patient's risk stratification [3].

Long-term prognosis has improved dramatically in the recent past, with 5-year survival rates between 50% and 80% now being reported [25,33–36]. Absence of metastatic disease and gross total surgical resection are associated with a better prognosis [25,27,35]. Patients with metastatic disease at diagnosis have worse outcomes [36,37]. Recurrence is common and is also associated with a poor prognosis [25].

Ependymomas

Ependymomas are the third most common pediatric brain tumor, accounting for 6%–15% of brain tumors in children [3,38–40]. They tend to occur in younger children with a mean age at presentation of approximately 3 years and reported median ages ranging from 4 to 6 years [38–40]. Although ependymomas may occur anywhere in the central nervous system, approximately two thirds of intracranial ependymomas are localized to the posterior fossa. Localization to the posterior fossa is, in fact, more common in children less than 3 years of age [3,38]. A supratentorial location accounts for the remaining one third of intracranial ependymomas and is more common in children over 3 years of age [38].

Posterior fossa ependymomas frequently present with symptoms related to obstructive hydrocephalus secondary to compression of the fourth ventricle, including headache, nausea, and vomiting [3,38]. Tumor compression of posterior fossa structures may also result in ataxia, hemiparesis, neck pain, torticollis, nuchal rigidity, visual disturbances including nystagmus, papilledema, and cranial nerve palsies [38]. The duration of symptoms is usually less than 6 months at diagnosis [38]. In contrast, supratentorial tumors tend to present with signs and symptoms related to ventricular compression and midline shift, including headache, nausea, vomiting, lethargy, papilledema, and cognitive decline or behavioral changes [38]. These tumors are usually well demarcated and distinct from adjacent areas of unaffected brain [3]. The degree of surgical resection appears to be a critical prognostic variable [3,38–45]. A gross total resection is associated with a substantially greater 5-year progression-free survival compared with a subtotal resection [3,38–45]. Younger age (≤3–5 years), metastatic disease, and higher histologic grade are associated with worse outcomes [38–49].

Craniopharyngiomas

Craniopharyngiomas are the most common tumor to affect the hypothalamic-pituitary region in children and account for approximately 6%–10% of all childhood intracranial tumors [4,50,51]. Craniopharyngiomas are thought to arise from epithelial cell remnants of Rathke's pouch at the junction of the infundibular stalk and the pituitary gland, although one case report documents de novo tumor occurrence in a 55-year-old woman [52]. The vast majority of these tumors have a cystic component, with less than 20% being totally solid [53]. Although the histology is benign and the overall survival rate is high, these tumors are associated with significant morbidity because of their proximity to the optic nerves and the hypothalamus [50,53]. The median age of presentation is 8 years, and presenting symptoms are usually related to the location of the tumor, including visual disturbances, headache, nausea, and vomiting [53,54]. Endocrine abnormalities and intellectual dysfunction are also common at presentation [53,54]. The median duration of symptoms has been reported to be 8 months, with a range of 1 week to 4 years, the wide range reflecting the nonspecific nature of the symptoms [54]. Neuroimaging is useful in determining the size, exact location, presence of calcification, and the cystic nature of the tumor as well as detecting the presence of hydrocephalus (seen in as many as 23% of patients) [53,54].

The optimal management of craniopharyngioma in children remains controversial because of the attempt to balance the risks of a slowly progressive disease with the potential for high morbidity associated with treatment [53–56]. Some combination of surgical resection with radiation remains the mainstay of therapy. Diabetes insipidus is a common complication in the immediate postoperative period, and the pediatric critical care provider should be prepared for this complication [54,57]. In a report of 46 surgical resections for craniopharyngioma, diabetes insipidus was observed preoperatively in 14 cases, intraoperatively in five others, and postoperatively within 18 hr of surgery in 25 of the 27 remaining cases [57]. Long-term replacement of other hormones is almost always required.

Perioperative Care of Brain Tumors

The pediatric intensivist plays a key role in the perioperative care of children with brain tumors. For example, these children often present with increased ICP and require emergent attention. The initial management may include controlling the airway in a neuroprotective manner, facilitating transport to the imaging center, and consulting with the neurosurgeon in a timely fashion. Increased ICP is often secondary to obstructive hydrocephalus requiring emergent placement of an external ventricular drain [3]. Shemie et al. have described a series of seven children who had sudden, unexpected death associated with acute hydrocephalus from a previously undiagnosed intracranial tumor, highlighting the need for a high index of suspicion and prompt intervention [58]. In addition to standard management of intracranial hypertension (see Chapter 5), intracranial tumors are often associated with local vasogenic edema and may benefit from administration of corticosteroids. Corticosteroids have been used for brain tumors since the 1960s, and a remarkable decline in perioperative mortality rates coincided with their implementation [59–61]. Several mechanisms for the observed corticosteroid-induced reduction in edema in this setting have been suggested, including reduced expression of the edema-producing factor vascular endothelial growth factor (VEGF) [59,62,63]. The edema-reducing effect of corticosteroids is rapid, with decreased capillary permeability being noted 1 hr after a single dose in an animal model [64]. In addition to decreasing edema around the tumor, corticosteroids have also been demonstrated to decrease the tumor volume itself [65,66]. According to the neurosurgical literature, dexamethasone appears to be the most commonly used corticosteroid.

In addition to emergent preoperative management, postoperative care may be critical for these patients. Intensive care monitoring has been recommended for ≥12–24 hours to detect serious postoperative complications and facilitate rapid intervention, as well as to optimize the reestablishment of systemic and neurologic homeostasis [67]. Immediately upon admission to the PICU, a baseline neurologic assessment of the patient must be made so that any subsequent, subtle deterioration may be identified promptly. A clinical deterioration from baseline is an indication for emergent CT imaging. Early postoperative complications that may result in a prolonged PICU course include cerebrospinal fluid leaks, diabetes insipidus, lower cranial nerve palsies, pneumocephalus, intracranial hemorrhage, and significant postoperative edema [68]. For example, in a study of 105 pediatric posterior fossa tumor resections between 1982 and 1992, one third of the patients were found to have an intra- or postoperative complication including hydrocephalus requiring shunt placement (N = 9), pseudomeningocele formation requiring additional treatment (N = 5), wound problems (N = 4), hematoma requiring craniotomy (N = 3), and gastrointestinal hemorrhage (N = 2) [69]. The association of gastrointestinal hemorrhage with intracranial pathology and posterior fossa resections has been long established [69–71]. Ross et al. described three children with posterior fossa tumors who developed massive exsanguinating upper gastrointestinal hemorrhage within 7 days of their primary neurosurgical procedure and recommended stress ulcer prophylaxis for this patient population [71].

The monitoring of other parameters such as blood pressure, cerebral perfusion pressure, fluid balance, serum sodium concentration (monitoring for central diabetes insipidus or cerebral salt wasting syndrome), and coagulation studies may be important in the postoperative care of these patients. The use of an arterial catheter may assist in blood pressure management. Although it is vital that an adequate cerebral perfusion pressure is maintained, it is also important to avoid potentially harmful hypertension. Consistent communication with the neurosurgeon and oncologist will facilitate care. Postoperative imaging, which may provide important prognostic and therapeutic information, is best performed within 24–48 hr of surgery to avoid the effect of normal postoperative changes that may be mistaken for residual disease and thus is often the responsibility of the critical care team [4,14].

Malignant Spinal Cord Compression

Acute spinal cord dysfunction is a neurologic emergency and, in a pediatric patient with cancer, is most likely secondary to metastatic cord compression [72]. Acute metastatic spinal cord compression occurs in approximately 3% of all children with cancer [72,73] and in 5% of those with solid tumors [74]. The most common tumors associated with malignant spinal cord compression in children include sarcomas, neuroblastomas, and leukemias/lymphomas [72–76]. Depending on the series, 8%–12% of patients with sarcoma, 7%–8% of patients with neuroblastoma, and 2%–4% of patients with lymphoma will develop spinal cord disease [72,74]. In one large series, 18% of children with Ewing sarcoma developed this complication [74].

Although often believed to be an end-stage problem, particularly in adults, as many as 33% of cases in children occur at presentation of their malignant disease with an additional proportion occurring at the time of relapse [72,76]. Moreover, children differ from adults

in both the cause and mechanism of their spinal cord compression [72,75,76]. The mechanism of compression in the child is more often direct spread from a paravertebral tumor through the vertebral foramen that impinges on the spinal cord directly, without significant bony involvement. The mass compressing the lesion is lateral, and spinal stability is usually not a factor [76]. This is in contrast to spinal cord compression in the adult, where metastasis more often invades the epidural space from a metastatic lesion in a vertebral body. This difference, and differences in tumor type (lung carcinoma, breast carcinoma, and prostate carcinomas being the most common causes in adults), suggest a need for a different approach to therapy for children [76]. In light of this, one report suggested that conclusions derived from the adult experience have led to recommendations that are inappropriate for children [74]. Moreover, there are data suggesting that children are more likely to have better outcomes than adults [74].

Pain is the most common symptom of malignant spinal cord compression and may be the only symptom at presentation [72,75,76]. Spinal tenderness and weakness are also common clinical findings [72,75,76]. The weakness occurs predominantly in the lower extremities, reflecting the most likely locations of the lesions; 6% cervical, 59% thoracic, and 35% sacral [72,75,76]. Loss of sphincter control and bowel/bladder dysfunction occur in approximately 50% of patients at presentation [72,76]. Sensory deficits are often the least useful clinical finding, as patients are frequently unaware of this finding and these deficits are difficult to ascertain in younger children [72,75–77].

The diagnosis of malignant spinal cord compression should be considered for any child with cancer (particularly those tumor types at highest risk, e.g., sarcomas) who presents with back pain, weakness, or sphincter disturbances. However, although metastatic spinal cord compression is the most likely cause of spinal cord dysfunction in children with cancer, accounting for 88% of the cases in one series, other conditions must be considered in the differential [72]. Infection or radiation-induced transverse myelitis, spinal cord stroke, intradural/extradural hematoma, or extradural abscess may all present with similar symptoms in this patient population. Cases may be misdiagnosed as Guillain-Barré syndrome, sciatica, myopathy, plexopathy, or hip pain from bony metastasis. Magnetic resonance imaging is the diagnostic test of choice because it is noninvasive, provides high soft tissue resolution, can image several planes, and allows for reconstructed images (Figure 4.2) [75]. Although plain radiographs and myelography are falling out of favor, computed tomography imaging is still useful for implantation and instrumentation that may accompany surgery and dose planning for radiotherapy.

Treatment requires timely recognition and prompt intervention. The initial therapy for any child suspected of having malignant spinal cord compression is intravenous dexamethasone [72,75,77]. Two large pediatric studies have retrospectively attempted to assess the impact of surgery with chemoradiotherapy to chemoradiotherapy alone [74,76]. Emergent radiotherapy may be useful; however, close proximity to the spinal cord limits the dose that may be administered, and tumor type influences radiosensitivity [74,75]. Surgery is indicated when neurologic dysfunction and an epidural mass are discovered in a child without a preexisting diagnosis [72,75]. Surgery may also be indicated if neurologic function deteriorates during radiation therapy [72]. Two large studies have retrospectively assessed the role of surgical intervention in treating malignant spinal cord compression [74,76]. In a series of 33 children, Raffel et al. reported that a decompressive laminectomy

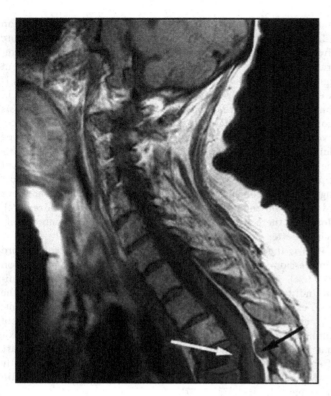

FIGURE 4.2. Magnetic resonance image of extradural malignant spinal cord compression at the T3–T4 level. The arrows depict both anterior and posterior compression of the spinal cord (Data from Prasad and Schiff [75]. © 2005 with permission from Elsevier.)

resulted in better neurologic outcomes, in terms of both motor function and sphincter control, than radiation therapy alone [76]. In that series, all patients who were ambulatory before surgery remained so, and 5 of 13 patients who were not became ambulatory after surgical intervention. Nine of 13 patients who were incontinent regained bladder control, and 10 of 13 regained normal bowel function. Similar results were not observed in the children who received radiation alone. The authors of this study also reported immediate improvement in back pain, reported no surgical mortality or morbidity (although fusions were required in two patients), and recommended that radiation therapy and chemotherapy follow the surgery [76].

In another report of 112 children with malignant spinal cord compression, Klein et al. recommended decompressive laminectomy for children with sarcomas (except for osteogenic sarcoma where it tends to be a late diagnosis and treatment may not be offered), but not for children with small cell tumors unless there was rapid neurologic deterioration or complete loss of motor function [74]. In that study, sarcoma patients treated surgically (N = 31) had a better improvement in neurologic status post-treatment than those only medically treated (N = 21) despite no difference in pre-treatment neurologic status. Among the 40 patients with small cell tumors (neuroblastoma, germ cell tumors, Hodgkin lymphoma), there was no difference in outcome independent of treatment modality. However, independent of tumor type, among the 31 patients with a complete motor and sensory level, there was a significant difference in post-treatment neurologic status between those treated with a decompressive laminectomy plus medical management (N = 18) and those treated with medical management

alone (N = 13) [74]. In fact, 50% of those treated with a laminectomy became ambulatory after the procedure. Because laminectomy and spinal radiation in children may ultimately result in anterior subluxation, scoliosis, and kyphosis, it appears best to use these therapies for those who will benefit most and to avoid these treatments and their complications whenever possible [74].

The prognosis of malignant spinal cord compression is most related to the degree of disability at diagnosis, which is associated with the duration of symptoms and the time to diagnosis, emphasizing the need for early detection and intervention [72,75,78]. In one small series, 80% of children who were paraplegic for <24 hr regained function compared with only 43% of those who were paraplegic for >24 hr [72]. Early and aggressive intervention can lead to improved neurologic outcomes. Available data suggest that, with appropriate and timely intervention, a majority of children who have loss of bowel or bladder function or who are unable to ambulate will regain these abilities [72,74,76]. Even in cases of a complete motor and sensory level, as many as 50% of children will regain the ability to ambulate, further underscoring the need for aggressive therapy [74].

References

1. American Cancer Society. Facts and Figures. Surveillance Research. Atlanta, GA: American Cancer Society; 2003.
2. Gurney JG, Smith MA, Bunin GR. CNS and miscellaneous intracranial and intraspinal neoplasms. In: Ries LAG, Smith MA, Gurney JG, Linet M, Tamra T, Young JL, Bunin GR, eds. Cancer Incidence and Survival Among Children and Adolescents: United States SEER Program 1975–1995, NIH Publ. No. 99-4649. Bethesda, MD: National Cancer Institute; 1999:51–63.
3. Rutka JT, Kuo JS. Pediatric surgical neuro-oncology: current best care practices and strategies. J Neurooncol 2004;69:139–·50.
4. Kline NE, Sevier N. Solid tumors in children. J Pediatr Nurs 2003; 18:96–102.
5. Ross JA, Severson RK, Pollack BH, Robinson LL. Childhood cancer in the United States. A geographical analysis of cases from the Pediatric Cooperative Clinical Trials groups. Cancer 1996;77:201–208.
6. Ullrich NJ, Pomeroy SL. Pediatric brain tumors. Neurol Clin 2003;21: 897–902.
7. Central Brain Tumor Registry of the United States: 2004–2005 Statistical Report Tables. Available online at: http://www.cbtrus.org/2004-2005/tables/2005.table13.pdf. Accessed June 20, 2005.
8. Saran F. Recent advances in paediatric neuro-oncology. Curr Opin Neurol 2002;15:671–677.
9. Pollack IF. Pediatric brain tumors. Semin Surg Oncol 1999;16:73–90.
10. Rilliet B, Vernet O. Gliomas in children: a review. Childs Nerv Syst 2000;16:735–741.
11. Freeman CR, Farmer JP, Montes J. Low-grade astrocytomas in children: evolving management strategies. Int J Radiat Oncol Biol Phys 1998;41:979–987.
12. Fernandez C, Figarella-Branger D, Girard N, et al. Pilocytic astrocytomas in children: prognostic factors—a retrospective study of 80 cases. Neurosurgery 2003;53:544–553.
13. Broniscer A, Gajjar A. Supratentorial high-grade astrocytoma and diffuse brainstem glioma: two challenges for the pediatric oncologist. Oncologist 2004;9:197–206.
14. Campbell JW, Pollack IF, Martinez AJ, Shultz BL. High grade astrocytomas in children: radiologically complete resection is associated with an excellent long-term prognosis. Neurosurgery 1996;38:258–264.
15. Finlay JL, Boyett JM, Yates AJ, Wisoff JH. Randomized phase III trial in childhood high-grade astrocytoma comparing vincristine, lomustine and prednisone with the eight-drugs-in-1-day regimen. J Clin Oncol 1995;13:112–123.

16. Wisoff JH, Boyett JM, Berger MS, et al. Current neurosurgical management and the impact of the extent of resection in the treatment of malignant gliomas of childhood: a report of the Children's Cancer Group Trial No. CCG-945. J Neurosurg 1998;89:52–59.

17. Heideman RL, Kuttesch J Jr, Gajjar AJ, et al. Supratentorial malignant gliomas in childhood: a single institution perspective. Cancer 1997;80: 497–504.

18. Wolff JE, Gnekow AK, Kortmann RD, et al. Preradiation chemotherapy for pediatric patients with high-grade glioma. Cancer 2002;94:264–271.

19. Sanford RA, Freeman CR, Burger P, Cohen ME. Prognostic criteria for experimental protocols in pediatric brainstem gliomas. Surg Neurol 1988;30:276–280.

20. Pollack IF. Brain tumors in children. N Engl J Med 1994;331:1500–1507.

21. Guillamo JS, Doz F, Delattre JY. Brain stem gliomas. Curr Opin Neurol 2001;14:711–715.

22. Walker DA, Punt JA, Sokal M. Clinical management of brain stem glioma. Arch Dis Child 1999;80:558–564.

23. Molloy PT, Bilaniuk LT, Vaughan SN, et al. Brainstem tumors in patients with neurofibromatosis type 1: a distinct clinical entity. Neurology 1995;45:1897–1902.

24. Milstein JM, Geyer JR, Berger MS, Bleyer WA. Favorable prognosis for brainstem gliomas in neurofibromatosis. J Neurooncol 1989;7:367–371.

25. Koeller KK, Rushing EJ. From the archives of the AFIP: medulloblastoma: a comprehensive review with radiologic-pathologic correlation. Radiographics 2003;23:1613–1637.

26. Kaatsch P, Rickert CH, Kuhl J, Schuz J, Michaelis J. Population-based epidemiologic data on brain tumors in German children. Cancer 2001;92:3155–3164.

27. Roberts RO, Lynch CF, Jones MP, Hart MN. Medulloblastoma: a population-based study of 532 cases. J Neuropathol Exp Neurol 1991;50: 134–144.

28. Park TS, Hofman HJ, Hendrick EB, Humphreys RP, Becker LE. Medulloblastoma: clinical presentation and management—experience at the Hospital for Sick Children, Toronto, 1950–1980. J Neurosurg 1983;58: 543–552.

29. Al-Mefty O, Jinkins JR, El-Senoussi M, El-Shaker M, Fox JL. Medulloblastomas: a review of modern management with a report on 75 cases. Surg Neurol 1985;24:606–624.

30. Pomeroy SL, Tamayo P, Gaasenbeek M, et al. Prediction of central nervous system embryonal tumour outcome based on gene expression. Nature 2002;415:436–442.

31. Sutton LN, Phillips PC, Molloy PT. Surgical management of medulloblastoma. J Neurooncol 1996;29:9–21.

32. Pollack IF, Polinko P, Albright AL, Towbin R, Fitz C. Mutism and pseudobulbar symptoms after resection of posterior fossa tumors in children: incidence and pathophysiology. Neurosurgery 1995;37:885–893.

33. Packer RJ, Sutton LN, Elterman R, et al. Outcome for children with medulloblastoma treated with radiation and cisplatin, CCNU, and vincristine chemotherapy. J Neurosurg 1994;81:690–698.

34. Rutkowski S, Bode U, Deinlein F, et al. Treatment of early childhood medulloblastoma by postoperative chemotherapy alone. N Engl J Med 2005;352:978–986.

35. Zeltzer PM, Boyett JM, Finlay JL, et al. Metastasis stage, adjuvant treatment, and residual tumor are prognostic factors for medulloblastoma in children: conclusions from the Children's Cancer Group 921 randomized phase III study. J Clin Oncol 1999;17:832–845.

36. David KM, Casey AT, Hayward RD, Harkness WF, Phipps K, Wade AM. Medulloblastoma: is the 5-year survival rate improving? A review of 80 cases from a single institution. J Neurosurg 1997;86:13–21.

37. Miralbell R, Bieri S, Huguenin P, et al. Prognostic value of cerebrospinal fluid cytology in pediatric medulloblastoma. Swiss Pediatric Oncology Group. Ann Oncol 1999;10:239–241.

38. Smyth MD, Horn BN, Russo C, Berger MS. Intracranial ependymomas of childhood: current management strategies. Pediatr Neurosurg 2000;33:138–150.

39. Figarella-Branger D, Civatte M, Bouvier-Labit C, et al. Prognostic factors in intracranial ependymomas in children. J Neurosurg 2000;93: 605–613.

40. Agaoglu FY, Ayan I, Dizdar Y, Kebudi R, Gorgun O, Darendeliler E. Ependymal tumors in childhood. Pediatr Blood Cancer 2005;45: 298–303.

41. Jaing TH, Wang HS, Tsay PK, et al. Multivariate analysis of clinical prognostic factors in children with intracranial ependymomas. J Neurooncol 2004;68:255–261.

42. Horn B, Heideman R, Geyer R, et al. A multi-institutional retrospective study of intracranial ependymoma in children: identification of risk factors. J Pediatr Hematol Oncol 1999;21:203–211.

43. Massimino M, Gandola L, Giangaspero F, et al. Hyperfractionated radiotherapy and chemotherapy for childhood ependymoma: final results of the first prospective AIEOP (Associazione Italiana di Ematologia-Oncologia Pediatrica) study. Int J Radiat Oncol Biol Phys 2004; 58:1336–1345.

44. Perilongo G, Massimino M, Sotti G, et al. Analyses of prognostic factors in a retrospective review of 92 children with ependymoma: Italian Pediatric Neuro-oncology Group. Med Pediatr Oncol 1997;29:79–85.

45. Timmermann B, Kortmann RD, Kuhl J, et al. Combined postoperative irradiation and chemotherapy for anaplastic ependymomas in childhood: results of the German prospective trials HIT 88/89 and HIT 91. Int J Radiat Oncol Biol Phys 2000;46:287–295.

46. Gambarelli D, Raquin MA, Couanet D, et al. Postoperative chemotherapy without irradiation for ependymoma in children under 5 years of age: a multicenter trial of the French Society of Pediatric Oncology. J Clin Oncol 2001;19:1288–1296.

47. Palma L, Celli P, Mariottini A, Zalaffi A, Schettini G. The importance of surgery in supratentorial ependymomas: long-term survival in a series of 23 cases. Childs Nerv Syst 2000;16:170–175.

48. Pollack IF, Gerszten PC, Martinez AJ, et al. Intracranial ependymomas of childhood: long-term outcome and prognostic factors. Neurosurgery 1995;37:655–666.

49. Vinchon M, Soto-Ares G, Riffaud L, Ruchoux MM, Dhellemmes P. Supratentorial ependymoma in childhood. Pediatr Neurosurg 2001;34: 77–87.

50. Srinivasan S, Ogle GD, Garnett SP, Briody JN, Lee JW, Cowell CT. Features of the metabolic syndrome after childhood craniopharyngioma. J Clin Endocrinol Metab 2004;89:81–86.

51. Petito CK, DeGirolami U, Earle KM. Craniopharyngiomas: a clinical and pathological review. Cancer 1976;37:1944–1952.

52. Arginteanu MS, Hague K, Zimmerman R, et al. Craniopharyngioma arising de novo in middle age. Case report. J Neurosurg 1997;86:1046–1048.

53. Lena G, Paredes AP, Scavarda D, Giusiano B. Craniopharyngioma in children: Marseille experience. Childs Nerv Syst 2005;21:778–784.

54. Merchant TE, Kiehna EN, Sanford RA, et al. Craniopharyngioma: the St. Jude Children's Research Hospital experience 1984–2001. Int J Radiat Oncol Biol Phys 2002;53:533–542.

55. Scott RM, Hetelekidis S, Barnes PD, et al. Surgery, radiation, and combination therapy in the treatment of childhood craniopharyngioma—A 20-year experience. Pediatr Neurosurg 1994;21(Suppl 1):75–81.

56. Sosa IJ, Krieger MD, McComb JG. Craniopharyngiomas of childhood: the CHLA experience. Childs Nerv Syst 2005;21:785–789.

57. Lehrnbecher T, Muller-Scholden J, Danhauser-Leistner I, Sorensen N, von Stockhausen HB. Perioperative fluid and electrolyte management in children undergoing surgery for craniopharyngioma. A 10-year experience in a single institution. Childs Nerv Syst 1998;14:276–279.

58. Shemie S, Jay V, Rutka J, Armstrong D. Acute obstructive hydrocephalus and sudden death in children. Ann Emerg Med 1997;29:524–528.

59. Kaal EC, Vecht CJ. The management of brain edema in brain tumors. Curr Opin Oncol 2004;16:593–600.

60. Ruderman N, Hall T. Use of glucocorticoids in the palliative treatment of metastatic brain tumors. Cancer 1965;18:298–306.

61. Jelsma R, Bucy PC. The treatment of glioblastoma multiforme of the brain. J Neurosurg 1967;27:388–400.

62. Heiss JD, Papavassiliou E, Merrill MJ, et al. Mechanism of dexamethasone suppression of brain tumor-associated vascular permeability in rats. Involvement of the glucocorticoid receptor and vascular permeability factor. J Clin Invest 1996;98:1400–1408.

63. Machein MR, Kullmer J, Ronicke V, et al. Differential downregulation of vascular endothelial growth factor by dexamethasone in normoxic and hypoxic rat glioma cells. Neuropathol Appl Neurobiol 1999;25: 104–112.

64. Shapiro WR, Hiesiger EM, Cooney GA, et al. Temporal effects of dexamethasone on blood-to-brain and blood-to-tumor transport of 14C-alpha-aminoisobutyric acid in rat C6 glioma. J Neurooncol 1990;8: 197–204.

65. Leiguarda R, Sierra J, Pardal C, et al. Effect of large doses of methylprednisolone on supratentorial intracranial tumors. A clinical and CAT scan evaluation. Eur Neurol 1985;24:23–32.

66. Hatam A, Bergstrom M, Yu ZY, et al. Effect of dexamethasone treatment on volume and contrast enhancement of intracranial neoplasms. J Comput Assist Tomogr 1983;7:295–300.

67. Kelly DF. Neurosurgical postoperative care. Neurosurg Clin North Am 1994;5:789–810.

68. Ziai WC, Varelas PN, Zeger SL, Mirski MA, Ulatowski JA. Neurologic intensive care resource use after brain tumor surgery: an analysis of indications and alternative strategies. Crit Care Med 2003;31:2782–2787.

69. Cochrane DD, Gustavsson B, Poskitt KP, Steinbok P, Kestle JR. The surgical and natural morbidity of aggressive resection for posterior fossa tumors in childhood. Pediatr Neurosurg 1994;20: 19–29.

70. Lewis EA. Gastroduodenal ulceration and haemorrhage of neurogenic origin. Br J Surg 1973;60:279–283.

71. Ross AJ 3rd, Siegel KR, Bell W, Templeton JM Jr, Schnaufer L, Bishop HC. Massive gastrointestinal hemorrhage in children with posterior fossa tumors. J Pediatr Surg 1987;22:633–636.

72. Lewis DW, Packer RJ, Raney B, Rak IW, Belasco J, Lange B. Incidence, presentation, and outcome of spinal cord disease in children with systemic cancer. Pediatrics 1986;78:438–443.

73. Ch'ien LT, Kalwinsky DK, Peterson G, et al. Metastatic epidermal tumors in children. Med Pediatr Oncol 1982;10:455–462.

74. Klein SL, Sanford RA, Muhlbauer MS. Pediatric spinal epidural metastases. J Neurosurg 1991;74:70–75.

75. Prasad D, Schiff D. Malignant spinal-cord compression. Lancet Oncol 2005;6:15–24.

76. Raffel C, Neave VC, Lavine S, McComb JG. Treatment of spinal cord compression by epidural malignancy in childhood. Neurosurgery 1991;28:349–352.

77. Kelly KM, Lange B. Oncologic emergencies. Pediatr Clin North Am 1997;44:809–830.

78. Byrne TN. Spinal cord compression from epidural metastases. N Engl J Med 1992;327:614–619.

5
Intracranial Hypertension

Steven G. Kernie and Samuel M. Lehman

Historical Perspective

The fact that increases in intracranial pressure (ICP) often result in significant mortality if left untreated has been recognized for centuries. Alexander Monro (1733–1817), a Scottish anatomist, published a paper in 1783 describing certain aspects of brain anatomy that also incorporated principles of physics [1]. He described the brain as being enclosed in nonexpandable bone and that the brain itself is essentially incompressible. Therefore, there must be balanced inflow and outflow of blood within the brain to keep the volume constant. A pupil of Monro, George Kelli, studied the venous blood in animals and humans who had died from various causes and noted that the blood volume in the brain remains constant even in deaths caused by hanging where venous drainage from the head and neck is severely impaired [2]. Thus, these observations serve as the basis for the often-quoted Monro-Kelli doctrine (or hypothesis). Interestingly, neither scientist acknowledged the existence of cerebrospinal fluid (CSF). Dating back to Galen's writings in the second century is the notion that the cerebral ventricles were filled with *spiritus animalus*. It was François Magendie, a French physiologist in the 19th century, who convinced his colleagues that the cerebral ventricles were actually filled with fluid by tapping the cisterna magna in animals and performing rudimentary analysis of CSF [3].

Pathophysiology of the Intracranial Vault

Cerebrospinal Fluid

The clinical consequences of raised ICP based on the Monro-Kelli doctrine were first widely recognized by Cushing in 1926 [4]. He incorporated the existence of CSF as a vital component of intra-cranial hypertension contributing to brain pathology following injury. He offered a more precise formula for the Monro-Kelli doctrine that indicated that, with an intact skull, the sum of the volume of the brain with the CSF and intracranial blood is constant. Therefore, an increase in one should cause a reduction in one or both of the remaining two [3].

Cerebral spinal fluid production and subsequent absorption is, like cerebral blood flow, quite dynamic. The choroid plexus accounts for at least 70% of the brain's production of CSF, and the transependymal movement of fluid from the brain parenchyma to the ventricular system accounts for the rest. The average volume of CSF in children 4–13 years of age is 90 mL, and the rate of formation is approximately 500 mL per day, resulting in an hourly turnover of about 14% of the total volume. The rate of production remains fairly constant and declines only slightly with increased ICP, but the rate of absorption increases linearly as the pressure exceeds approximately 15 mm Hg to approximately 40 mm Hg to where the rate of absorption is triple the rate of production [5].

Cerebral Blood Flow

The morbidity associated with increasing ICP largely centers on its effects on cerebral blood flow. Clinically, it is difficult to accurately gauge changing cerebral hemodynamics, so most attention is centered on cerebral blood flow and its surrogate, cerebral perfusion pressure (CPP). The CPP is simply the ICP subtracted from the mean arterial blood pressure (MAP).

$$CPP = MAP - ICP \text{ or } CPP = MAP - CVP$$

Unfortunately, the optimal CPP in children is extrapolated from adult guidelines that have been subject to considerable change. Cerebral autoregulation refers to a unique property of the brain's vasculature that enables it to maintain constant perfusion despite fluctuating blood pressure (Figure 5.1) [6]. This constant perfusion comes at the expense of variable blood volume, and therefore the perfusion state of the brain is intimately linked to ICP. Cerebral autoregulation in mammals was first established in the 1930s by Mogens Fog who created a window in the skulls of cats to directly observe vessel changes in response to various stimuli [7]. What he and subsequently others described in other species, including humans, was the ability of cerebral vessels to dilate in response to lower systemic blood pressure and to constrict in response to higher pressures, thereby maintaining constant blood flow to the

D.S. Wheeler et al. (eds.), *The Central Nervous System in Pediatric Critical Illness and Injury*,
DOI 10.1007/978-1-84800-993-6_5, © Springer-Verlag London Limited 2009

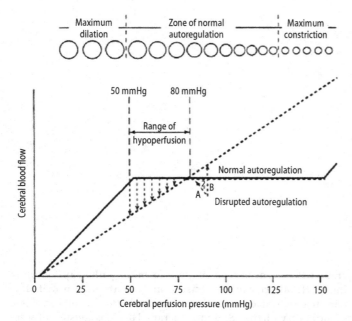

FIGURE 5.1. Cerebral autoregulation under normal conditions and after head injury. With autoregulation intact, cerebral blood flow is maintained over a range of systemic blood pressures (50 to 150 torr). In injuries that disrupt autoregulation, such as traumatic brain injury, the curve is shifted (arrows, dashed line), and cerebral blood flow is not maintained between 50 and 80 torr, thus creating a range of hypoperfusion. The degree to which autoregulation is disrupted depends on the degree of head injury and may vary significantly among individuals. (From Lang and Chestnut [6]. © 1994 W.B. Saunders, with permission from Elsevier).

brain [8]. In normal adults, therefore, cerebral blood flow remains constant at a CPP above 40 mm Hg, but, below this threshold, ischemia occurs as autoregulation cannot compensate for further decreases in systemic pressure. In children who normally have lower mean arterial blood pressure or those who have hypertension, these cerebral threshold values are altered.

In the setting of brain injury, autoregulation becomes disrupted and ischemia may occur at CPPs greater than 40 mm Hg [9]. If autoregulation becomes completely disrupted, it is unclear what the optimal CPP then becomes, although it is clearly greater than 40 mm Hg, and currently adult guidelines place it at 60 mm Hg [10]. For children, it becomes less clear. Cerebral autoregulation is disrupted in response to many forms of brain injury, and the optimal CPP becomes an age-dependent phenomenon with secondary ischemia likely occurring at a higher CPP with advancing age until normal systemic blood pressures matches that of adults.

Herniation Syndromes

When intracranial hypertension exceeds the limited ability of the brain to compensate, the structural rigidity of the intracranial vault in noninfants plays a critical role in directing outcome following various brain insults. The brain itself is divided into anterior, middle, and posterior fossae. The anterior and middle fossae are separated from the posterior fossa by the tentorium cerebelli, an inflexible fibrous dural lamina that contains the tentorial notch, the opening through which pass the brainstem, the posterior cerebral artery and the third cranial nerve and where communication between the anterior and posterior fossa occurs (Figure 5.2) [11]. When intracranial pressure rises due to a variety of causes, herniation typically occurs through the tentorial notch by downward displacement of middle fossa contents into the posterior fossa. Critical structures that are compromised by this downward displacement include the oculomotor nerve (the third cranial nerve) and the posterior cerebral arteries. The parasympathetic components that control pupillary constriction are the most vulnerable part of the oculomotor nerve when increased pressure causes nerve impingement; thus, ipsilateral papillary dilatation is a precursor to herniation.

Herniation syndromes include *unilateral (or uncal) transtentorial herniation* in the case of unilateral mass-occupying lesions whereby the ipsilateral temporal lobe displaces the uncus or hippocampus on that side through the tentorial notch. This is typically

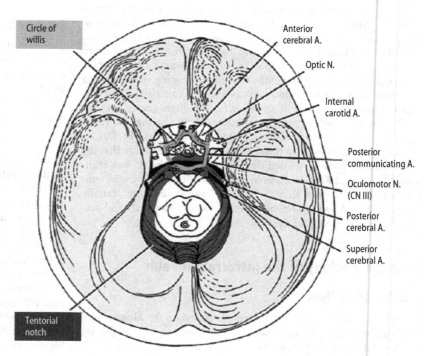

FIGURE 5.2. The floor of the anterior and middle cerebral fossae illustrating the tentorial notch (dark gray) and the contents that pass through it. Note that the sections of the circle of Willis (light gray) that is most at risk during downward tentorial herniation are the posterior cerebral arteries. These run adjacent to both branches of the oculomotor nerve (cranial nerve III) that controls papillary dilatation. (Adapted from Plumb and Posner [11].)

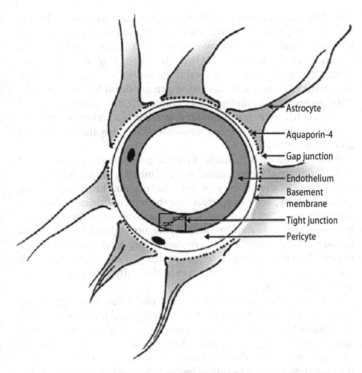

FIGURE 5.3. Cross-sectional schematic of the blood–brain barrier. This transverse section demonstrates the tight junctions of the endothelium (boxed area) and their close proximity to ensheathing pericytes and basement membrane. Astrocytic foot processes that express the water channel aquaporin-4 regulate water flow into the brain.

accompanied by an increase in blood pressure, a decrease in heart rate, and a unilateral fixed and dilated pupil. *Central transtentorial herniation* is associated with generalized cerebral edema whereby both hemispheres are displaced downward and both the diencephalons and the midbrain are pushed caudad through the tentorial notch and results in rapidly evolving coma, pupil constriction, and then dilatation followed by death [5,11].

Cerebral Edema

Cerebral edema itself is caused by a variety of factors that have commonly been divided into vasogenic, cytotoxic, and interstitial edema. Vasogenic edema is caused by increased capillary permeability and disruption of the blood–brain barrier (BBB) following injury. It is seen with brain tumors, abscesses, hemorrhage, and trauma. Cytotoxic edema results from the swelling of neurons, glia, and endothelial cells and is caused by hypoxic–ischemic insults, infection, and trauma. Although this classification system is useful in understanding individual disease processes, it is likely that elements of cytotoxic and vasogenic edema take place in all disease states.

Interstitial edema occurs when the usual flow of transependymal fluid into the ventricular system is altered or impeded [5]. This occurs either when CSF absorption is blocked or when production is increased beyond the brain's ability to reabsorb it. Much of the pathology associated with the development of cerebral edema centers on the BBB. The BBB is a diffusion barrier unique to the brain and required for its proper functioning. The endothelial cells within the brain are a critical component of the BBB and differ from endothelial cells in other organs by their lack of fenestrations and more extensive tight junctions. In addition to endothelial cells, the BBB is composed of the capillary basement membrane, pericytes

embedded within the basement membrane, and astrocytic end-feet that ensheath the blood vessels (Figure 5.3) [12].

The aquaporins are a family of water channels that regulate water permeability across microvessels. In the brain, aquaporin-4 is the most abundantly expressed member of this family and is found primarily on the astrocytic foot processes that contribute to the BBB (13). In mice deficient for aquaporin-4, cytotoxic edema caused by simulated stroke or water intoxication is diminished, whereas vasogenic edema caused by parenchymal water infusion or a freeze injury worsens outcome and causes increased pressure [13]. Thus, it appears that aquaporin-4–mediated transcellular water movement is critical for the development of a mouse model of cytotoxic edema and is also needed for the resolution of experimental models of vasogenic edema.

Evaluation and Monitoring of the Patient with Intracranial Hypertension

The clinical features of raised ICP vary with age in the pediatric population. Newborns and infants with open fontanelles can partially vent increased ICP by expanding the volume of the skull. The rate of change of ICP is a primary determinant in its clinical presentation. Slow changes are tolerated relatively well, particularly in children whose sutures can reopen in response to increases in volume. Sudden changes are intolerable, and children with a rapid rise in ICP present with headache, confusion, and decreasing consciousness.

The Glasgow Coma Scale (GCS) is the best known and most validated of all neurologic assessment scales in trauma. It was developed to quantify the level of arousal states following head trauma. It can be used to predict children at highest risk for significant intracranial hypertension. It is divided into three areas: eye opening, verbal response, and motor response. Of these the motor component is the most reliable and the strongest predictor of outcome [14]. The original GCS was adopted for adults but has been modified for use with young children and infants (Table 5.1)

TABLE 5.1. Glasgow Coma Scale and modified Glasgow Coma Scale for infants and children.

Best response	Adults and children	Infants	Score
Eye	Spontaneous	Spontaneous	4
	To verbal stimuli	To verbal stimuli	3
	To pain only	To pain only	2
	No response	No response	1
Verbal	Oriented, appropriate	Coos and babbles	5
	Confused	Irritable cries	4
	Inappropriate words	Cries to pain	3
	Incomprehensible sounds	Moans to pain	2
	No response	No response	1
Motor	Obeys commands	Moves spontaneously and purposefully	6
	Localizes pain	Withdraws to touch	5
	Withdrawal from pain	Withdraws to pain	4
	Flexion to pain	Abnormal flexion in response to pain (decorticate)	3
	Extension to pain	Abnormal extension in response to pain (decerebrate)	2
	No response	No response	1

Note: Total score is 3 to 15.
Source: Data are from Chameides and Hazinski [15] and Teasdale and Jennett [16].

[15,16]. Glasgow Coma Scale scores range from 3 to 15, where a score of 13–15 represents mild injury, 9–12 is moderate injury, and 3–8 is severe injury. There is obviously overlap in the true degree of injury based on other clinical and radiologic findings as well as the rate of improvement or deterioration in the GCS. Similarly, GCS at the time of admission is more predictive of outcome than GCS in the field [14].

The neurologic evaluation of the patient with a severe rise in ICP depends greatly on a properly performed assessment. Often the etiology of the altered patient is not due to intracranial hypertension alone but can also be secondary to hypoxia, ingestions, tumors, and metabolic factors that can all present in the setting of trauma or other etiologies that result in altered consciousness. Evaluation of coma status is self-explanatory for the eye and verbal portions of the GCS, but the motor component is the most difficult to properly evaluate. If a painful stimulus is administered, it should be done along the cutaneous distribution of a cranial nerve and not on the limbs or torso where it may elicit spinal reflexes that can mimic a central response. The Cushing reflex occurs when brain stem ischemia results in systemic hypertension and reactive bradycardia. It is still unclear whether this reflex is a normal regulator of blood pressure when the brain is at rest and baroreceptor afferents are not activated, or it only occurs in response to pathologic ischemia of the brainstem [17]. In any event, it clinically represents an attempt during periods of brain compromise to overcome cerebral hypoperfusion by supraphysiologic increases in systemic blood pressure.

Computed tomography (CT) remains the primary radiologic method for evaluating the presence of intracranial hypertension, particularly in the setting of trauma where speed of diagnosing intracranial pathology is particularly important. In addition, CT scans of the head are also quite sensitive in detecting extrabrain pathology involving the skull and soft tissues. Computed tomography scans with intravenous contrast are usually not needed and may in fact obscure acute pathology. Drawbacks to CT include its inferior resolution compared with magnetic resonance imaging (MRI), missed pathology such as small bleeds because of inappropriate window level and width, and difficulty identifying some low-density acute hemorrhages in the setting of severe anemia [18].

All children in the intensive care unit with suspected intracranial hypertension should undergo a CT scan primarily for identification of potentially reversible etiologies. It is less clear in the emergency department setting which clinical criteria best predict which patients might benefit from a CT scan. Diffuse brain swelling that leads to intracranial hypertension can be caused by many etiologies and is manifest on CT by obliteration of cerebral sulci and basal cisterns, effacement of the gray matter–white matter interface, and small ventricles. Other lesions more commonly associated with trauma are intracranial bleeds and fluid collections. A commonly used clinical rating scale was published by Marshall et al. that categorizes acute CT abnormalities in head injury from diffuse injury I (no visible intracranial pathology) to IV (greater than 5 mm midline shift and presence of nonspecific edema) [19].

If CT findings are not consistent with the clinical course, then MRI should be performed. Magnetic resonance imaging and CT appear to have equivalent sensitivities for detecting hemorrhagic lesions, but MRI is much more sensitive in detecting nonhemorrhagic and brain stem lesions in the setting of trauma [18]. In the setting of traumatic brain injury, intracranial hypertension often manifests along with diffuse axonal injury. Diffuse axonal injury can occur in either white matter or subcortical gray matter and is one of the most common findings that correlate with poor clinical outcome. In practice, diffuse axonal injury is actually many small shearing injuries at the gray matter–white matter interface, and MRI is much better than CT at their detection. Magnetic resonance imaging is also superior at detecting extraaxial fluid collections, and, unlike CT, it is able to distinguish subdural blood from subdural hygromas (pathologic collections of CSF). Other causes of increased ICP that are secondary to trauma or hypoxia such as vascular lesions and venous sinus clots are also much easier to detect with MRI.

As discussed earlier, much of the long-term sequelae associated with intracranial hypertension are attributed to impaired cerebral blood flow. In the absence of overt herniation, brain injury and intracranial hypertension affect how the metabolic demands of the brain are met. The most widespread surrogate of brain metabolic demands are measured by quantifying both global and regional cerebral blood flows. There are now many modalities to detect impaired cerebral blood flow in the setting of raised ICP, although none has gained uniform acceptance clinically, and each has significant drawbacks.

Imaging methods to detect cerebral blood flow have significant advantages because they can detect both global and regional disruptions in blood flow. Magnetic resonance imaging can be used to determine cerebral blood flow (CBF) (perfusion MRI) but has not gained acceptance within the intensive care unit setting because of the long time for each examination and the need for invasive monitoring equipment to be in the presence of high-powered magnetic fields. Xenon-CT is more widely used and is considered accurate and reliable, although it is limited by the fact that xenon produces anesthesia at high doses, and at the low doses that are used there is a relatively low signal-to-noise ratio. Single photon emission tomography (SPECT) allows qualitative determinations of cerebral perfusion and is much easier to use and less expensive than positron emission tomography, although it has not been useful at providing quantitative measurements of cerebral blood flow. Positron emission tomography is considered the gold standard for determining CBF. Using ^{15}O-labeled water, a real-time global indicator of cerebral blood flow can be obtained quickly. Its disadvantages include its relatively low spatial resolution, high cost, lack of availability, and, particularly for young children, exposure to ionizing radiation [20].

There are also numerous nonimaging modalities to detect both global and regional impairments of cerebral blood flow. In 1945, Kety and Schmidt published the first quantitative method to detect cerebral blood flow using N_2O as an inert tracer gas and Fick's principle to calculate cerebral blood flow from the arteriovenous difference [21]. A modified version with argon[25] is still used today, although it is quite labor intensive and not widely practiced [20]. Another version of the Kety-Schmidt technique is to use [133]xenon by either injection or inhalation and then calculate by measuring its washout. This method is also not practical and gives fairly limited information based on its ability to measure mainly cortical blood flow. There are also several techniques available that are more commonly used in the intensive care unit setting, although they are nonquantitative. Jugular bulb oximetry gives global data concerning the adequacy of cerebral blood flow in relation to metabolic demand. It has been widely studied, and correlations are found between the number of desaturations and clinical outcome, although it has not proved useful in managing patients with impaired cerebral blood flow [20]. Transcranial Doppler is easy to use and noninvasive but measures blood flow velocity and may not give a true indication of cerebral blood flow. Near-infrared spectroscopy (NIRS) measures the average cerebral saturation in an area that cannot be clearly defined. It is controversial because of the large number of contradictory results that have appeared in the literature, although it appears to be promising because it is noninvasive, it monitors continuously, and it is relatively inexpensive.

Brain tissue PO_2 monitoring using an invasive probe that can be inserted through existing pressure monitors appears to give relatively reliable data regarding regional oxygen saturations at the end capillary level. In the injury setting, however, the difference between tissue saturation and end capillary saturations does not correlate as well [20]. Microdialysis is a promising technology used to monitor tissue biochemistry, although it has not been shown to be useful in measuring cerebral blood flow [22]. It is still unclear what to do with data suggesting impairment of cerebral blood flow. Meaningful interventions directed at optimizing brain perfusion and meeting changing metabolic demands in the injured brain necessitates that uniform and accurate standards are validated before such interventions can be reliably assessed.

Treatment of Intracranial Hypertension

The purpose of treating intracranial hypertension is to avoid further brain injury caused by elevated ICP. Injury can be from focal or global brain ischemia caused by decreased blood flow. The ultimate and most severe form of ischemia takes place during a herniation event that causes compression of the arterial supply to the brain. The following sections outline a variety of therapies aimed at lowering the ICP. These therapies are listed in Table 5.2, and each is reviewed in this section. The therapies listed are effective in lowering ICP by a variety of mechanisms. There are limited therapies, however, that are proven to be beneficial when studied long term, and there are fewer yet that have data supporting improved outcomes in children. Use of these therapies for many disease processes are often extrapolated from the trauma literature, sometimes with little scientific support. The sections that follow describe pertinent data as they relate to disease-specific therapy. Table 5.3 summarizes the evidence that serves as the basis for published guidelines.

There is more known about intracranial hypertension resulting from traumatic brain injury than perhaps all the other causes of intracranial hypertension combined. There have been excellent reviews of the current literature and publication of scientific statements for the management of traumatic brain injury in both adults and children (Figure 5.4) [10,23]. In addition to reviewing the current state of knowledge about traumatic head injury, these reviews offer a critical pathway for the management of intracranial hypertension in traumatic brain injury. There are a number of causes of Intracranial hypertension in patients with traumatic brain injury: space-occupying lesions from extraaxial bleeding, hydrocephalus from edema or mass lesions around the third or fourth ventricles, vasogenic edema from direct brain injury, alteration in the intracranial vault from a depressed skull fracture, and cytotoxic brain edema from ischemia, which can occur as a primary or secondary mode of injury.

Traumatic brain injury–induced intracranial hypertension is defined as an ICP of greater than 20 mm Hg. This threshold is based on five studies assigned as class III data from adults, and the pediatric guidelines state that it is optional to treat ICP greater than 20 mm Hg. There are no prospective randomized studies that

TABLE 5.2 Intracranial hypertension therapies.

Therapy	Onset of action	Proposed mechanisms of action
Avoiding ICH exacerbation Midline positioning Reverse Trendelenburg Seizure treatment Avoiding hypoxia, hyperthermia, hypotension, hypercapnia	Variable	Various
Hyperventilation Hypocapnia Alkalosis	Seconds to minutes	Decreased CBF Decreased CBV
Osmotic agents Mannitol Hypertonic Saline Glycerol	Minutes	Decreased cerebral water content Improved CBF Decreased CBV
Barbiturates	Minutes	Decreased cerebral oxygen demand leading to decreased CBF/CBV
Sedation and Neuromuscular blockade	Minutes	Decreased metabolic demand and CBF
Hypothermia	Hours	Decreased cerebral oxygen consumption and decreased CBF and CBV
Corticosteroids	Hours	Restoring altered BBB permeability Reduction of CSF production
Acetazolamide	Hours	Reduction of CSF production
Surgical removal of mass lesions	Variable	Decreased cerebral contents
Decompressive craniotomy	Variable	Increasing volume of intracranial vault
Ventricular drain	Variable	Removal of CSF

BBB, blood–brain barrier; CBF, cerebral blood flow; CBV, cerebral blood volume; CSF, cerebrospinal fluid; ICH, intracerebral hemorrhage.

directly compare treatment threshold to outcomes. Although there may be a lower threshold for younger children or those with open sutures and fontanelle, there are no data that supports this. It should be noted, however, that brain ischemia and herniation can occur at pressures lower than 20 mm Hg, depending on the location of edema and the presence of mass lesions. Factors that are known to exacerbate cerebral edema should be avoided. These include hyperthermia, hypoxia, hypotension, and hypercarbia [23].

Sedation and neuromuscular blockade are often used to treat elevated ICP caused by increases in cerebral metabolism due to

TABLE 5.3 Evidence requirements and certainty classification based on the pediatric and adult guidelines for severe traumatic brain injury.

Recommendation	Degree of certainty	Evidence required
Standard	High degree of clinical certainty	Randomized controlled trials with outcome data
Guideline	Moderate degree of clinical certainty	Weaker data from controlled trials Prospectively collected data with retrospective analysis (case control, cohort, etc.) Preponderance of retrospective data
Option	Unclear clinical certainty	Retrospective reviews without controls: case reports, case series and expert opinion

Source: Data are from the Brain Trauma Foundation [10] and from Adelson et al. [23].

noxious stimuli and pain [23,24]. There are several reports of mild increases in ICP with narcotic use and decreases in ICP with ketamine, diazepam, and propofol [25–28]. It should be noted, however, that ketamine has been considered contraindicated for patients with intracranial hypertension, and continuous propofol infusion is not recommended for pediatric patients. Although commonly used for patients with traumatic brain injury and intracranial hypertension, there are no studies with children that demonstrate an improvement in outcome from use of sedation or neuromuscular blockade.

Drainage of CSF via an external ventricular drain for reduction in total intracranial contents is an effective means of reducing ICP. In the pediatric guidelines, however, there is only enough scientific support to make CSF drainage an option; there is only one small retrospective pediatric study and some outcome data extrapolated from the adult guidelines [10,29]. In addition to CSF drainage through ventricular access, there has been some success with lumbar drains. Two case series of pediatric head injury from the same institution demonstrated significant reduction in ICP with the institution of lumbar CSF drainage [30,31]. Although there

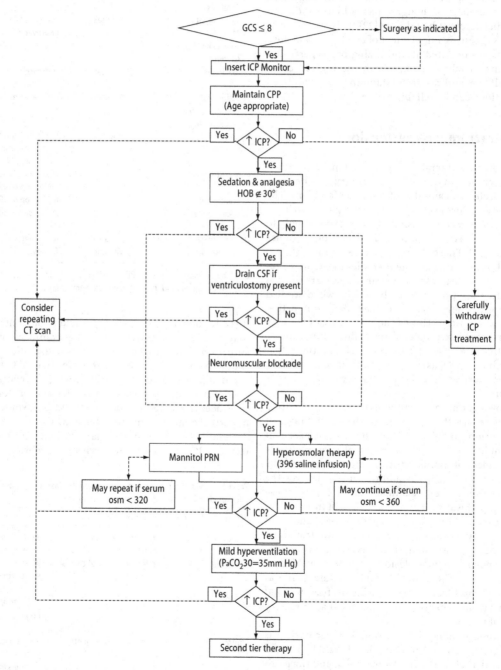

Figure 5.4. First tier therapy for the management of pediatric traumatic brain injury. CPP, cerebral perfusion pressure; CSF, cerebrospinal fluid; CT, computed tomography; GSC, Glasgow Coma Score; HOB, head of bed; ICP, intracranial pressure; PRN, as needed. (From Adelson et al. [23]. © 2003 with permission from Lippincott Williams & Wilikins.)

is theoretical concern of potentiating transtentorial or tonsillar herniation by using lumbar drains, this risk appears to be minimized by selecting patients with open basilar cisterns and no mass lesions [32].

Hyperosmolar therapy with either mannitol or hypertonic saline has been a mainstay of treatment for elevated intracranial hypertension for decades. Mannitol is an osmotic diuretic based on a six-carbon sugar that was first used for decreasing elevated ICP by Wise and Chater in the 1950s [33]. Mannitol's effect on intracranial hypertension is probably related to several different functional properties [34]. It has historically been thought to be clinically efficacious because of its osmotic effects that promote movement of extravascular fluid into the capillaries and then out of the intracranial vault. This "brain dehydration" effect of mannitol may certainly be a factor in its ICP-lowering properties, although changes in cerebral blood flow and volume may be more important. Mannitol induces a rheologic effect on blood and blood flow by altering blood viscosity from changes in erythrocyte cell compliance [35,36]. There have been several studies on the effects of mannitol on cerebral blood flow, ICP, blood viscosity, and vessel diameter in both animals and humans. It appears from a subset of these studies that the decrease in ICP may be from cerebral vasoconstriction. This vasoconstriction does not occur in patients with defective autoregulation, and thus there was a less pronounced effect on lowering ICP [37,38].

Hypertonic saline solutions for the treatment of intracranial hypertension was first described by Weed and McKibben in 1919 and were the first osmotic agents studied for this purpose [23]. Like mannitol, the mechanisms of action of hypertonic saline on intracranial hypertension are probably multifactorial. Hypertonic saline not only acts to lower ICP but is also a volume expander acting to increase cardiac output and increase mean arterial blood pressure [39–41]. In addition to its effects on ICP and CPP, hypertonic saline appears to have immunomodulatory and neurochemical effects [42]. Animal studies of hypertonic saline treatment in experimental (cryogenic) brain injury tend to show decreases in contralateral cortical water, decreased ICP, and increased CPP. In addition to pressure differences, animal studies have demonstrated increased cerebral blood flow and oxygen delivery compared with isotonic resuscitation fluids [42]. Although the observed effects of hypertonic saline may be secondary to fluid shifts that occur because of its osmotic effect, it is likely that there are additional effects similar to mannitol's on cerebral blood flow and vessel diameter accounting for these findings. Hypertonic saline does have the benefit over mannitol of elimination of the rebound hypovolemia and possible hypotension seen with osmotic and nonosmotic diuretics.

Initial reports on the use of hypertonic saline for traumatic brain injury were case reports and case series of patients who had failed conventional management strategies and had persistent intracranial hypertension [43–45]. Since then there have been several prospective trials evaluating hypertonic saline in the treatment of intracranial hypertension. These studies have shown that the hypertonic saline group had lower ICPs and higher CPPs, required less interventions, demonstrated fewer complications, and had shorter intensive care unit stays [46,47]. The use of hypertonic saline to induce hypernatremia has also been evaluated to control intracranial hypertension. In children refractory to conventional ICP therapy, it appears that increased serum Na induced by hypertonic saline may be beneficial in managing intracranial hypertension [48,49]. Although mannitol is more accepted as an osmolar

therapy for intracranial hypertension, there is more evidence supporting the use of hypertonic saline in pediatric traumatic brain injury [23]. The pediatric guidelines have no *standards* for osmolar therapy but do offer the *option* of using either mannitol or hypertonic saline, with suggested limits of an osmolarity of 320 mOsm/L for mannitol and 360 mOsm/L for hypertonic saline [23]. Although deemed effective by most investigators, future studies of osmolar therapy in intracranial hypertension need to better define the optimal dosing, method of administration (continuous vs. bolus), and use of induced hypernatremia compared with other second and third tier therapies.

Hyperventilation had previously been a cornerstone of treatment of intracranial hypertension in traumatic brain injury based on Bruce's data implicating hyperemia as the cause of intracranial hypertension in pediatric brain trauma [50]. More recent studies have challenged the idea that hyperventilation is beneficial for traumatic brain injury and have conveyed concern over brain ischemia and decreased brain oxygenation caused by hypocapnia [23]. Hyperventilation leads to hypocapnia and CSF alkalosis, which results in vasoconstriction, decreased cerebral blood flow, decreased cerebral blood volume, decreased oxygen delivery, and cerebral ischemia [51]. Over time the extracellular fluid pH normalizes by buffering mechanisms resulting in return of cerebral blood flow to normal levels. The return toward normocapnia in a buffered extracellular cerebral fluid can cause rebound intracranial hypertension and hyperperfusion [52,53]. Although hyperventilation does transiently lower ICP, it does so at the expense of cerebral blood flow, and in patients with altered cerebral autoregulation it can cause regional mismatches in oxygen supply to metabolic demand. The pediatric guidelines for the use of hyperventilation to treat intracranial hypertension offer only treatment options, noting insufficient data for guidelines or standards. The four options are that prophylactic hyperventilation should be avoided, mild hyperventilation may be considered for refractory intracranial hypertension, aggressive hyperventilation (PaCO$_2$ < 30) may be considered as a second tier option with monitoring for cerebral ischemia, and aggressive hyperventilation may be used in the setting of impending herniation. Although hyperventilation for control of intracranial hypertension was once the standard of care, there is little evidence to support its use, and there is a growing body of evidence to suggest that it may be harmful. There is still not enough pediatric evidence to demonstrate a direct association between worse outcomes and hyperventilation. There may be a role for hyperventilation in the setting of acute neurologic deterioration because this is often the most rapidly applicable therapy for the herniating patient. In addition, there may be a role for hyperventilation as a second tier therapy for refractory intracranial hypertension (Figure 5.5).

Barbiturates can be effective agents in lowering ICP in patients with intracranial hypertension. It is likely that barbiturates act therapeutically by lowering cerebral oxygen consumption. Decreased oxygen demand will lead to decreased cerebral blood flow in those areas of the brain that can couple supply and demand, thus leading to a decrease in ICP [54]. In addition to their ICP-lowering effects, barbiturates have been shown to have direct neuroprotective effects, including inhibition of free radical–mediated lipid peroxidation [23]. Use of high-dose barbiturates, however, has also been associated with systemic complications of myocardial depression and immune suppression. Thiopental and pentobarbital have both been described for control of intracranial hypertension, but presumably other barbiturates may be as effective. The

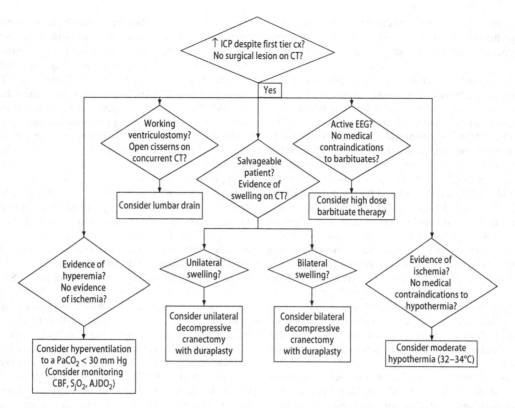

Figure 5.5. Second tier therapy in the management of pediatric traumatic brain injury. AJDO2, arterial, jugular venous difference in oxygen content; CBF, cerebral blood flow; CT, computed tomography; EEG, electroencephalogram; ICP, intracranial pressure; SjO2, jugular oxygen saturation. (From Adelson et al. [23]. © 2003 with permission from Lippincott Williams & Wilikins.)

benefit to adverse effect ratio decreases as the patients reach burst suppression on electroencephalography, and there is little more reduction in cerebral metabolism achieved with higher doses [55]. Although the adult traumatic head injury guidelines suggest barbiturate therapy to treat refractory intracranial hypertension, there is not as much support in the pediatric literature. A Cochrane review of barbiturates used for traumatic head injury found there to be no evidence of improvement in outcome and suggested that their hypotensive effects offset any improvement in ICP that they may confer [55]. The pediatric guidelines do give the option of high-does barbiturate therapy for refractory intracranial hypertension, although high-dose barbiturate therapy falls into the second tier therapy group [23].

Hypothermia has both neuroprotective and ICP-lowering effects. It has been well established that hypothermia lowers cerebral metabolism and will thus reduce cerebral oxygen demand [56]. The resultant decreased cerebral blood flow and volume contribute to the ICP-lowering effect of therapeutic hypothermia. In addition, hypothermia is neuroprotective, resulting in less inflammation, less cytotoxicity, and less lipid peroxidation. Hypothermia does have adverse effects that may counteract the beneficial effects of neuroprotection. Hypotension, cardiac arrhythmias, and immune suppression are three of the more significant drawbacks. The incidence of adverse effects in children compared with adults is not clear. Initial phase II clinical trials of therapeutic hypothermia for adult traumatic brain injury looked quite promising; however, a large multicenter study found no beneficial effect on outcome [57–59]. Any beneficial effect of hypothermia may have been negated by the complications seen with its use. It may be possible that children

who do not have as much preexisting organ dysfunction may be more resistant to these serious adverse effects. There is one small randomized, controlled study of hypothermia in pediatrics that did demonstrate significant trends toward ICP control without significant adverse effects [60]. There are few pediatric data to support the use of therapeutic hypothermia, and thus the pediatric guidelines give no standards but only the options to avoid hyperthermia and to potentially use hypothermia in the setting of refractory intracranial hypertension despite lack of clinical data [23].

For managing intracranial hypertension, corticosteroids have the putative beneficial effects of decreasing edema, limiting free radical production, limiting lipid peroxidation, decreasing vasoactive and chemoattractive factors, restoring altered vascular permeability, and decreasing inflammatory response [61]. The positive experience of glucocorticoids in edema surrounding brain tumors promoted their use in other disease states [62]. Use of corticosteroids for traumatic brain injury has been widespread, with as many as 64% of U.S. trauma centers using them routinely as recently as 10 years ago [63]. There have been multiple studies of adult head injury and steroid use, with outcome data that demonstrate no beneficial effect of steroids [64–67]. Based on existing evidence, the Brain Trauma Foundation published a standard to not recommend using steroids to improve outcome or reduce ICP in patients with severe traumatic head injury [10]. The CRASH trial (corticosteroid randomization after significant head injury) included over 10,000 patients and was stopped early as mortality was increased in the steroid treatment group [68]. There are insufficient pediatric data to make guideline or standard recommendations for using steroids in traumatic head injury, although, given the strong adult data, it is unlikely that steroids will be evaluated for pediatric traumatic brain injury.

An area of emerging use in the treatment of both adults and children with traumatic brain injury is decompressive craniectomy. Small case-controlled and randomized studies have confirmed the ICP-relieving effect of decompressive craniectomy and have shown a trend toward improved outcomes in these patients. There are insufficient data for standards or guidelines to be established for the use of this operative technique, although options for its use include the setting of severe traumatic brain injury with diffuse swelling and intracranial hypertension refractory to medical management, refractory intracranial hypertension in abusive traumatic brain injury, and cases with indicators of "recoverable" brain injury [23]. As with all incompletely studied therapies for severe traumatic brain injury and intracranial hypertension, it is possible that decompressive craniectomy will result in decreased mortality by increasing the incidence of vegetative and severely disabled survivors. Timing, patient selection, and operative technique are three areas that need further study for this therapy that is rapidly gaining popularity.

Selected Disease States with Intracranial Hypertension

The differential diagnosis of intracranial hypertension is quite variable. Table 5.4 lists some of the etiologies. In this section, we review selected causes of intracranial hypertension and what is known about disease-specific treatments.

Hepatic Encephalopathy, Hyperammonemia, and Brain Edema

Several metabolic causes of intracranial hemorrhage and brain edema are seen in the pediatric intensive care unit. Two of the most common are fulminant hepatic failure and inborn errors of metabolism associated with hyperammonemia (such as urea cycle defects). Reye's syndrome and Reye-like syndromes were common causes of hyperammonemia and intracranial hypertension but are now almost nonexistent. Although it is known that brain edema and intracranial hypertension are associated with hepatic failure and hyperammonemia, the exact underlying mechanisms are unclear. It is likely that there is not just one unifying mechanism for the etiology of the brain edema but rather a group of mechanisms that may be more or less important in individual patients and in different diseases. One of the most important factors in the development of intracranial hypertension is the increased water content of the brain [69].

Ammonia, once thought to be the sole cause of the cerebral edema, is still recognized as a key player in its development. Hyperammonemia seems to be required for brain herniation in acute liver failure, and there are no reports of brain edema in acute liver failure with normal ammonia levels [70,71]. Hyperammonemia is associated with increased brain glutamine as its route of detoxification, and this may contribute an osmotic force in the development of brain edema. Ammonia may play a roll in the development of oxygen free radicals as demonstrated in animal studies of hyperammonemia [72]. Glutamate accumulation in the extracellular fluid of the brain has also been demonstrated in hepatic failure, although the exact role of this excitatory amino acid in the develop-

TABLE 5.4 Etiology of intracranial hypertension.

Trauma
  Vasogenic edema
  Traumatic hydrocephalus
  Hematoma (epidural, subdural, intra parenchymal)
  Alteration of cranial vault (depressed skull fracture)
Metabolic disease
  Diabetic ketoacidosis
  Hepatic encephalopathy
  Hyperammonemia
Neoplastic disease
  Malignant tumors
  Nonmalignant tumors
Hydrocephalus
  Communicating
  Noncommunicating
Hypoxic–ischemic injury
  Near drowning
  Seizures
  Cardiac arrest
  Severe anemic hypoxia
  Severe hypoxic hypoxia
Vascular
  Arteriovenous malformation
  Vascular aneurysm
  Stoke
    Hemorrhagic
    Nonhemorrhagic
Infectious
  Meningitis
    Bacterial
    Viral
    Fungal
  Brain abscess
Miscellaneous
  Pseudotumor cerebri
  Malignant hypertension

ment on cerebral edema is unclear [73]. Cerebral blood flow is altered in the setting of hyperammonemia and fulminate hepatic failure. Both pressure-regulated and carbon dioxide-responsive cerebral vasomotor control is lost in the setting of fulminant hepatic failure [74,75].

Treatment of intracranial hypertension in the setting of hyperammonemia and/or acute liver failure is mostly based on adult data. Intracranial pressure catheters are an accepted way of monitoring these patients; however, those with fulminant hepatic failure may be at increased risk from complications [76]. Mannitol has been the mainstay of treatment of increased ICP for both its effects on cerebral blood flow and its possible reduction of cerebral water content through osmotic effects. A small randomized controlled trail of mannitol for treatment of cerebral edema demonstrated more frequent resolution and better survival in the mannitol treatment group [77]. The same trial also demonstrated no difference in the incidence or survival of patients who were treated with dexamethasone. Hypertonic saline may also have a role in treatment and prevention of intracranial hypertension in patients with acute liver failure, as one small prospective randomized study in adults showed decreases in ICP and less need for inotropic support [78].

Hyperventilation has been found to decrease ICP, reduce the cerebral glutamine efflux, and restore cerebral blood flow autoregulation, although its role for treating liver failure–related intra-cranial hypertension remains unclear [74,75,79–81]. Use of barbiturates for control of hepatic encephalopathy–induced intracranial hypertension has not been studied in a randomized and controlled fashion, although it has been used in several small trials [79,82,83]. There is a growing body of evidence that use of moderate hypothermia in adult patients with hepatic encephalopathy and intracranial hypertension has favorable results. A rat model of hepatic encephalopathy demonstrated that moderate hypothermia reduced the amount of deposition of select osmolytes [84]. Moderate hypothermia appears to restore cerebral blood flow autoregulation and reactivity to carbon dioxide, in addition to the case series demonstrating improvements in intracranial hypertension. There are, however, no randomized and controlled trials of hypothermia in hepatic or metabolic disease-induced intracranial hypertension.

Future treatment of intracranial hypertension in metabolic and liver disease will need to rely on examining the effects of osmotic agents, hypothermia, barbiturates, and hyperventilation in controlled trials. Ammonia detoxification strategies, including ultra-filtration and ornithine-L-aspartate, play current and future roles in the treatment of these patients. In addition, there are some data that indomethacin may be a future therapeutic option for hepatic encephalopathy–induced intracranial hypertension [85].

Diabetic Ketoacidosis and Cerebral Edema

Cerebral edema and resultant intracranial hypertension is the major cause of mortality in pediatric patients with diabetes [86]. Cerebral edema in diabetic ketoacidosis (DKA) patients is more common in new presentations of diabetes [87]. Early studies have suggested that there is an increased incidence of cerebral edema in younger children and infants; however, more recent large patient studies have found no association between age and its development [87,88]. In addition to the obvious cases of DKA-associated cerebral edema, there appears to be evidence of subclinical cerebral edema that can be noted on CT scans of patients with only mild or no central nervous system symptoms, a phenomenon not seen in all patients [89–91]. The mechanism of development of cerebral edema in patients with DKA is not entirely clear. It is likely that the cerebral edema is a result of osmotic forces that cause increased intracellular fluid and swelling. These osmotic changes are most likely seen during the treatment phase, but there are examples of cerebral edema occurring before institution of therapy [87,88]. A consensus statement on DKA in children compiled the following proposed mechanisms for development of cerebral edema: cerebral ischemia–hypoxia, generation of inflammatory mediators, increased cerebral blood flow, disruption of cell membranes and ion transport, aquaporin channels, and generation of intracellular organic osmolytes [92]. Recent data using perfusion-weighted MRI suggests that cerebral edema results from expansion of the extracellular space (vasogenic edema) and not from cell swelling [93].

Identification of risk factors for the development of cerebral edema in DKA has been derived from retrospective cohort studies and case series. In Glaser's study of 61 cases of cerebral edema out of 6,977 hospitalizations for DKA, they found that low $PaCO_2$, high serum urea nitrogen, and treatment with sodium bicarbonate in patients presenting with DKA were at increased risk for cerebral edema [88]. Although the changes in serum osmolality that occur with the initiation of treatment have long been thought to be a cause of DKA-associated cerebral edema, this rate of change may not be relevant [88,94,95].

There is little information on the treatment of cerebral edema associated with DKA, mostly because its infrequent nature does not lend itself to easy study of its treatment. There are only case reports and case series of patients who have been treated with mannitol or hypertonic saline [92,96,97]. One retrospective study of patients with DKA and cerebral edema noted worse outcomes in patients who were hyperventilated to a $PCO_2 < 22\,mm\,Hg$ [98]. It remains unclear what the optimal ventilation strategy is when mechanical ventilation is initiated in a patient who had been previously hypocarbic with $PvCO_2$ values of 10–20 or even lower secondary to Kusmal respirations [99,100]. There are case reports of patients improving with CSF drainage and use of ventriculostomy for ICP monitoring [101]. There are no data on the use of barbiturates, glucocorticoids, hypothermia, or other ICP therapies [92].

Mass Lesions: Tumors and Hydrocephalus

Hydrocephalus and abnormal CSF collections are the result of abnormal CSF flow (obstructive/noncommunicating) or inadequate CSF absorption (communicating). Communicating hydrocephalus is usually caused by obstruction of the absorptive function of the arachnoid villi from intracranial hemorrhage, meningitis, cerebral venous thrombosis, or malignancy [102]. Noncommunicating hydrocephalus can result from a variety of processes that obstruct CSF outflow from the lateral ventricles, including aqueductal stenosis, neural tube defects, and lesions of the posterior fossa (tumors, arteriovenous malformations, Chiari malformation, Dandy-Walker syndrome). Infants with hydrocephalus usually present with an enlarged head, a large fontanelle, split sutures, deviation of eyes downward (sun-setting eyes), and long tract signs [103]. Older children tend to present more with signs of increasing ICP.

The treatment of obstructive hydrocephalus and increased ICP is surgical decompression with an extracranial shunt or drain. With the exception of supportive care, medical management of intracranial hypertension in a patient with impending herniation and hydrocephalus is rarely helpful, although it may be of use in preventing herniation until definitive neurosurgical decompression is possible. Treatment of communicating hydrocephalus also focuses on removal of CSF; however, the temporary measure of CSF removal via lumbar puncture is an option. Use of acetazolamide and furosemide for decreasing the CSF production is not substantiated with meaningful data [104].

Brain tumors in children are a well-recognized cause of increased ICP. There reasons for the increased ICP in these patients include the mass of the tumor itself, the edema surrounding the tumor, and hydrocephalus from impingement of the third and fourth ventricles from infratentorial tumors. Although treatment most often requires resection of the tumor and/or ventricular drainage of CSF, there may be some value to initial medical management. Seizure prophylaxis and use of glucocorticoids for treatment of vasogenic edema associated with brain tumors are the mainstays of medical management [105]. Acute management of increased ICP relies on supportive care, airway and blood pressure management, osmotic therapy, and hyperventilation.

Hypoxic–Ischemic Brain Injury

Severe hypoxic–ischemic brain injury occurs from lack of oxygen delivery to the brain from severe hypotension, cardiac arrest, severe hypoxia, or severe anemia. There are several mechanisms by which neuronal injury occurs [106]. Glutamate and other excitatory amino acids accumulate and are associated with calcium release. The resultant calcium and excitatory amino acids are associated with activation of neuronal proteolysis. In addition, oxygen free radical generation, inducible nitric oxide synthase activation, and granulocyte accumulation all lead to energy depletion and cell death by either necrosis or apoptosis. The cerebral edema that takes place after a hypoxic–ischemic brain injury is initially described as cytotoxic edema as a result of swelling of glial cells and neurons [107]. After reperfusion takes place there is increased BBB permeability from pinocytosis and opening of endothelial tight junctions. This leads to vasogenic edema that also plays a significant role in the development of cerebral edema.

If the cerebral edema of hypoxic–ischemic injury is severe, it will cause intracranial hypertension. Treatment of intracranial hypertension from hypoxic–ischemic injury is controversial [108,109]. There were several small studies of patients with cardiac arrest from near drowning in the 1980s that looked at ICP monitoring, ICP therapy, and outcomes [110–113]. Although the numbers were not large (the largest series included 66 patients), increased ICP in any patient whose primary insult was hypoxic–ischemic damage was associated with death or a vegetative state despite any therapy. It is generally accepted that monitoring and treating raised ICP following ischemic brain injury does not improve outcome and has thus fallen out of favor.

Infectious Causes of Intracranial Hypertension

The association between cerebral edema, intracranial hypertension, and infectious meningitis is clear to any pediatric intern who has measured an opening pressure when performing a lumbar puncture on a patient with meningitis. The mechanism of the development of cerebral edema in these patients is multifactorial and caused by cytotoxic or cellular swelling, disruption of the BBB and thus increased permeability, loss of cerebral blood flow autoregulation, and hydrocephalus caused by abnormal CSF resorption across inflamed arachnoid villi [114]. Cerebral edema, intracranial hypertension, and brain stem herniation can lead to exacerbation of ongoing brain injury and death. Although it seems reasonable that preventing or treating intracranial hypertension may be beneficial, there have been no controlled studies evaluating outcomes using monitoring or intracranial hypertension treatments. Unlike hypoxic–ischemic brain injury, intracranial hypertension is common in patients who have both good and poor outcomes, and it is unclear if attempts at attenuating intracranial hypertension result in improved perfusion and outcome. Monitoring and treatment of intracranial hypertension in pediatric patients with meningitis is not standard care. In pediatric critical care practiced in training programs throughout the United States, a recent informal poll revealed that about one third of centers routinely monitor and treat intracranial hypertension in infectious meningitis, about one third do so on occasion, and another one third never do so.

Vascular Accidents and Intracranial Hypertension

Stroke and spontaneous cerebral hemorrhage (an arteriovenous malformation or aneurysm) can lead to cerebral edema and increased ICP. Cytotoxic edema occurs 3–5 days after cerebral infarction and if large enough can lead to intracranial hypertension from both the edema itself and the hydrocephalus caused by compromised flow of CSF. Stroke is a relatively common disease process in adults and quite infrequent in children. In addition, the etiology of stroke in children is much more diverse and much less likely to be caused by an embolic phenomenon, which is seen more commonly in adults. Most information about intracranial hypertension in stroke patients comes from adult studies and series. Even though the disease process is different and therefore the therapy may need to be quite different, at this point we can only extrapolate from adult data.

The American Stroke Association's scientific statement on the management of stroke complications addresses the issue of cerebral edema and its treatment [115]. The only strong recommendation they make is the avoidance of corticosteroids following ischemic stroke. They give a moderate recommendation for use of osmotherapy and hyperventilation in patients who have neurologic deterioration and have evidence of brain stem herniation. The recommendations backed up by less rigorous data include surgical interventions (decompression, CSF drainage, infarct evacuation) and treatment of seizures. It is not clear if ICP monitoring and management of intracranial hypertension improves outcome after stroke in adults, much less in children. Despite this lack of evidence, use of ICP monitoring and therapy for certain types of stroke with intracranial hypertension remains an option.

Treatment Strategies

Intracranial hypertension is a medical emergency that if not treated properly may result in morbidity or death. Although the data are not clear as to the best treatment strategies or if any treatment strategy is helpful at all, some general principles of management can be followed. We divide treatment into the categories of emergency, etiology based, and global ICP based.

It is important to consider the onset of action in addition to the mechanism of action of each therapy. For emergency treatment, often the goal is to prevent herniation with any means possible until definitive therapy can be performed. Although osmotic agents and hyperventilation may not be as effective or beneficial in the long term for an intracranial mass, these therapeutic modalities can be instituted quickly. For a patient with severe intracranial hypertension these measures can be effective in temporarily preventing permanent injury while awaiting the definitive neurosurgical procedure. Intubation, sedation, mannitol, hypertonic saline, and hyperventilation should be instituted in the case of impending herniation.

Etiology-based treatment is often the most effective at relieving intracranial hypertension. This is treatment aimed at removing the offending agent. In the case of hydrocephalus, it would be removal of CSF by means of a ventricular drain. In the case of a tumor, it would be surgical resection of the tumor. For hemorrhage, it would involve evacuation of the blood clot causing the mass effect. In the case of seizures, it would mean abolishing the seizure and its associated increased metabolic demands. For hyperthermia, it would be cooling the patient to relieve the increased metabolic demand. These are just some of the more common examples of etiology-based treatment; treatments can include any that are aimed toward the removal of an intracranial mass that is causing the intracranial hypertension. After emergency treatment, this should be the first treatment modality addressed.

Global ICP-based treatment in the setting of intracranial hypertension can be done using a variety of methods as outlined in this chapter. Because most experience in managing intracranial hypertension is found in both the adult and pediatric traumatic brain injury populations, the proposed guidelines for intracranial hypertension management for traumatic brain injury are the most reasonable data available for other disease processes that result in intracranial hypertension. Exceptions include etiology-specific rationales for deviating from the standards for traumatic brain injury, such as the use of steroids for brain tumor edema.

Finally, it is important to make a note about cerebral perfusion and its management. The newer methods of measuring and monitoring cerebral blood flow and substrate delivery have yet to be systematically evaluated. Cerebral perfusion pressure, although a crude measurement of ischemia and brain perfusion, has the most information behind it. Study of the adult Traumatic Data Coma Bank date has found levels of CPP that correlate with outcome, and the original Brain Trauma Foundation recommendations suggested a minimum CPP of 70 mm Hg in adults [10]. These have since been modified to target CPP in adults to 60 mm Hg, with the recognition that the development of acute respiratory distress syndrome is likely related to increased CPP [116,117]. There is not the same CPP versus outcome distribution for children, although the number of pediatric study patients evaluated is much fewer than those included in adult studies. It is evident that children with CPPs of less than 40 mm Hg have worse outcomes in traumatic brain injury, and it is likely that there is a continuum of optimal CPP between 40 mm Hg for infants and 60 mm Hg for older children and adults [23].

References

1. Monro A. Observations on Structure and Functions of the Nervous System. Edinburgh: Creech and Johnson; 1783.
2. Kelli G. Appearances Observed in the Dissection of Two Individuals; Death from Cold and Congestion of the Brain. Transcripts Medical-Surgical Society of Edinburgh 1824;1:84.
3. Mokri B. The Monro-Kellie hypothesis: applications in CSF volume depletion. Neurology 2001;56(12):1746–1748.
4. Cushing H. The Third Circulation in Studies in Intracranial Physiology and Surgery. London: Oxford University Press; 1926.
5. Fenichel M. Clinical Pediatric Neurology, 2nd ed. Philadelphia: W.B. Saunders Company; 1993.
6. Lang EW, Chestnut RM. Intracranial pressure monitoring and management. Neurosury Clin N Am 1994;5(4):573–605.
7. Fog M. Cerebral circulation II. The reaction of the pial arteries to an increase in blood pressure. Arch Neurol Psychiatry 1939(41):260–268.
8. Anthony MY. Cerebral autoregulation in sick infants. Pediatr Res 2000;48(1):3–5.
9. Golding EM, Robertson CS, Bryan RM, Jr. The consequences of traumatic brain injury on cerebral blood flow and autoregulation: a review. Clin Exp Hypertens 1999;21(4):299–332.
10. Foundation TBT. Management and Prognosis of Severe Traumatic Brain Injury. Brain Trauma Foundation; 2000.
11. Plum F, Posner JB. The Diagnosis of Stupor and Coma, 3rd ed. New York: Oxford University Press; 2000.
12. Ballabh P, Braun A, Nedergaard M. The blood–brain barrier: an overview: structure, regulation, and clinical implications. Neurobiol Dis 2004;16(1):1–13.
13. Kobayashi H, Yanagita T, Yokoo H, Wada A. Molecular mechanisms and drug development in aquaporin water channel diseases: aquaporins in the brain. J Pharmacol Sci 2004;96(3):264–270.
14. Marcin JP, Pollack MM. Triage scoring systems, severity of illness measures, and mortality prediction models in pediatric trauma. Crit Care Med 2002;30(11 Suppl):S457–S467.
15. Chameides L, Hazinski MF, eds. Pediatric Advanced Life Support, 3rd ed. Dallas: American Heart Association; 1997.
16. Teasdale G, Jennett B. Assessment of coma and impaired consciousness. A practical scale. Lancet 1974;2(7872):81–84.
17. Guyenet PG. Neural structures that mediate sympathoexcitation during hypoxia. Respir Physiol 2000;121(2-3):147–162.
18. Cihangiroglu M, Ramsey RG, Dohrmann GJ. Brain injury: analysis of imaging modalities. Neurol Res 2002;24(1):7–18.
19. Marshall LF, Marshall SB, Klauber MR, Van Berkum Clark M, Eisenberg H, Jane JA, et al. The diagnosis of head injury requires a classification based on computed axial tomography. J Neurotrauma 1992;9 Suppl 1:S287–S292.
20. Steiner LA, Czosnyka M. Should we measure cerebral blood flow in head-injured patients? Br J Neurosurg 2002;16(5):429–439.
21. Kety SS, Schmidt CF. The determination of cerebral blood flow in man by the use of nitrous oxide in low concentrations. Am J Physiol 1945(143):53.
22. Johnston AJ, Gupta AK. Advanced monitoring in the neurology intensive care unit: microdialysis. Curr Opin Crit Care 2002;8(2):121–127.
23. Adelson PD, Bratton SL, Carney NA, Chesnut RM, du Coudray HE, Goldstein B, et al. Guidelines for the acute medical management of severe traumatic brain injury in infants, children, and adolescents. Chapter 19. The role of anti-seizure prophylaxis following severe pediatric traumatic brain injury. Pediatr Crit Care Med 2003;4(3 Suppl): S72–S75.
24. Kerr ME, Sereika SM, Orndoff P, Weber B, Rudy EB, Marion D, et al. Effect of neuromuscular blockers and opiates on the cerebrovascular response to endotracheal suctioning in adults with severe head injuries. Am J Crit Care 1998;7(3):205–217.
25. Cotev S, Shalit MN. Effects on diazepam on cerebral blood flow and oxygen uptake after head injury. Anesthesiology 1975;43(1):117–122.
26. Albanese J, Arnaud S, Rey M, Thomachot L, Alliez B, Martin C. Ketamine decreases intracranial pressure and electroencephalographic activity in traumatic brain injury patients during propofol sedation. Anesthesiology 1997;87(6):1328–1334.
27. Spitzfaden AC, Jimenez DF, Tobias JD. Propofol for sedation and control of intracranial pressure in children. Pediatr Neurosurg 1999;31(4):194–200.
28. Tobias JD. Increased intracranial pressure after fentanyl administration in a child with closed head trauma. Pediatr Emerg Care 1994;10(2):89–90.
29. Shapiro K, Marmarou A. Clinical applications of the pressure-volume index in treatment of pediatric head injuries. J Neurosurg 1982;56(6): 819–825.
30. Baldwin HZ, Rekate HL. Preliminary experience with controlled external lumbar drainage in diffuse pediatric head injury. Pediatr Neurosurg 1991;17(3):115–120.
31. Levy DI, Rekate HL, Cherny WB, Manwaring K, Moss SD, Baldwin HZ. Controlled lumbar drainage in pediatric head injury. J Neurosurg 1995;83(3):453–460.
32. Munch EC, Bauhuf C, Horn P, Roth HR, Schmiedek P, Vajkoczy P. Therapy of malignant intracranial hypertension by controlled lumbar cerebrospinal fluid drainage. Crit Care Med 2001;29(5):976–981.
33. Wise B, Chater N. The value of hypertonic mannitol solution in decreasing brain mass and lowering cerebrospinal-fluid pressure. J Neurosurg 1963;19:1038–1043.
34. Dias MS. Traumatic brain and spinal cord injury. Pediatr Clin North Am 2004;51(2):271–303.
35. Schrot RJ, Muizelaar JP. Mannitol in acute traumatic brain injury. Lancet 2002;359(9318):1633–1634.
36. Burke AM, Quest DO, Chien S, Cerri C. The effects of mannitol on blood viscosity. J Neurosurg 1981;55(4):550–553.
37. Muizelaar JP, Wei EP, Kontos HA, Becker DP. Mannitol causes compensatory cerebral vasoconstriction and vasodilation in response to blood viscosity changes. J Neurosurg 1983;59(5):822–828.
38. Muizelaar JP, Lutz HA, 3rd, Becker DP. Effect of mannitol on ICP and CBF and correlation with pressure autoregulation in severely head-injured patients. J Neurosurg 1984;61(4):700–706.

39. Holcroft JW, Vassar MJ, Turner JE, Derlet RW, Kramer GC. 3% NaCl and 7.5% NaCl/dextran 70 in the resuscitation of severely injured patients. Ann Surg 1987;206(3):279–288.

40. Kien ND, Reitan JA, White DA, Wu CH, Eisele JH. Cardiac contractility and blood flow distribution following resuscitation with 7.5% hypertonic saline in anesthetized dogs. Circ Shock 1991;35(2):109–116.

41. Landau EH, Gross D, Assalia A, Feigin E, Krausz MM. Hypertonic saline infusion in hemorrhagic shock treated by military antishock trousers (MAST) in awake sheep. Crit Care Med 1993;21(10):1554–1562.

42. Doyle JA, Davis DP, Hoyt DB. The use of hypertonic saline in the treatment of traumatic brain injury. J Trauma 2001;50(2):367–383.

43. Einhaus SL, Croce MA, Watridge CB, Lowery R, Fabian TC. The use of hypertonic saline for the treatment of increased intracranial pressure. J Tenn Med Assoc 1996;89(3):81–82.

44. Suarez JI, Qureshi AI, Bhardwaj A, Williams MA, Schnitzer MS, Mirski M, et al. Treatment of refractory intracranial hypertension with 23.4% saline. Crit Care Med 1998;26(6):1118–1122.

45. Worthley LI, Cooper DJ, Jones N. Treatment of resistant intracranial hypertension with hypertonic saline. Report of two cases. J Neurosurg 1988;68(3):478–481.

46. Fisher B, Thomas D, Peterson B. Hypertonic saline lowers intracranial pressure in children after head trauma. J Neurosurg Anesthesiol 1992;4:4–10.

47. Simma B, Burger R, Falk M, Sacher P, Fanconi S. A prospective, randomized, and controlled study of fluid management in children with severe head injury: lactated Ringer's solution versus hypertonic saline. Crit Care Med 1998;26(7):1265–1270.

48. Peterson B, Khanna S, Fisher B, Marshall L. Prolonged hypernatremia controls elevated intracranial pressure in head-injured pediatric patients. Crit Care Med 2000;28(4):1136–1143.

49. Khanna S, Davis D, Peterson B, Fisher B, Tung H, O'Quigley J, et al. Use of hypertonic saline in the treatment of severe refractory posttraumatic intracranial hypertension in pediatric traumatic brain injury. Crit Care Med 2000;28(4):1144–1151.

50. Bruce DA, Raphaely RC, Goldberg AI, Zimmerman RA, Bilaniuk LT, Schut L, et al. Pathophysiology, treatment and outcome following severe head injury in children. Childs Brain 1979;5(3):174–191.

51. Fortune JB, Feustel PJ, deLuna C, Graca L, Hasselbarth J, Kupinski AM. Cerebral blood flow and blood volume in response to O_2 and CO_2 changes in normal humans. J Trauma 1995;39(3):463–472.

52. Laffey JG, Kavanagh BP. Hypocapnia. N Engl J Med 2002;347(1):43–53.

53. Gleason CA, Short BL, Jones MD, Jr. Cerebral blood flow and metabolism during and after prolonged hypocapnia in newborn lambs. J Pediatr 1989;115(2):309–314.

54. Kassell NF, Hitchon PW, Gerk MK, Sokoll MD, Hill TR. Alterations in cerebral blood flow, oxygen metabolism, and electrical activity produced by high dose sodium thiopental. Neurosurgery 1980;7(6):598–603.

55. Roberts I. Barbiturates for acute traumatic brain injury. Cochrane Database Syst Rev 2000(2):CD000033.

56. Polderman KH. Application of therapeutic hypothermia in the ICU: opportunities and pitfalls of a promising treatment modality. Part 1: Indications and evidence. Intensive Care Med 2004;30(4):556–575.

57. Clifton GL, Allen S, Barrodale P, Plenger P, Berry J, Koch S, et al. A phase II study of moderate hypothermia in severe brain injury. J Neurotrauma 1993;10(3):263–273.

58. Clifton GL, Miller ER, Choi SC, Levin HS, McCauley S, Smith KR Jr, et al. Lack of effect of induction of hypothermia after acute brain injury. N Engl J Med 2001;344(8):556–563.

59. Marion DW, Penrod LE, Kelsey SF, Obrist WD, Kochanek PM, Palmer AM, et al. Treatment of traumatic brain injury with moderate hypothermia. N Engl J Med 1997;336(8):540–546.

60. Biswas AK, Bruce DA, Sklar FH, Bokovoy JL, Sommerauer JF. Treatment of acute traumatic brain injury in children with moderate hypothermia improves intracranial hypertension. Crit Care Med 2002;30(12):2742–2751.

61. Hardman JG, Limbird LE, eds. Goodman and Gilman's The Pharmacological Basis of Therapeutics, 10th ed. New York: McGraw-Hill; 2001.

62. French LA, Galicich JH. The use of steroids for control of cerebral edema. Clin Neurosurg 1964;••(10):212–223.

63. Ghajar J, Hariri RJ, Narayan RK, Iacono LA, Firlik K, Patterson RH. Survey of critical care management of comatose, head-injured patients in the United States. Crit Care Med 1995;23(3):560–567.

64. Cooper PR, Moody S, Clark WK, Kirkpatrick J, Maravilla K, Gould AL, et al. Dexamethasone and severe head injury. A prospective double-blind study. J Neurosurg 1979;51(3):307–316.

65. Dearden NM, Gibson JS, McDowall DG, Gibson RM, Cameron MM. Effect of high-dose dexamethasone on outcome from severe head injury. J Neurosurg 1986;64(1):81–88.

66. Giannotta SL, Weiss MH, Apuzzo ML, Martin E. High dose glucocorticoids in the management of severe head injury. Neurosurgery 1984;15(4):497–501.

67. Grumme T, Baethmann A, Kolodziejczyk D, Krimmer J, Fischer M, von Eisenhart Rothe B, et al. Treatment of patients with severe head injury by triamcinolone: a prospective, controlled multicenter clinical trial of 396 cases. Res Exp Med (Berl) 1995;195(4):217–229.

68. Roberts I, Yates D, Sandercock P, Farrell B, Wasserberg J, Lomas G, et al. Effect of intravenous corticosteroids on death within 14 days in 10,008 adults with clinically significant head injury (MRC CRASH trial): randomised placebo-controlled trial. Lancet 2004;364(9442):1321–1328.

69. Cordoba J, Blei AT. Brain edema and hepatic encephalopathy. Semin Liver Dis 1996;16(3):271–280.

70. Clemmesen JO, Larsen FS, Kondrup J, Hansen BA, Ott P. Cerebral herniation in patients with acute liver failure is correlated with arterial ammonia concentration. Hepatology 1999;29(3):648–653.

71. Vaquero J, Chung C, Blei AT. Brain edema in acute liver failure. A window to the pathogenesis of hepatic encephalopathy. Ann Hepatol 2003;2(1):12–22.

72. Kosenko E, Felipo V, Montoliu C, Grisolia S, Kaminsky Y. Effects of acute hyperammonemia in vivo on oxidative metabolism in nonsynaptic rat brain mitochondria. Metab Brain Dis 1996;12(1):69–82.

73. Tofteng F, Jorgensen L, Hansen BA, Ott P, Kondrup J, Larsen FS. Cerebral microdialysis in patients with fulminant hepatic failure. Hepatology 2002;36(6):1333–1340.

74. Larsen FS, Ejlersen E, Hansen BA, Knudsen GM, Tygstrup N, Secher NH. Functional loss of cerebral blood flow autoregulation in patients with fulminant hepatic failure. J Hepatol 1995;23(2):212–217.

75. Larsen FS, Adel Hansen B, Pott F, Ejlersen E, Secher NH, Paulson OB, et al. Dissociated cerebral vasoparalysis in acute liver failure. A hypothesis of gradual cerebral hyperaemia. J Hepatol 1996;25(2):145–151.

76. Blei AT, Olafsson S, Webster S, Levy R. Complications of intracranial pressure monitoring in fulminant hepatic failure. Lancet 1993;341(8838):157–158.

77. Canalese J, Gimson AE, Davis C, Mellon PJ, Davis M, Williams R. Controlled trial of dexamethasone and mannitol for the cerebral oedema of fulminant hepatic failure. Gut 1982;23(7):625–629.

78. Murphy N, Auzinger G, Bernel W, Wendon J. The effect of hypertonic sodium chloride on intracranial pressure in patients with acute liver failure. Hepatology 2004;39(2):464–470.

79. Daas M, Plevak DJ, Wijdicks EF, Rakela J, Wiesner RH, Piepgras DG, et al. Acute liver failure: results of a 5-year clinical protocol. Liver Transplant Surg 1995;1(4):210–219.

80. Strauss G, Hansen BA, Knudsen GM, Larsen FS. Hyperventilation restores cerebral blood flow autoregulation in patients with acute liver failure. J Hepatol 1998;28(2):199–203.

81. Strauss GI, Knudsen GM, Kondrup J, Moller K, Larsen FS. Cerebral metabolism of ammonia and amino acids in patients with fulminant hepatic failure. Gastroenterology 2001;121(5):1109–1119.

82. Forbes A, Alexander GJ, O'Grady JG, Keays R, Gullan R, Dawling S, et al. Thiopental infusion in the treatment of intracranial hypertension complicating fulminant hepatic failure. Hepatology 1989;10(3): 306–310.

83. Marshall LF, Shapiro HM, Rauscher A, Kaufman NM. Pentobarbital therapy for intracranial hypertension in metabolic coma. Reye's syndrome. Crit Care Med 1978;6(1):1–5.

84. Zwingmann C, Chatauret N, Rose C, Leibfritz D, Butterworth RF. Selective alterations of brain osmolytes in acute liver failure: protective effect of mild hypothermia. Brain Res 2004;999(1):118–123.

85. Larsen FS, Hansen BA, Blei AT. Intensive care management of patients with acute liver failure with emphasis on systemic hemodynamic instability and cerebral edema: a critical appraisal of pathophysiology. Can J Gastroenterol 2000;14 Suppl D:105D–111D.

86. Edge JA, Ford-Adams ME, Dunger DB. Causes of death in children with insulin dependent diabetes 1990-96. Arch Dis Child 1999;81(4): 318–323.

87. Edge JA, Hawkins MM, Winter DL, Dunger DB. The risk and outcome of cerebral oedema developing during diabetic ketoacidosis. Arch Dis Child 2001;85(1):16–22.

88. Glaser N, Barnett P, McCaslin I, Nelson D, Trainor J, Louie J, et al. Risk factors for cerebral edema in children with diabetic ketoacidosis. The Pediatric Emergency Medicine Collaborative Research Committee of the American Academy of Pediatrics. N Engl J Med 2001;344(4):264–269.

89. Hoffman WH, Steinhart CM, el Gammal T, Steele S, Cuadrado AR, Morse PK. Cranial CT in children and adolescents with diabetic ketoacidosis. AJNR Am J Neuroradiol 1988;9(4):733–739.

90. Krane EJ, Rockoff MA, Wallman JK, Wolfsdorf JI. Subclinical brain swelling in children during treatment of diabetic ketoacidosis. N Engl J Med 1985;312(18):1147–1151.

91. Smedman L, Escobar R, Hesser U, Persson B. Sub-clinical cerebral oedema does not occur regularly during treatment for diabetic ketoacidosis. Acta Paediatr 1997;86(11):1172–1176.

92. Dunger DB, Sperling MA, Acerini CL, Bohn DJ, Daneman D, Danne TP, et al. ESPE/LWPES consensus statement on diabetic ketoacidosis in children and adolescents. Arch Dis Child 2004;89(2):188–194.

93. Glaser NS, Wootton-Gorges SL, Marcin JP, Buonocore MH, Dicarlo J, Neely EK, et al. Mechanism of cerebral edema in children with diabetic ketoacidosis. J Pediatr 2004;145(2):164–171.

94. Bello FA, Sotos JF. Cerebral oedema in diabetic ketoacidosis in children. Lancet 1990;336(8706):64.

95. Hale PM, Rezvani I, Braunstein AW, Lipman TH, Martinez N, Garibaldi L. Factors predicting cerebral edema in young children with diabetic ketoacidosis and new onset type I diabetes. Acta Paediatr 1997;86(6):626–631.

96. Kamat P, Vats A, Gross M, Checchia PA. Use of hypertonic saline for the treatment of altered mental status associated with diabetic ketoacidosis. Pediatr Crit Care Med 2003;4(2):239–242.

97. Curtis JR, Bohn D, Daneman D. Use of hypertonic saline in the treatment of cerebral edema in diabetic ketoacidosis (DKA). Pediatr Diabetes 2001;2(4):191–194.

98. Marcin JP, Glaser N, Barnett P, McCaslin I, Nelson D, Trainor J, et al. Factors associated with adverse outcomes in children with diabetic ketoacidosis-related cerebral edema. J Pediatr 2002;141(6):793–797.

99. Garcia E, Abramo TJ, Okada P, Guzman DD, Reisch JS, Wiebe RA. Capnometry for noninvasive continuous monitoring of metabolic status in pediatric diabetic ketoacidosis. Crit Care Med 2003;31(10): 2539–2543.

100. Wood EG, Go-Wingkun J, Luisiri A, Aceto T Jr. Symptomatic cerebral swelling complicating diabetic ketoacidosis documented by intraventricular pressure monitoring: survival without neurologic sequela. Pediatr Emerg Care 1990;6(4):285–288.

101. Eskandar EN, Weller SJ, Frim DM. Hydrocephalus requiring urgent external ventricular drainage in a patient with diabetic ketoacidosis and cerebral edema: case report. Neurosurgery 1997;40(4):836–839.

102. Zitelli BJ, Davis HW, eds. Atlas of Pediatric Physical Diagnosis, 2nd ed. St. Louis: Mosby; 1992.

103. Behrman, ed. Nelson Textbook of Pediatrics, 11th ed. 2004.

104. Kennedy CR, Ayers S, Campbell MJ, Elbourne D, Hope P, Johnson A. Randomized, controlled trial of acetazolamide and furosemide in posthemorrhagic ventricular dilation in infancy: follow-up at 1 year. Pediatrics 2001;108(3):597–607.

105. Weissman DE. Glucocorticoid treatment for brain metastases and epidural spinal cord compression: a review. J Clin Oncol 1988;6(3): 543–551.

106. Biagas K. Hypoxic–ischemic brain injury: advancements in the understanding of mechanisms and potential avenues for therapy. Curr Opin Pediatr 1999;11(3):223–228.

107. Xiao F, Zhang S, Arnold TC, Alexander JS, Huang J, Carden DL, et al. Mild hypothermia induced before cardiac arrest reduces brain edema formation in rats. Acad Emerg Med 2002;9(2):105–114.

108. Conn AW, Edmonds JF, Barker GA. Near-drowning in cold fresh water: current treatment regimen. Can Anaesth Soc J 1978;25(4): 259–265.

109. Sachdeva RC. Near drowning. Crit Care Clin 1999;15(2):281–296.

110. Allman FD, Nelson WB, Pacentine GA, McComb G. Outcome following cardiopulmonary resuscitation in severe pediatric near-drowning. Am J Dis Child 1986;140(6):571–575.

111. Bohn DJ, Biggar WD, Smith CR, Conn AW, Barker GA. Influence of hypothermia, barbiturate therapy, and intracranial pressure monitoring on morbidity and mortality after near-drowning. Crit Care Med 1986;14(6):529–534.

112. Dean JM, McComb JG. Intracranial pressure monitoring in severe pediatric near-drowning. Neurosurgery 1981;9(6):627–630.

113. Sarnaik AP, Preston G, Lieh-Lai M, Eisenbrey AB. Intracranial pressure and cerebral perfusion pressure in near-drowning. Crit Care Med 1985;13(4):224–227.

114. Scheld WM, Dacey RG, Winn HR, Welsh JE, Jane JA, Sande MA. Cerebrospinal fluid outflow resistance in rabbits with experimental meningitis. Alterations with penicillin and methylprednisolone. J Clin Invest 1980;66(2):243–253.

115. Adams HP, Jr., Adams RJ, Brott T, del Zoppo GJ, Furlan A, Goldstein LB, et al. Guidelines for the early management of patients with ischemic stroke: a scientific statement from the Stroke Council of the American Stroke Association. Stroke 2003;34(4):1056–1083.

116. Contant CF, Valadka AB, Gopinath SP, Hannay HJ, Robertson CS. Adult respiratory distress syndrome: a complication of induced hypertension after severe head injury. J Neurosurg 2001;95(4):560–568.

117. Juul N, Morris GF, Marshall SB, Marshall LF. Intracranial hypertension and cerebral perfusion pressure: influence on neurological deterioration and outcome in severe head injury. The Executive Committee of the International Selfotel Trial. J Neurosurg 2000;92(1):1–6.

6

Nonaccidental Trauma and Shaken Baby Syndrome

Robert C. Tasker

Introduction

This chapter presents the science and clinical evidence that form the basis for rational therapeutic strategies in the intensive care treatment of infants suffering nonaccidental head injury (NAHI) or shaken baby syndrome (SBS). This chapter is not about forensic investigation of suspected inflicted injuries, nor is it focused on the medicolegal aspects of such investigation. Accounts of appropriate professional practice, with these perspectives in mind, can be found in reports from the American Academy of Pediatrics [1,2]. The Royal College of Paediatrics and Child Health [3], and in standard textbooks [4,5].

Definition

In general, in clinical reports of NAHI the condition is defined as including one or more of the following features: shaking injury, cerebral lesions as a result of direct impact, compression, and penetrating injuries [6,7]. Shaking injury, or SBS, is the most frequent form of NAHI in infancy (i.e., birth to 12 months) [8]. Population-based studies indicate that, in Scotland, the annual incidence is 24.6 per 100,000 children younger than 1 year (95% confidence interval 14.9 to 38.5) [6], and, in North Carolina, the incidence is 17 per 100,000 per person-year in the first 2 years of life (95% confidence interval 13.3 to 20.7) [9]. Many of these patients die, and, in survivors, severe neurologic sequelae (e.g., cerebral palsy, blindness, epilepsy, cognitive and behavioral disturbances) are commonplace. In the acute phase, seizures and the presence of raised intracranial pressure (ICP) appear to be the key intensive care–related factors that are of adverse prognostic significance.

Clinical Best Evidence

In recent years, there has been a move toward basing medical practice and opinions on the best available medical and scientific evidence [10]. In 2003, Mark Donohoe used these methods and rated the quality of evidence regarding SBS [11]. In the process, he identified three areas where there exist major data gaps in the medical literature.

Donohoe searched the Biomednet database for articles related to the pathogenesis, diagnosis, or management of SBS, using the search term "shaken baby syndrome" (http://www.biomednet.com/db/medline). Letters, brief correspondence, and articles in non-English journals that lacked an English abstract were excluded from the assessment. Fifty-four remaining publications were then categorized into one of four types: (1) randomized controlled trial (one report), (2) case series (26 reports), (3) single case reports (12 reports), and (4) other—reviews, opinion, and articles on social implication (15 reports). Table 6.1 summarizes the key features of these reports, which were published between 1966 and 1998. The largest experience has been with case series, where all but one was retrospective and all but five had no control population with which to compare. In total, 307 SBS cases were assessed among 23 papers. In those reports where the numbers of SBS cases were provided, there was a median of 7 cases per series [12–34]. Donohoe found that there were three major gaps in the literature regarding SBS, which were as follows:

- Lack of clear definition of cases (Donohoe proposed that there is an urgent need for standard criteria with which to identify cases for the purpose of homogeneity in trials and for identification of unique features of SBS as opposed to other abuse, medical conditions, and controls.)
- Lack of diagnostic markers of SBS
- Lack of a checklist or management tool to assess cases and to quantify index of suspicion of shaking

In the following sections, SBS is discussed with a focus on issues related to critical care and on the literature published since 1998. However, the reader should be aware that, even in these reports, there remains a *gap* with regard to method of diagnosis and, therefore, a problem of clinical inhomogeneity.

D.S. Wheeler et al. (eds.), *The Central Nervous System in Pediatric Critical Illness and Injury,*
DOI 10.1007/978-1-84800-993-6_6, © Springer-Verlag London Limited 2009

TABLE 6.1. Results of clinical evidence search, 1966–1998.

Report	Total	Notes
Controlled trial	1	Randomized assessment of electroretinograph in diagnosis
Case series	26	• 25/26 studies are retrospective studies
		• 12/26 studies did not state the selection criteria for shaken baby syndrome
		• 21/26 studies had no control group
Case reports	12	Eclectic
Other reports	15	• 10/15 papers are historical reviews
		• 3/15 papers are opinion pieces

Source: Donohoe [11].

Outcome of Shaken Baby Syndrome

Survival and Category of Outcome

Our knowledge of morbidity and mortality among infant victims of SBS is derived from relatively small populations of injured children in the United States or the United Kingdom. Barlow et al. have recently reviewed the 16 case series reporting the outcomes of NAHI that fall into this category [35]. The median number (and interquartile range) of patients in these series was 23 (and 14 to 28) cases. The mortality rate in individual reports in the literature ranged from 13% to 36%. The overall mortality rate when these studies, including the cases put forward by Barlow et al. [35] are combined is 20.6% (112 out of 544 cases). Morbidity in survivors ranged from 59% to 100%. In all, the reports provide a total of 317 survivors of NAHI with outcome documented, and 74% of these cases are neurologically abnormal, with only 26% being *normal* on follow-up examination.

An extensive and comprehensive population-based study of clinical characteristics and outcomes of hospital cases of SBS was reported by King et al. in 2003 (36). This Canadian group evaluated all the cases of SBS for the years 1988 to 1998 that were referred to the child protection teams at 11 tertiary care pediatric hospitals. These hospitals were responsible for a large part of pediatric care in Canada with over 90,000 admissions annually (i.e., 85% of tertiary care pediatric beds). The authors defined SBS as *any form of intracranial, intraocular, or cervical spine injury as a result of a substantial or suspected shaking, with or without impact, in a child aged less than 5 years.* The researchers relied on the diagnosis assigned by the physicians responsible for child protection at each hospital. Out of 364 children identified according to these criteria, 69 (19%) died; of those who survived, 162 (55%) had ongoing neurologic injury, and 192 (65%) had visual impairment. Only 65 (22%) of those who survived were considered to show no signs of health or developmental impairment at the time of discharge.

Outcome in Relation to Severity of Acute Encephalopathy

Children with NAHI are often pale and shocked upon admission to the hospital. In addition to a primary brain insult, such patients are also at risk of secondary insults resulting from physiologic derangement outside normal ranges (e.g., hypoxia, hypotension, hypertension, bradycardia, and tachycardia). In this context, there are two clinical indicators of poor outcome: comatose state and absent pupil response.

Outcome is worse in infants who are comatose on presentation—the majority die or survive with profound mental retardation, spastic quadriplegia, or severe motor dysfunction [35,37]. Outcome is also worse in those children with absent pupil response, although, by definition, this is not independent of coma. For example, in 30 consecutive SBS cases (meeting the authors' ophthalmologic criteria for review, i.e., bilateral retinal hemorrhages), McCabe and Donahue found that nonreactive pupils and midline shift of brain structures at presentation correlate highly with mortality (38). With regard to outcome of vision, it is best predicted by the need for mechanical ventilation rather than visual acuity on presentation, again reiterating that it is the global encephalopathic state that determines outcome.

Brain Imaging

Brain imaging gives some insight into the evolving mechanism of injury in the acute encephalopathic stage of NAHI. For example, cranial computed tomography (CT) scans of patients with acute subdural (interhemispheric or convexity) hemorrhage can be categorized as those with diffuse cerebral hypoattenuation or those with focal cerebral hypoattenuation [39]. Gilles and Nelson found that, on follow-up, such patterns of infarction fell into three groups: (1) total hemisphere necrosis following acute hemisphere swelling subjacent to an ipsilateral convexity subdural hematoma; (2) infarction related to acute brain swelling with CT findings of infarction either in the posterior cerebral artery distribution or in the distribution of the callosomarginal branch of the anterior cerebral artery; and (3) infarction related to hypoperfusion—arterial border zone distribution between anterior and middle and middle and posterior cerebral arteries [39]. Interestingly, the authors found that acute seizures were a common finding in these patients. The significance of this problem is discussed later, but the reader should be aware that, as with other causes of infantile encephalopathy [40], seizures may be a symptom of underlying vascular pathology.

Diffusion-weighted imaging (DWI) and apparent diffusion coefficient (ADC) maps—forms of magnetic resonance imaging data sensitive to ischemia and cytotoxic edema—reveal nonhemorrhagic infarction (i.e., similar to that seen in CT). This type of investigation, however, can identify it much earlier than CT, in fact within hours [41]. Suh et al. found DWI/ADC abnormalities in 16 of 18 (89%) NAHI patients [41]. These changes were more likely to involve posterior aspects of the cerebral hemispheres, and, on review, severity of abnormality correlated significantly with poor outcome.

Seizures and Poor Cerebral Perfusion

Imaging points to some ischemia- or hypoperfusion-induced pathology that not only leads to symptomatic seizures but also results in poor outcome. Recently, these phenomena have been studied explicitly, and there is an indication that unfavourable outcome results from the severity of early post-traumatic seizures and lower perfusion pressures of the brain. The standard definition for an early post-traumatic seizure is that it has to occur within 1 week of trauma [42]. Barlow et al. found that 32 of 44 cases (73%) of NAHI met this criterion and had early seizures, and the mortality rate in these children was 6% [43]. The authors classified seizures as being either responsive to medication without episodes of status epilepticus or unresponsive to medication (i.e., failure to respond to at least two anticonvulsant agents) with or without episodes of status epilepticus. In general, seizures occurred within 24 hr of admission, reached a peak severity and frequency by day 2, and resolved by 1 week. One third of the patients had seizures

TABLE 6.2. Range of neurologic sequelae of shaken baby syndrome.

Morbidity	Notes
Cranial nerve	• Rare • Sensorineural deafness • Brain stem lower motor cranial nerves—III, VII, XII
Speech and language	• Common, ~67% • Usually associated with other abnormalities
Epilepsy	Common, ~60%
Vision	• Common, ~40%: cortical or optic radiation injury are the major causes • Include in descending order: cortical blindness, visual field deficits, visual agnosia, and decreased visual acuity
Neuromotor	Hemiparesis, ataxia, tetraplegia

Source: Barlow et al. [35].

that were refractory to treatment. At follow up, neurodevelopmental outcome correlated significantly with the presence and severity of the seizures. The authors' conclusion was that severity of primary brain injury was reflected in the severity of early seizures. That is, the seizures were symptomatic of underlying pathology.

Raised ICP has been described in four case series of NAHI [44–47]. The most recent report is from Barlow and Minns, who retrospectively reviewed level of ICP and cerebral perfusion pressure (CPP, which is mean blood pressure minus ICP) in relation to outcome in 17 children [47]. The authors found that neurodevelopmental outcome was associated with lowest CPP and MAP, but not maximum ICP. However, on inspection of the data in the report, there does not appear to be a relationship between quality of survival and level of CPP. In fact, blood pressure appears to be the major problem.

Range of Neurologic Sequelae and Cerebral Abnormalities

A variety of neurologic sequelae have been reported in survivors of SBS [35,36]. It is important to consider each of these, because our understanding of their pathophysiologies may give insight into how best to manage acute critical care (Table 6.2). Based on the above information, a number of potential candidates causing problems for critical care can be inferred, and these are listed in Table 6.3. The pathophysiology of SBS involves cerebral hypoxia, cerebral edema, raised ICP, vaso-occlusion, subdural hematoma, and brain tissue shifts or herniation caused by general swelling or space-occupying lesion.

After critical care another problem may evolve—cerebral atrophy. There have been four case series suggesting an interference with head and brain growth following SBS [48–51]. The two largest series showed that 15 of 34 survivors of NAHI developed

TABLE 6.3. Potential causes of secondary brain injury in shaken baby syndrome and nonaccidental head injury.

Secondary cause	Effects
Cerebral edema	Brain swelling Raised intracranial pressure Tissue shifts and herniation Infarction
Intracranial hemorrhage	Tissue shifts Seizures
Tissue herniation	Infarction in vascular territory Seizures

cerebral atrophy [50], and 15 of 16 NAHI children acquired microcephaly after injury [51].

Neuropathology

In 2001, Geddes et al. reported macroscopic neuropathology in 53 cases of NAHI [52]. The authors analyzed patterns of neuropathology in children of different ages (i.e., up to 8 years). The cases came from the files of two neuropathologists, and the authors carefully described what the cases comprised: (1) 7 head injuries where there had been a confession by the perpetrator; (2) 19 cases where NAHI had been established as a result of conviction in a criminal court and in which there were also unexplained extracranial injuries to support this diagnosis; (3) 8 cases with unexplained injuries elsewhere in the body, in addition to the head injury, but no conviction; (4) 12 cases where the carer was tried and convicted of injuring the child but in which there were no extracranial injuries; and (5) 7 cases where there was a major discrepancy between the explanation of the incident given by the carer and significant injuries such as a skull fracture, or if the history was developmentally incompatible. The principal finding was that diffuse traumatic axonal injury occurred infrequently (i.e., 3 of 53 cases, 95% confidence interval 1% to 16%). In all, 45 out of 53 cases were found to have signs of impact to the head at autopsy in the form of either subscalp bruising or skull fracture. In the remaining 8 cases, all infants, neither bruising nor fracture was found at autopsy. These 8 infants were assumed victims of SBS, and in one case the carer had confessed to having been responsible. In a second report from Geddes et al. [53], in 37 infants under 9 months of age (using similar diagnostic criteria to their first study), the authors found that the predominant histologic abnormality was diffuse hypoxic brain damage. Also, there was epidural cervical hemorrhage and focal axonal damage to the brain stem and spinal roots in 11 cases, but not controls.

The authors' principal conclusion from these data was that the craniocervical junction is vulnerable in infant NAHI, the neuropathology being that of stretch injury from cervical hyperextension and flexion. (This finding has also been reported by a group from Canada [54].) Geddes et al. also concluded that the presence of diffuse hypoxic brain damage, rather than diffuse axonal injury, could be explained either by resistance to traumatic damage of unmyelinated axons in the immature brain or by the fact that shaking-type injuries are not of sufficient force to produce diffuse axonal injury [52,53]. Instead, the authors suggested that craniocervical injury could lead to apnea and global hypoxia. This problem may be pertinent in infants without evidence of cerebral contusion or cranial impact injuries. Eleven of 37 infants in the second report had either trivial or no subscalp bruising and no skull fracture or contemporaneous extracranial injury. Three of these 11 infants had craniocervical axonal injury of varying severity [53,55,56]. The remaining 8 had no evidence of such injury, implying either that the authors were unable to detect it or that their terminal hypoxic-cell encephalopathy was not caused by trauma. Taken together with the above imaging and clinical reports, these findings are in keeping with a hypoxia- or ischemia-related problem. Geddes et al. have discussed this pathophysiology in their most recent work and proposed a nontraumatic etiology in cases of SBS without impact [55]. These issues have been debated in the literature by those who disagree with the nontraumatic hypothesis [57,58], and Geddes et al. [56] and others [59] have responded to this critique.

Neurochemistry

Neuron-specific enolase—an enzyme involved in glycolysis localized in neurons and axonal processes—potentially escapes into the blood and cerebrospinal fluid (CSF) at the time of neural injury (It should be noted, however, that this enzyme is also found in erythrocytes). S100β protein, a calcium-binding protein localized to astroglial cells, may also be released from cells at the time of cerebral damage. However, this protein is also contained within non-nervous tissue, such as fat, cartilage, and skin. Recently, Kleine et al. monitored a range of serum *damage markers* of brain and non-nervous tissue injury in 401 acute care patients [60]. They also examined CSF of patients in coma or convulsive state. The data revealed that the most relevant sample to monitor brain damage was CSF and the presence of raised NSE and/or S100β in this fluid reflected injury. Furthermore, raised serum S100β with normal serum NSE indicates release from non-nervous tissue and points to other organ dysfunction, the implication being that studies where serum S100β is measured in isolation are not interpretable.

Traumatic Brain Injury

In traumatic brain injury there has been growing interest in the neurochemical markers that are concerned with broadly assessing tissue- and cell-specific injury in patients. A number of clinical monitoring studies of S100β and NSE have been undertaken in adults with head injury but, as discussed later, in the main they follow serum levels and not CSF. The results should therefore be interpreted with caution because they may reflect co-morbid, nonhead injury (not reported by most authors).

In patients with mild traumatic brain injury, de Kruijk et al. found that in blood samples taken shortly after trauma the median and range of NSE levels were similar in patients (N = 104) and controls (N = 92) [61]. However, the authors found that S100β levels were significantly higher, in patients particularly in those trauma patients who were also vomiting. Ingebrigtsen and colleagues selected a similar group of 50 patients (i.e., with a Glasgow Coma Scale [GCS] score of 13 to 15 and CT scan showing no abnormalities) and found that serum S100β protein levels were highest immediately after the trauma and then declined each hour thereafter such that the level was undetectable 6 hr postinjury [62]. Interestingly, four of the five patients with a magnetic resonance imaging (MRI)—detectable brain contusion had detectable levels of S100β.

In patients with more severe injuries (GCS score ≤8), Raabe et al. found that the level of S100β in venous blood was higher in non-survivors, and on logistic regression the S100β level was an independent predictor of outcome along with age, GCS score, ICP, and CT scan findings [63]. Importantly, these authors also reported that persistent elevation of S100β for 3 to 5 days occurred even in patients with favorable outcome and no signs of secondary insults [63,64]. Finally, in this class of patient, venous NSE appears to perform poorly as a diagnostic marker of severity [65]. Its level rises acutely in both favorable and unfavorable outcome patients; and, using a cut-off level of >100 μg/L, the likelihood ratio for positively identifying unfavorable outcome is ~2 (i.e., specificity 0.96 and sensitivity 0.09), which is of indeterminate diagnostic impact.

Nontraumatic Encephalopathy

There are reports of monitoring serum NSE and S100β in a variety of nontraumatic encephalopathic conditions. For children with sei-zures, there are studies of those with febrile convulsion [66], non-complicated tonic-clonic seizure [67], and West syndrome [68]. None of these studies shows a significant elevation in serum NSE concentration in patients with acute seizures [66–68]. Serum S100β level was equally uninformative in the two studies that have measured it [67,68], and CSF levels in these two studies were also not different from those of controls.

In contrast to the neurochemical findings following seizure, levels of S100β and NSE are altered in newborn infants with hypoxic–ischemic encephalopathy [69–71]. For example, Thorn-gren-Jerneck et al. found that infants with moderate and severe hypoxic–ischemic encephalopathy had significantly higher serum levels of S100β on postnatal days 1 and 2; a level above 12 μg/L on the first day was significantly more frequent in infants who died or developed cerebral palsy than in infants with no impairment at follow up [69]. Gazzolo et al. found that, in the first sample of urine after birth, a cut-off value of 0.41 μg/L had a high diagnostic impact for predicting the development of hypoxic–ischemic encephal-opathy (i.e., likelihood ratio ~17, sensitivity of 0.91, and specificity of 0.95) [70]. Finally, with regard to serum NSE, Celtik et al. found higher acute levels in more severe hypoxic–ischemic encephal-opathy [71]. However, by using a cut-off value of 45.4 g/L the likeli-hood ratio for positively identifying poor outcome is ~3 (i.e., specificity 0.70 and sensitivity 0.84), which is of indeterminate diagnostic impact. Taken together, these biochemical data indicate that, in infants, hypoxic–ischemic encephalopathy rather than sei-zures results in alterations in S100β. However, given the limitations of serum sampling and the discrepancy between S100β and NSE, it remains possible that the results in hypoxic–ischemic encephalop-athy reflect systemic insult where the extent of brain injury is accompanied by a similar degree of other organ injury.

Shaken Baby Syndrome and Nonaccidental Head Injury

A variety of neurochemical derangements have been observed in the CSF of infants with NAHI. These include markers of cell stress response [72], inflammation and macrophage activation [73], and apoptosis [74]. In general, the findings are more pronounced in patients with NAHI than in patients with accidental head injury. Almost all off this work has come from one group of investigators, and their findings support the idea that NAHI is not the same as accidental head injury. That is, NAHI is different because of differences in age at occurrence (NAHI and SBS are seen in infants); injury frequency, duration, and severity; or mechanism.

With regard to levels of S100β and NSE, Berger et al. studied serial values of the CSF of individuals with NAHI as well as those with noninflicted head injury [75]. Of note, these authors found that in both mechanisms of trauma there was a single peak in S100β at ~27 hr after injury, but there was a difference in the profile for NSE. After an initial or transient peak in NSE (around 11 hr after injury) in both forms of insult, NAHI had the additional feature of a sustained and delayed peak at around 63 hr after injury.

Collating these facts about neurochemical protein markers of injury, we are therefore left with a dilemma. Does the very nature of sustaining a head injury initiate a "normal," yet insignificant, transient release (albeit marked in CSF) of NSE and S100β into the circulation? Alternatively, are we failing to identify patterns of injury with varying mechanisms such as cerebral contusion in the case of S100β and unappreciated hypoxia–ischemia or diffuse injury in the case of NSE?

Treatment

The outcomes of NAHI and SBS and features of their encephalopathy, neuropathology, and neurochemistry have been reviewed in this chapter. Treatment for this population has not been studied. Physicians are therefore left with adapting principles of neurocritical care—hopefully basing specific treatments on reason. However, this lack of data presents a problem.

Nonaccidental head injury and SBS are unlike traumatic brain injuries seen in older children and adults. The evidence indicates that these are conditions with a much poorer prognosis, more severe brain swelling and vaso-occlusion, and more deranged neurochemistry. In fact, they have features more typical of hypoxic–ischemic encephalopathy. Here is the dilemma: do we treat comatose NAHI and SBS patients according to our therapies for traumatic brain injury or according to our current management of comatose postcardiac arrest or near-drowning victims? In traumatic brain injury of later childhood, we use a variety of therapies aimed at maintaining cerebral perfusion and limiting secondary brain insults. In hypoxic–ischemic brain injury we take a less intensive course with limited neurocritical care. At present there are no clear evidence-based guidelines for the management of NAHI or SBS.

Traumatic Brain Injury Guidelines

With regard to managing the consequences of traumatic brain injury in infants, there are now guidelines endorsed by the American Association for the Surgery of Trauma, the Child Neurology Society, the International Society for Pediatric Neurosurgery, the International Trauma Anesthesia and Critical Care Society, the Society of Critical Care Medicine, and the World Federation of Pediatric Intensive and Critical Care Societies [76]. These guidelines are summarized in Table 6.4; in general, intensivists follow these recommendations. (Specific management strategies for traumatic brain injury are covered elsewhere in this textbook, and the reader is referred to Chapters 5, 7.)

Other Therapies for Infantile Encephalopathy

Another aspect of critical care for NAHI and SBS is how best to manage refractory seizures. Barlow et al. found one third of their patients had such seizures [43]. For these patients, anticonvulsant treatment should be given according to a standard protocol [77–79]. Continuous infusion of midazolam features most in the recent pediatric intensive care literature on refractory status epilepticus [80,81]. The alternatives are high-dose pentobarbital [82] or anes-

TABLE 6.4. A summary of guidelines for acute medical management of traumatic brain injury.

Guideline	A. Standard: accepted principles with certainty; B. Guide: Notes moderate clinical certainty	(Infants)
Pediatric trauma center (PTC)	A. Insufficient data	
	B. Metropolitan area: transport to PTC	
Prehospital airway management	A. Insufficient data	
	B. Avoid hypoxia, correct immediately, and use supplemental	
	O_2. Endotracheal intubation is not better than bag-valve-mask ventilation	
Prehospital resuscitation of blood pressure and oxygenation	A. Insufficient data	Use infant-specific values
	B. Rapidly correct hypotension with fluid	
Indications for intracranial pressure (ICP) monitoring	A. Insufficient data	Normal computed tomography scan and open
	B. Insufficient data	fontanelles and/or sutures do not rule out raised ICP
Treatment threshold for raised ICP	A. Insufficient data	Herniation can occur at 25 mm Hg
	B. Insufficient data	
ICP monitoring	A. Insufficient data	
	B. Insufficient data	
Cerebral perfusion pressure (CPP)	A. Insufficient data	There are likely to be age-related differences in
	B. A CPP >40 mm Hg in children	optimal CPP goals
Sedation and neuromuscular blockade	A. Insufficient data	
	B. Insufficient data	
Cerebrospinal fluid drainage	A. Insufficient data	
	B. Insufficient data	
Hyperosmolar therapy	A. Insufficient data	
	B. Insufficient data	
Hyperventilation	A. Insufficient data	
	B. Insufficient data	
Barbiturate coma	A. Insufficient data	May have deleterious effects on
	B. Insufficient data	neurodevelopment
Temperature control	A. Insufficient data	
	B. Insufficient data	
Surgical treatment of ICP	A. Insufficient data	
	B. Insufficient data	
Corticosteroids	A. Insufficient data	Recent adult study indicates worse outcome
	B. Insufficient data	with steroids

Source: Lai et al. [72].

thesia with short-acting barbiturates [83]. The main problems with the barbiturates are the zero order kinetics once treatment is prolonged and the inability to assess clinical neurology [40,83] (the specific management of seizures and status epilepticus is covered elsewhere in this textbook).

One other therapy is a potential candidate for the future—induced hypothermia. To date, the weight of evidence points to no effect of induced hypothermia in improving outcome after traumatic brain injury in adults [84] (the reader should be aware that the results of a pediatric hypothermia study in traumatic brain injury are pending). In contrast to this result, there are now two studies of adults that indicate that mild therapeutic hypothermia improves neurologic outcome after cardiac arrest [85,86]. Also, there is a suggestion that selective head cooling with mild systemic hypothermia could improve survival without severe neurodevelopmental disability in infants with moderate neonatal hypoxic–ischemic encephalopathy [87]. Taken together with the previous discussion on pathophysiology (i.e., a significant hypoxic component and similarity with hypoxic–ischemic encephalopathy), infants with SBS may be the next appropriate group for a randomized controlled trial of hypothermia.

Conclusion

The pediatric critical care clinician should be aware of the possibility of NAHI in children and infants presenting with unexplained encephalopathy and subdural and retinal hemorrhages. Recent literature provides practical guidance in three key areas of management. First, to aid diagnosis, Kemp has reviewed the essential baseline assessment of an infant or child in this category (Table 6.5)

TABLE 6.5. Essential baseline medical assessment of an infant with subdural hemorrhage.

Assessment	Notes
Clinical history	• Full case history
	• Full documentation of all possible explanations for injury
	• Identification of any previous concerns about unexplained injury
	• Identification of relevant criminal record of caregivers
Examination	• Thorough general examination
	• Documentation and clinical photographs of coexisting injury
	• Head circumference, weight, and length plotted on percentiles
Eyes	Ophthalmologist to examine both eyes through dilated pupils
Radiology	• Initial cranial computed tomography scan
	• Repeated neuroimaging at 7 and 14 days
	• Neuroradiologic report of all imaging
	• Full skeletal survey; repeat at 10 and 14 days
Serology	• Full blood count repeated over first 24–48 hr
	• Coagulation screen
	• Urea and electrolytes, liver function tests, blood cultures
Follow-up investigations indicated by tests above	• Exclude glutamic aciduria in cases with frontotemporal atrophy
	• Lumbar puncture where meningitis is possible
	• Save serum for viral serology

Source: Kemp [88].

[88]. Second, in relation to medical and legal issues, Zenel and Goldstein have summarized the critical care perspective [89]. Finally, concerning limitation of or forgoing life-sustaining treatment, the American Academy of Pediatrics Committee on Child Abuse and Neglect has provided recommendations to be used for abused children [90].

Beyond these issues, there is the question of best treatment and how we can improve outcomes of critically ill infants and children with NAHI or SBS. Central to this discussion must be better diagnosis and better understanding of mechanism and pathophysiology. The conclusion of Kemp et al.—*Coma at presentation, apnea, and diffuse brain swelling or hypoxic ischaemia all predict poor outcome.... There is evidence of associated violence in the majority of infants with NAHI. At this point in time however we do not know the minimum forces necessary to cause NAHI*—highlights an issue that is the central question for future research [37]. What are the relative contributions of traumatic brain injury and hypoxic–ischemic encephalopathy, and on which of these components should we be focusing our therapy?

References

1. American Academy of Pediatrics Committee on Child Abuse and Neglect. Shaken baby syndrome: inflicted cerebral trauma. Pediatrics 1993;92:872–875.
2. Kairys SW, Alexander RC, Block RW, Everett VD, Hymel KP, Johnson CF, Kanda MB, Malinkovich P, Bell WC, Cora-Bramble D, DuPlessis HM, Handal GA, Holmberg RE, Lavin A, Tayloe DT Jr, Varrasso DA, Wood DL. American Academy of Pediatrics. Committee on Child Abuse and Neglect and Committee on Community Health Services. Investigation and review of unexpected infant and child deaths. Pediatrics 1999;104:1158–1160.
3. Royal College of Paediatrics and Child Health Working Group on Sudden Unexpected Death in Infancy. London: RCPCH; 2004.
4. Hobbs CJ, Hanks HGI, Wynne JM. Child Abuse and Neglect: A Clinician's Handbook, 2nd ed. New York: Churchill Livingstone; 2000.
5. Byard RW. Sudden Death in Infancy, Childhood, and Adolescence, 2nd ed. Cambridge: Cambridge University Press; 2004.
6. Barlow KM, Minns RA. Annual incidence of shaken impact syndrome in young children. Lancet 2000;356:1571–1572.
7. Bonnier C, Nassogne MC, Saint-Martin C, Mesples B, Kadhim H, Sebire G. Neuroimaging of intraparenchymal lesions predicts outcome in shaken baby syndrome. Pediatrics 2003;112:808–814.
8. Duhaime AC, Christian CW, Rorke LB, Zimmerman RA. Nonaccidental head injury in infants–the "shaken-baby syndrome." N Engl J Med 1998;338:1822–1829.
9. Keenan HT, Runyan DK, Marshall SW, Nocera MA, Merten DF, Sinal SH. A population-based study of inflicted traumatic brain injury in young children. JAMA 2003;290:621–626.
10. Sackett DL, Straus SE, Richardson WS, Rosenberg W, Haynes RB. Evidence-Based Medicine: How to Practice and Teach EBM, 2nd ed. New York: Churchill Livingstone; 2000.
11. Donohoe M. Evidence-based medicine and shaken baby syndrome: part I: literature review, 1966–1998. Am J Forensic Med Pathol 2003; 24:239–242.
12. Ludwig S, Warman M. Shaken baby syndrome: a review of 20 cases. Ann Emerg Med 1984;13:104–107.
13. Bass M, Kravath RE, Glass L. Death-scene investigation in sudden infant death. N Engl J Med 1986;315:100–105.
14. Apolo JO. Bloody cerebrospinal fluid: traumatic tap or child abuse? Pediatr Emerg Care 1987;3:93–95.
15. Duhaime AC, Gennarelli TA, Thibault LE, Bruce DA, Margulies SS, Wiser R. The shaken baby syndrome: a clinical, pathological, and biomechanical study. J Neurosurg 1987;66:409–415.

16. Roussey M, Dabadie A, Betremieux P, Lefrancois MC, Journel H, Gandon Y. [Not-always-apparent abuse: the shaken baby syndrome.] Arch Fr Pediatr 1987;44:441–444.

17. Gaynon MW, Koh K, Marmor MF, Frankel LR. Retinal folds in the shaken baby syndrome. Am J Ophthalmol 1988;106:423–425.

18. Teyssier G, Rayet I, Miguet D, Damon G, Freycon F. [Cerebro-meningeal hemorrhage in infants: shaken children? Abuse or accidents? 3 cases.] Pediatrie 1988;43:535–538.

19. Brenner SL, Fischer H, Mann-Gray S. Race and the shaken baby syndrome: experience at one hospital. J Natl Med Assoc 1989;81:183–184.

20. Hadley MN, Sonntag VK, Rekate HL, Murphy A. The infant whiplash-shake injury syndrome: a clinical and pathological study. Neurosurgery 1989;24:536–540.

21. Wilkinson WS, Han DP, Rappley MD, Owings CL. Retinal hemorrhage predicts neurologic injury in the shaken baby syndrome. Arch Ophthalmol 1989;107:1472–1474.

22. Alexander R, Sato Y, Smith W, Bennett T. Incidence of impact trauma with cranial injuries ascribed to shaking. Am J Dis Child 1990;144: 724–726.

23. Han DP, Wilkinson WS. Late ophthalmic manifestations of the shaken baby syndrome. J Pediatr Ophthalmol Strabismus 1990;27:299–303.

24. Closset M, Leclerc F, Hue V, Martinot A, Vallee L, Pruvo JP. [Is pericerebral hemorrhage a cause of severe malaise in infants?] Pediatrie 1992;47:459–465.

25. Munger CE, Peiffer RL, Bouldin TW, Kylstra JA, Thompson RL. Ocular and associated neuropathologic observations in suspected whiplash shaken infant syndrome. A retrospective study of 12 cases. Am J Forensic Med Pathol 1993;14:193–200.

26. Budenz DL, Farber MG, Mirchandani HG, Park H, Rorke LB. Ocular and optic nerve hemorrhages in abused infants with intracranial injuries. Ophthalmology 1994;10:559–565.

27. Starling SP, Holden JR, Jenny C. Abusive head trauma: the relationship of perpetrators to their victims. Pediatrics 1995;95:259–262.

28. Betz P, Puschel K, Miltner E, Lignitz E, Eisenmenger W. Morphometrical analysis of retinal hemorrhages in the shaken baby syndrome. Forensic Sci Int 1996;78:71–80.

29. Haseler LJ, Arcinue E, Danielsen ER, Bluml S, Ross BD. Evidence from proton magnetic resonance spectroscopy for a metabolic cascade of neuronal damage in shaken baby syndrome. Pediatrics 1997;99:4–14.

30. Kapoor S, Schiffman J, Tang R, Kiang E, Li H, Woodward J. The significance of white-centered retinal hemorrhages in the shaken baby syndrome. Pediatr Emerg Care 1997;13:183–185.

31. Odom A, Christ E, Kerr N, Byrd K, Cochran J, Barr F, Bugnitz M, Ring JC, Storgion S, Walling R, Stidham G, Quasney MW. Prevalence of retinal hemorrhages in pediatric patients after in-hospital cardiopulmonary resuscitation: a prospective study. Pediatrics 1997;99:E3.

32. Jayawant S, Rawlinson A, Gibbon F, Price J, Schulte J, Sharples P, Sibert JR, Kemp AM. Subdural haemorrhages in infants: population based study. BMJ 1998;317:1558–1561.

33. Loh JK, Chang DS, Kuo TH, Howng SL. Shaken baby syndrome. Kaohsiung J Med Sci 1998;14:112–116.

34. Shannon P, Smith CR, Deck J, Ang LC, Ho M, Becker L. Axonal injury and the neuropathology of shaken baby syndrome. Acta Neuropathol (Berl) 1998;95:625–631.

35. Barlow K, Thompson E, Johnson D, Minns RA. The neurological outcome of non-accidental head injury. Pediatr Rehabil 2004;7: 195–203.

36. King WJ, MacKay M, Sirnick A; Canadian Shaken Baby Study Group. Shaken baby syndrome in Canada: clinical characteristics and outcomes of hospital cases. CMAJ 2003;168:155–159.

37. Kemp AM, Stoodley N, Cobley C, Coles L, Kemp KW. Apnoea and brain swelling in non-accidental head injury. Arch Dis Child 2003;88: 472–476.

38. McCabe CF, Donahue SP. Prognostic indicators for vision and mortality in shaken baby syndrome. Arch Ophthalmol 2000;118:373–377.

39. Gilles EE, Nelson MD Jr. Cerebral complications of nonaccidental head injury in childhood. Pediatr Neurol 1998;19:119–128.

40. Tasker RC, Boyd SG, Harden A, Kendall B, Harding B, Matthew DJ. The clinical significance of seizures in critically ill young infants. Neuropediatrics 1991;22:129–138.

41. Suh DY, Davis PC, Hopkins KL, Fajman NN, Mapstone TB. Nonaccidental pediatric head injury: diffusion-weighted imaging findings. Neurosurgery 2001;49:309–318.

42. Jennett B, Teasdale G. Trauma as a cause of epilepsy in childhood. Dev Med Child Neurol 1973;15:56–72.

43. Barlow KM, Spowart JJ, Minns RA. Early posttraumatic seizures in non-accidental head injury: relation to outcome. Dev Med Child Neurol 2000;42:591–594.

44. Frank Y, Zimmerman R, Leeds NMD. Neurological manifestations in abused children who have been shaken. Dev Med Child Neurol 1985;27:312–316.

45. Bonnier C, Nassogne MC, Evrard P. Outcome and prognosis of whiplash shaken infant syndrome: late consequences after a symptom-free period. Dev Med Child Neurol 1995;37:943–956.

46. Cho DY, Wang YC. Decompressive craniectomy for acute shaken/impact baby syndrome. Pediatric Neurosurg 1996;24:292–298.

47. Barlow KM, Minns RA. The relation between intracranial pressure and outcome in non-accidental head injury. Dev Med Child Neurol 1999;41:220–225.

48. Oliver JE. Microcephaly following baby battering and shaking. BMJ 1975;2:262–264.

49. Bonnier C, Nassogne MC, Evrard P. Outcome and prognosis of whiplash shaken infant syndrome; late consequences after a symptom-free interval. Dev Med Child Neurol 1995;37:943–956.

50. Rao P, Carty H, Pierce A. The acute reversal sign: comparison of medical and non-accidental injury patients. Clin Radiol 1999;54: 495–501.

51. Lo TY, McPhillips M, Minns RA, Gibson RJ. Cerebral atrophy following shaken impact syndrome and other non-accidental head injury (NAHI). Pediatr Rehabil 2003;6:47–55.

52. Geddes JF, Hackshaw AK, Vowles GH, Nickols CD, Whitwell HL. Neuropathology of inflicted head injury in children. I. Patterns of brain damage. Brain 2001;124:1290–1298.

53. Geddes JF, Vowles GH, Hackshaw AK, Nickols CD, Scott IS, Whitwell HL. Neuropathology of inflicted head injury in children. II. Microscopic brain injury in infants. Brain 2001;124:1299–1306.

54. Shannon P, Smith CR, Deck J, Ang LC, Ho M, Becker L. Axonal injury and the neuropathology of shaken baby syndrome. Acta Neuropathol 1998;95:625–631.

55. Geddes JF, Tasker RC, Hackshaw AK, Nickols CD, Adams GGW, Whitwell HL. Dural haemorrhage in non-traumatic infant deaths: does it explain the bleeding in "shaken baby syndrome"? Neuropath Appl Neurobiol 2003;29:14–22.

56. Geddes JF, Tasker RC, Adams GGW, Whitwell HL. Violence is not necessary to produce subdural and retinal haemorrhage: a reply to Punt et al. Pediatr Rehabil 2004;7:261–265.

57. Punt J, Bonshek RE, Jaspan T, McConachie NS, Punt N, Ratcliffe JM. The "unified hypothesis" of Geddes et al. is not supported by the data. Pediatric Rehabilitation 2004;7:173–184.

58. Block RW. Fillers. Pediatrics 2004;113:432–433.

59. Miller M, Leestma J, Barnes P, Carlstrom T, Gardner H, Plunkett J, Stephenson J, Thibault K, Uscinski R, Niedermier J, Galaznik J. A sojourn in the abyss: hypothesis, theory, and established truth in infant head injury. Pediatrics 2004;114:326.

60. Kleine TO, Benes L, Zofel P. Studies of the brain specificity of S100B and neuron-specific enolase (NSE) in blood of acute care patients. Brain Res Bull 2003;15:265–279.

61. de Kruijk JR, Leffers P, Menheere PP, et al. S-100B and neuron-specific enolase in serum of mild traumatic brain injury patients. A comparison with healthy controls. Acta Neurol Scand 2001;103:175–179.

62. Ingebrigtsen T, Waterloo K, Jacobsen EA, et al. Traumatic brain damage in minor head injury: relation of serum S-100 protein measurements to magnetic resonance imaging and neurobehavioural outcome. Neurosurgery 1999;45:468–475.

63. Raabe A, Grolms C, Sorge O, et al. Serum S-100B protein in severe head injury. Neurosurgery 1999;45:477–483.

64. Raabe A, Menon DK, Gupta S, et al. Jugular venous and arterial concentrations of serum S-100B protein in patients with severe head injury: a pilot study. J Neurol Neurosurg Psychiatry 1998;65:930–932.

65. Raabe A, Grolms C, Seifert V: Serum markers of brain damage and outcome prediction in patients after severe head injury. Br J Neurosurg 1999;13:56–59.

66. Borusiak P, Herbold S. Serum neuron-specific enolase in children with febrile seizures: time profile and prognostic implications. Brain Dev 2003;25:272–274.

67. Palmio J, Peltola J, Vuorinen P, Laine S, Suhonen J, Keranen T. Normal CSF neuron-specific enolase and S-100 protein levels in patients with recent non-complicated tonic-clonic seizures. J Neurol Sci 2001;183: 27–31.

68. Suzuki Y, Toribe Y, Goto M, Kato T, Futagi Y. Serum and CSF neuron-specific enolase in patients with West syndrome. Neurology 1999;53: 1761–1764.

69. Thorngren-Jerneck K, Alling C, Herbst A, Amer-Wahlin I, Marsal K. S100 protein in serum as a prognostic marker for cerebral injury in term newborn infants with hypoxic ischemic encephalopathy. Pediatr Res 2004;55:406–412.

70. Gazzolo D, Marinoni E, Di Iorio R, Bruschettini M, Kornacka M, Lituania M, Majewska U, Serra G, Michetti F. Urinary S100B protein measurements: tool for the early identification of hypoxic–ischemic encephalopathy in asphyxiated full-term infants. Crit Care Med 2004; 32:131–136.

71. Celtik C, Acunas B, Oner N, Pala O. Neuron-specific enolase as a marker of the severity and outcome of hypoxic ischemic encephalopathy. Brain Dev 2004;26:398–402.

72. Lai Y, Kochanek PM, Adelson PD, Janesko K, Ruppel RA, Clark RS. Induction of the stress response after inflicted and non-inflicted traumatic brain injury in infants and children. J Neurotrauma 2004;21: 229–237.

73. Berger RP, Heyes MP, Wisniewski SR, Adelson PD, Thomas N, Kochanek PM. Assessment of the macrophage marker quinolinic acid in cerebrospinal fluid after pediatric traumatic brain injury: insight into the timing and severity of injury in child abuse. J Neurotrauma 2004;21: 1123–1130.

74. Satchell MA, Lai Y, Kochanek PM, Wisniewski SR, Fink EL, Siedberg NA, Berger RP, Dekosky ST, Adelson PD, Clark RS. Cytochrome c, a biomarker of apoptosis, is increased in cerebrospinal fluid from infants with inflicted brain injury from child abuse. J Cereb Blood Flow Metab 2005;25:919–927 (advance online publication, 2 March;doi:10.1038/sj. jcbfm.9600088).

75. Berger RP, Pierce MC, Wisniewski SR, et al.: Neuron-specific enolase and S100B in cerebrospinal fluid after severe traumatic brain injury in infants and children. Pediatrics 2002;109:E31.

76. Carney NA, Chesnut R, Kochanek PM; American Association for Surgery of Trauma; Child Neurology Society; International Society for Pediatric Neurosurgery; International Trauma Anesthesia and Critical Care Society; Society of Critical Care Medicine; World Federation of Pediatric Intensive and Critical Care Societies. Guidelines for the acute medical management of severe traumatic brain injury in infants, children, and adolescents. Pediatr Crit Care Med 2003;4: S1–S75.

77. Tasker RC. Emergency treatment of acute seizures and status epilepticus. Arch Dis Child 1998;79:78–83.

78. Tasker RC. Neurological critical care. Curr Opin Pediatr 2000;12:222–226.

79. Appleton R, Choonara I, Martland T, Phillips B, Scott R, Whitehouse W. The treatment of convulsive status epilepticus in children. The Status Epilepticus Working Party, Members of the Status Epilepticus Working Party. Arch Dis Child 2000;83:415–419.

80. Koul R, Chacko A, Javed H, Al Riyami K. Eight-year study of childhood status epilepticus: midazolam infusion in management and outcome. J Child Neurol 2002;17:908–910.

81. Ozdemir D, Gulez P, Uran N, Yendur G, Kavakli T, Aydin A. Efficacy of continuous midazolam infusion and mortality in childhood refractory generalized convulsive status epilepticus. Seizure 2005;14:129–132.

82. Crawford TO, Mitchell WG, Fishman LS, Snodgrass SR. Very-high-dose phenobarbital for refractory status epilepticus in children. Neurology 1988;38:1035–1040.

83. Tasker RC, Boyd SG, Harden A, Matthew DJ. EEG monitoring of prolonged thiopentone administration for intractable seizures and status epilepticus in infants and young children. Neuropediatrics. 1989;20: 147–153.

84. Clifton GL, Miller ER, Choi SC, Levin HS, McCauley S, Smith KR Jr, Muizelaar JP, Wagner FC Jr, Marion DW, Luerssen TG, Chesnut RM, Schwartz M. Lack of effect of induction of hypothermia after acute brain injury. N Engl J Med 2001;344:556–563.

85. Hypothermia After Cardiac Arrest Study Group. Mild therapeutic hypothermia to improve the neurologic outcome after cardiac arrest. N Engl J Med 2002;346:549–556.

86. Bernard SA, Gray TW, Buist MD, Jones BM, Silvester W, Gutteridge G, Smith K. Treatment of comatose survivors of out-of-hospital cardiac arrest with induced hypothermia. N Engl J Med 2002;346:557–563.

87. Gluckman PD, Wyatt JS, Azzopardi D, Ballard R, Edwards AD, Ferriero DM, Polin RA, Robertson CM, Thoresen M, Whitelaw A, Gunn AJ. Selective head cooling with mild systemic hypothermia after neonatal encephalopathy: multicentre randomised trial. Lancet 2005;365: 663–670.

88. Kemp AM. Investigating subdural haemorrhage in infants. Arch Dis Child 2002;86:98–102.

89. Zenel J, Goldstein B. Child abuse in the pediatric intensive care unit. Crit Care Med 2002;30:S515–S523.

90. American Academy of Pediatrics Committee on Child Abuse and Neglect. Forgoing life-sustaining medical treatment in abused children. Pediatrics 2000;106:1151–1153.

7
Evaluation of Coma

David J.J. Michelson and Stephen Ashwal

Normal and Impaired Consciousness

In the medical context, normal consciousness is determined by the presence of arousal and of awareness, easily recognizable in healthy individuals who are fully awake and responsive, with whom physicians can easily interact and identify. Patients with severe motor or sensory impairments may be fully conscious, but recognizing this may be difficult. Identifying states of impaired consciousness, suspected when alertness or responsiveness is incomplete or inconsistent, is of great importance in making medical and ethical decisions. The physiology of arousal depends on stimulation of the ascending reticular activating system (ARAS), which transmits sensory information from the spinal cord and brain stem to the hypothalamus, thalamus, and cerebral cortex. Awareness is thought to have a less linear pathway, arising from a network of connections between the cerebral cortex and the major subcortical nuclei [1]. Impaired consciousness can be the result of diminished arousal or awareness, although awareness is not possible without at least partial arousal. Coma is a state of deep and sustained (over 1 hr) unconsciousness. A patient in a coma appears to be asleep but cannot be aroused, unlike a person who is in fact asleep [2].

Patients can be found to have levels of arousal and awareness anywhere along a continuum from heightened to absent. This has led to the introduction (and often imprecise use) of various descriptive terms. Patients with diminished alertness can be lethargic (sleepy when unstimulated but easily awakened), obtunded (abnormally drowsy even when stimulated), or stuporous (responsive only with vigorous and frequent stimulation). A state of heightened arousal, which can be manifested by hypervigilance and decreased need for sleep, can be seen in patients with delirium.

Coma may be transient or may persist for days, months, or years. There are, however, other states of severely impaired consciousness, or mimics thereof, from which coma must be differentiated. These include brain death, the vegetative state, the minimally conscious state (MCS), the locked-in state, and akinetic mutism (Table 7.1). Patients may transition between various states as consciousness improves or worsens.

Patients in a vegetative state have sufficient hypothalamic and brain stem (vegetative) function to allow for normal sleep–wake cycles, with spontaneous eye opening during periods of arousal and prolonged survival with supportive care [3]. Such patients often have simple vocalizations (sounds but not words), facial expressions, and movements that can easily be misinterpreted by hopeful observers as reflecting awareness. In this unconscious state, however, such movements are random or reflexive, and prolonged observations by trained clinicians find that such patients do not have awareness of their internal or external environment. A vegetative state is considered permanent, with little chance of improvement, if it lasts longer than 12 months after traumatic injury or longer than 3 months after nontraumatic injury [4].

In contrast, patients in a minimally conscious state can at least occasionally demonstrate purposeful movements or responses. These can include following simple commands, making gestural or verbal responses to questions, making intelligible verbalizations, smiling or crying in response to evocative sounds or images, reaching accurately toward the location of an object, or fixating on and pursuing visual stimuli [5]. Accurate differentiation of minimally conscious patients from vegetative patients often requires repeated assessments by a multidisciplinary team with experience in the management of complex disabilities [6]. In the future, functional magnetic resonance imaging studies may be helpful in differentiating these conditions [7].

Patients in a locked-in state have normal arousal and awareness but little to no ability to respond to stimuli because of profound paralysis. This condition is rare, especially in children, but can occur with anterior brain stem injuries sparing the ARAS, and it has previously been described in patients with head trauma [8], pontine glioma [9], and basilar artery occlusion [10]. Paralysis sufficient to cause a locked-in state can also result from peripheral nervous system diseases such as Guillain-Barré syndrome [11], spinal muscular atrophy [12], botulism, and organophosphate toxicity [13].

Akinetic mutism is another state with preserved arousal and awareness but in which responses are impaired by what is best described as profound apathy. Patients appear awake and are attentive to visual stimuli but have slow and inconsistent movements and little to no speech. This state has been seen in patients with

D.S. Wheeler et al. (eds.), *The Central Nervous System in Pediatric Critical Illness and Injury*,
DOI 10.1007/978-1-84800-993-6_7, © Springer-Verlag London Limited 2009

TABLE 7.1. Disorders of consciousness and related conditions.

State	Awareness	Alertness	Purposeful movements	Spontaneous breathing
Brain death	Absent	Absent	Absent	Absent
Coma	Absent	Absent	Absent	Variable
Vegetative	Absent	Present	Absent	Present
Minimally conscious	Present	Present	Limited	Present
Akinetic mutism	Present	Present	Limited	Present
Locked-in	Present	Present	Limited	Variable

bilateral injuries to the more distal components of the ARAS, including the paramedian midbrain, basal diencephalon, and inferior frontal lobes. Injuries to these areas, with resulting akinetic mutism, have been seen in children as the result of head trauma [14], hydrocephalus [15], central nervous system infections [16], tumors [17], and tumor resection surgery [18]. Brain death is defined as complete loss of consciousness and of all brain stem reflexes that is caused by an irreversible brain injury. Variations exist among countries as to the extent of damage that must be present and the extent of confirmatory testing that is necessary [19].

Causes of Coma

Coma, with complete loss of arousal, is a nonspecific consequence of ARAS dysfunction caused by a localized process within the brain stem, a mutifocal process that affects ARAS targets within both cerebral hemispheres, or a global process affecting all areas of the central nervous system. Coma resulting from head trauma, for example, may be due to hemorrhage within the brain stem, diffuse axonal injury and edema within both cerebral hemispheres, global hypoxia, hypotension, and iatrogenic sedation [2]. The most common etiologies of coma are listed in Table 7.2. Annually, traumatic and nontraumatic causes of coma have roughly equal incidences of about 30 per 100,000 children. Nontraumatic causes are seen more frequently in infancy and early childhood, when congenital heart malformations and inborn errors of metabolism are most likely to become symptomatic. In a prospective, population-based study of nontraumatic coma in children, infection (38% of cases) was the most common etiology, followed by exogenous toxins (accidental and deliberate intoxication), seizures, congenital heart or brain malformations, hypoxic–ischemic injury, and endogenous toxins (diabetes, inborn errors of metabolism) [20].

History and Physical Examination

The evaluation of a comatose patient must be both rapid and complete, as early identification of the underlying cause of coma is crucial for patient management. Coma may be the consequence of the expected progression or complication of a prior illness or injury [21]. Coma of abrupt, witnessed, and unexplained onset is suggestive of an intracranial hemorrhage, seizure, or cardiac arrhythmia. Unwitnessed but abrupt onset of coma in a previously healthy child may be due to trauma or intoxication. An etiology for coma may remain obscure until, or even after, a thorough assessment of the patient. Nonaccidental head trauma is rarely witnessed or confessed to but may be suspected on the basis of a vague, changing, or inconsistent history or unexplained signs of acute or prior trauma [22].

The evaluation of a comatose patient, as with any seriously ill patient, begins with assessment of airway patency, adequacy of oxygenation and ventilation, and adequacy of circulation. Vital signs must be measured and continuous monitoring should be instituted as soon as is possible. Many alterations of vital signs can suggest the etiology of coma. Hyperthermia is suggestive of infection, but is also seen with acute disseminated encephalomyelitis (ADEM), heat stroke, neuroleptic malignant syndrome, status epilepticus, and anticholinergic poisoning. Even when an extracranial infection is apparent, consideration should still be given to possible intracranial involvement, septic shock, seizures, Reye's syndrome, or exacerbation of an inborn error of metabolism. Hypothermia can also occur with infection, especially in infancy, but is more often caused by drug intoxication or environmental exposure and rarely by hypothyroidism. Tachycardia can occur with fever, pain, hypovolemia, cardiomyopathy, and tachyarrhythmia. Bradycardia occurs with hypoxic–ischemic myocardial injury and as part of the Cushing triad of increased intracranial pressure (ICP) along with hypertension and irregular respirations. Tachypnea can be seen with pain, hypoxia, metabolic acidosis, and pontine injury. Slow, irregular, or periodic respirations occur with metabolic alkalosis,

TABLE 7.2. Causes of coma.

A. Metabolic
  a. Electrolyte, acid–base, glucose, water, or thermal disturbances
  b. Nutritional—thiamine, pyridoxine, or niacin deficiency
  c. Toxins—accidental or intentional ingestion, overdose, or inhalation
  d. Medications—overdose or adverse reaction
  e. Inborn errors of metabolism
    i. Organic acidurias and amino acidemias
    ii. Urea cycle defects
    iii. Carbohydrate disorders
    iv. Mitochondrial and carnitine disorders
    v. Fatty acid oxidation defects
    vi. Leukodystrophies
B. Organ dysfunction
  a. Endocrine—pituitary, thyroid, pancreas, adrenal
  b. Renal failure—uremia
  c. Hepatic failure—hyperammonemia, Reye's syndrome
  d. Cardiorespiratory failure—shock, hypoxia, CO_2 narcosis
C. Infectious
  a. Systemic
  b. Cerebral—meningitis, encephalitis, cerebritis, empyema, or abscess
D. Inflammatory
  a. Vasculitis
  b. Acute disseminated encephalomyelitis
E. Paroxysmal
  a. Seizure—convulsive, nonconvulsive, or postictal
  b. Migraine—"basilar"
F. Traumatic
  a. Intracranial hemorrhage or contusion
  b. Diffuse axonal injury
G. Neoplastic
  a. Infiltration or edema—herniation, hydrocephalus, seizures
  b. Chemotherapy or radiation therapy toxicity
H. Vascular
  a. Ischemia—thrombosis, embolism, strangulation, or arterial dissection
  b. Hemorrhage—arteriovenous malformation, aneurysm, coagulopathy, atrophy, or trauma
  c. Venous sinus thrombosis
I. Structural—communicating or noncommunicating hydrocephalus
J. Psychiatric—conversion, malingering, or Munchausen by proxy

diabetic ketoacidosis, sedative intoxication, and brain stem injuries. Hypotension suggests hypovolemic, septic, or cardiogenic shock, intoxication, and adrenal insufficiency. Hypertension may be caused by pain, intoxication, renal failure, and increased ICP.

A complete skin examination can be particularly helpful and requires carefully inspecting the scalp, removing all of the patient's clothing, and turning the patient to visualize the back. Abnormal skin color accompanies bruising (blue, purple, red, or yellow), hypoxia (blue), jaundice (yellow), anemia (white), and carbon-monoxide poisoning (cherry red). Bruising and swelling are suggestive of trauma, and the examination may reveal evidence of a basilar skull fracture such as periorbital bruising (raccoon eyes), mastoid bruising (battle sign), or cerebrospinal fluid (CSF) rhinorrhea or otorrhea. Bruises or burns of varying ages, unusual shapes, or unusual distributions should raise concerns regarding nonaccidental trauma. Rashes are often nonspecific but may suggest infection with herpes, measles, varicella, meningococci, or ricketsiae. Abnormally pigmented macules accompany tuberous sclerosis and neurofibromatosis, and generalized hyperpigmentation suggests primary adrenal insufficiency.

Neurologic Examination

The neurologic examination establishes the diagnosis of coma but can also provide invaluable clues as to its etiology. A fundoscopic examination showing papilledema can lead to early institution of measures to lower ICP. Findings consistent with meningeal irritation, such as passive resistance to neck flexion, involuntary knee flexion with forced hip flexion (Kernig's sign), or involuntary hip and knee flexion with forced neck flexion (Brudzinski's sign), can be seen with infectious meningitis, chemical meningitis (as with subarachnoid hemorrhage), and parameningeal inflammation.

As long as deep sedation and paralysis have not been induced iatrogenically, the cranial nerve examination can yield important information about brain stem function. The afferent arm of the pupillary reflex depends on intact transmission of light through the eye, activation of the retina, and transmission of impulses along a branch of the optic nerves to nuclei in the rostral midbrain. Signals from each eye are distributed to bilateral parasympathetic Edinger-Westphal nuclei, which affect pupillary constriction, and to bilateral sympathetic nuclei in the hypothalamus, which affect pupillary dilation. Lesions of one eye or optic nerve (CN II) result in a pupil that has little to no direct response to ipsilateral light but has a normal consensual response to contralateral light. Lesions of a parasympathetic nucleus or of its fibers (running along the surface of the ipsilateral third cranial nerve) results in ipsilateral pupillary dilation (mydriasis) and loss of both direct and consensual responses to light. Sympathetic efferents to the pupil originate in the hypothalamus, descend uncrossed through the brain stem and synapse with nuclei of the intermediolateral columns of the lower cervical and upper thoracic spinal cord. Second order axons then exit the spinal cord along with the ventral rami and synapse with nuclei of the paraspinal sympathetic chain. Third order axons then run along the surface of the internal carotid artery and the ophthalmic division of the trigeminal nerve to reach the ipsilateral radial pupillodilator muscles of the eye, the Muller's muscles of the upper and lower eyelids, and the sweat glands of the face. Compressive or destructive lesions anywhere along this pathway can result in an ipsilateral Horner syndrome, consisting of pupillary constriction (miosis), partial ptosis, and anhidrosis. Unequal pupil size (anisocoria) may be caused by direct injury to an iris, miosis of one

eye, or mydriasis of the other eye. Bilaterally miotic but reactive pupils can be seen with metabolic disorders, intoxications, and bilateral Horner syndrome. Fixed and mydriatic or midposition pupils can be seen with complete bilateral afferent defects but are most often seen with severe brain stem injuries that disrupt both the sympathetic and parasympathetic pupillary efferents.

The extraocular muscles controlling eye movements are innervated by the oculomotor (CN III), trochlear (CN IV), and abducens (CN VI) nuclei. Conjugate horizontal eye movement toward one side begins with activation of the ipsilateral parapontine reticular formation, which sends coordinated impulses to the ipsilateral abducens nucleus in the pons and contralateral oculomotor nucleus in the midbrain. Rapid horizontal eye movements to one side are directed by the contralateral prefrontal cortex. Smooth pursuit movements are influenced by coordination of visual, proprioceptive, and vestibular inputs by the cerebellum. The involuntary function of these pathways to maintain visual fixation during head movements can be tested with the oculocephalic (doll's eye) reflex. The oculocephalic reflex is abnormal when one or both eyes do not move in the opposite direction of rapid lateral or vertical head rotation. Such rapid neck movements are contraindicated in patients with diagnosed or suspected cervical spine injuries, but the oculovestibular (caloric) reflex tests the same pathways. Irrigation of the external ear canals with water can induce convection currents within the semicircular canals. Unilateral warm water irrigation (with 30° of head elevation) causes slow horizontal deviation of the eyes away from the irrigated ear, whereas cold water causes deviation toward the irrigated ear. Conscious patients will have saccadic eye movements that attempt to maintain visual fixation. It is from the direction of these saccades that the mnemonic COWS (Cold Opposite, Warm Same) is derived. In the unconscious patient, caloric testing is usually limited to cold water, saccades are not seen, and the mnemonic does not apply.

The corneal reflex tests the sensory function of the ophthalmic division of the ipsilateral trigeminal nerve (CN V), transmission of impulses within the pons from the trigeminal nucleus to bilateral facial nerve nuclei, and the motor function of the ophthalmic branches of the facial nerves to the orbicularis oculi muscles, which effect eyelid closure. An asymmetric response is suggestive of a compressive or destructive lesion interrupting one limb of the reflex arc. Closure of only one eye with stimulation of either cornea suggests an efferent defect. Lack of response to touching one cornea but not the other suggests an afferent defect. Bilateral absent corneal reflexes can be seen with more extensive structural lesions but also occur with metabolic disorders, intoxication, and paralysis.

The gag reflex depends on intact functioning of afferents and efferents from both the glossopharyngeal (CN IX) and vagal (CN X) nuclei within the medulla. The ideal test looks for palatal elevation with stimulation of each side of the posterior wall of the oropharynx. When a patient is tracheally intubated, as is often the case in the context of coma, eliciting a cough with endotracheal tube manipulation or suctioning is often used as an acceptable alternative. However, it should be noted that cough can also be elicited in these ways through reflexes involving the cervical spine.

Asymmetric limb movements or postures are also suggestive of lesions within the central nervous system. Flaccid weakness can occur with lesions of the medulla or spinal cord. Decerebrate posturing, with extension and internal rotation of both the arm and leg, can occur with lesions in the pons. Decorticate posturing, with flexion of the arm and extension of the leg, can occur with lesions

TABLE 7.3. Glasgow Coma Scale (GCS).

Sign	GCS*	GCS modified for children[†]	Score
Eye opening	Spontaneous	Spontaneous	4
	To command	To sound	3
	To pain	To pain	2
	None	None	1
Verbal response	Oriented	Age-appropriate vocalization, smile, or orientation to sound	5
	Confused, disoriented	Irritable, consolable, uncooperative, aware of the environment	4
	Inappropriate words	Irritable, inconsistently consolable	3
	Incomprehensible sounds	Inconsolable, unaware of the environment, restless, agitated	2
	None	None	1
Motor response	Obeys commands	Obeys commands, spontaneous movements	6
	Localizes pain	Localizes pain	5
	Withdraws	Withdraws	4
	Abnormal flexion to pain	Abnormal flexion to pain	3
	Abnormal extension to pain	Abnormal extension to pain	2
	None	None	1
Best total score			15

*Based on Teasdale and Jennett [83].
[†]Based on Simpson et al. [84].

of midbrain, thalamus, and cortex. Symmetric flaccid weakness or decorticate posturing is difficult to localize and can be associated with global metabolic insults, intoxication, and trauma. Asymmetric responses are particularly suggestive of focal compressive or destructive processes.

Rating scales such as the Glasgow Coma Scale and its modification for use in children (Table 7.3) are frequently used to summarize a patient's level of consciousness, using scores for motor, verbal, and eye opening responses. Such scales have proven descriptive and prognostic value, especially in the first hours and days of evaluation of coma, but it should be remembered that they do not reflect brain stem reflexes and other important aspects of a complete neurologic examination.

Herniation Syndromes

Beyond early infancy, when open fontanelles and sutures allow limited expansion, the skull is a fixed structure that cannot accommodate an increase in the overall volume of its contents. According to a principle known as the Monroe doctrine, an expansion of one of the three intracranial components (blood, CSF, and brain) will initially be compensated by a reciprocal decrease in the other components. Shifts of this kind normally occur throughout the day, with small changes in venous pressure and intracranial blood volume caused by position changes and valsalva maneuvers. Large increases in any of the components, as with a rapidly expanding hematoma, obstructive hydrocephalus, or cerebral edema, can overwhelm the capacity of the brain for compensation, induce rapid and dramatic increases in ICP, and result in herniation of brain contents past their usual boundaries, resulting in several well-characterized herniation syndromes (Figure 7.1).

Uncal herniation is a unilateral, downward transtentorial herniation caused by expansion within or above one temporal lobe, which pushes the mesial temporal lobe (uncus) and parahippocampal gyrus into the suprasellar cistern, through the tentorial notch, and onto the ipsilateral oculomotor nerve (Figure 7.2). Initial compression of this nerve affects the parasympathetic pupillomotor fibers running along its surface and results in a poorly reactive, then fixed and dilated pupil. Further compression causes the ptosis and outward and downward deviation of the ipsilateral eye (Figure 7.3). Ongoing uncal herniation can also lead to ipsilateral hemiparesis as the brain stem is pushed against the contralateral incisural notch, contralateral hemianopsia as the ipsilateral posterior cerebral artery is compressed, and apnea as the entire brain stem is pushed downward, causing hemorrhage and ischemia within the medulla.

Bilateral expansion of cranial contents, with a generalized increased in ICP, can result in *central herniation* of the thalamus and hypothalamus through the tentorial notch, downward movement of the brain stem, and eventual downward herniation of the cerebellar tonsils through the foramen magnum (Figure 7.4). Expansion within the posterior fossa alone can cause brain stem compression and downward herniation of the cerebellar tonsils or, rarely, upward transtentorial herniation of the cerebellum and brain stem.

Compression and ischemia of the diencephalon and brain stem can progress slowly in a rostrocaudal fashion or can occur abruptly. With a diencephalic level injury, patients show decorticate posturing, Cheyne-Stokes respirations, and small pupils but preserved brain stem reflexes and ability to localize noxious stimuli. With involvement of the midbrain and upper pons, posturing becomes

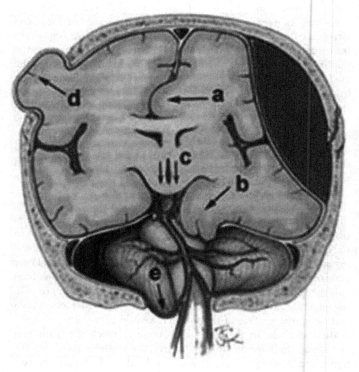

FIGURE 7.1. Herniation syndromes. **(A)** Subfalcine herniation. **(B)** Uncal herniation. **(C)** Central herniation. **(D)** Extracranial herniation. **(E)** Tonsillar herniation. (Copyright Harris and Troetscher, http://www.uth.tmc.edu/radiology/test/er_primer/skull_brain/skull.html.)

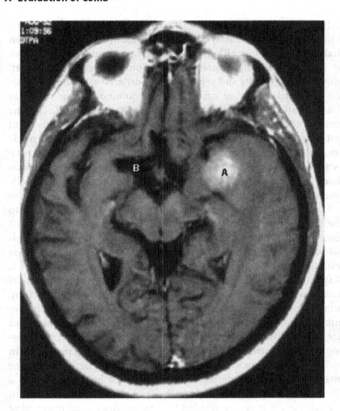

FIGURE 7.2. Uncal herniation. Axial T1-weighted magnetic resonance image of the brain, demonstrating increased intensity in the left medial temporal lobe from acute hemorrhage and swelling **(A)**, causing compression of the suprasellar cistern **(B)**. (Copyright H. Irvine and J.G. Smirniotopoulos, MD, rad.usuhs.mil/rad/herniation.)

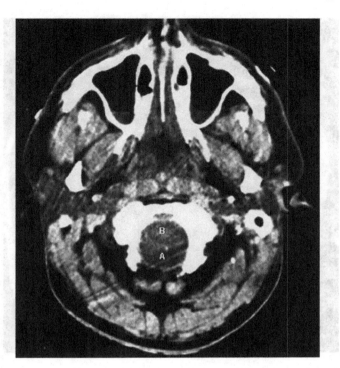

FIGURE 7.4. Tonsillar herniation. Axial computed tomography scan of the head of a patient whose cerebellar tonsils **(A)** have descended into the foramen magnum to compress the cervical spinal cord **(B)**. (Copyright H. Irvine and J.G. Smirniotopoulos, MD, rad.usuhs. mil/rad/herniation.)

decerebrate, pupils become midposition in size and sometimes irregular in shape, and there is a loss of pupillary, oculocephalic, and oculovestibular reflexes. Respirations may become rapid, leading to respiratory alkalosis. With involvement of the lower pons and medulla, all brain stem reflexes are lost, posturing is replaced with a flaccid paralysis, and respirations become ataxic, irregular, and slow before eventually ceasing.

Subfalcine herniation results from unilateral expansion of one hemisphere causing lateral movement of the ipsilateral cingulate gyrus underneath the anterior portion of the falx. The anterior horn of the ipsilateral ventricle is compressed by the local mass effect but the opposite lateral ventricle can become enlarged due to

obstruction of the foramen of Monroe (Figure 7.5). This type of herniation can also result in contralateral leg weakness as the ipsilateral anterior cerebral artery is pulled along with the cingulate gyrus and compressed by the falx.

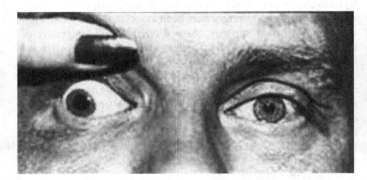

FIGURE 7.3. Oculomotor palsy. Total right third nerve palsy resulting in outward and downward deviation of the right eye with an efferent pupilary defect. (Copyright Jeremy Payne, www.neurology.arizona.edu/Training/c10.html.)

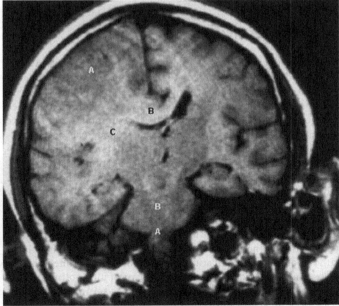

FIGURE 7.5. Subfalcine herniation. Coronal T1-weighted magnetic resonance image of the brain showing swelling of the right hemisphere **(A)** causing herniation of the right cingulate gyrus under the falx **(B)** and compression of the right lateral ventricle **(C)**. (Copyright H. Irvine and J.G. Smirniotopoulos, MD, rad.usuhs.mil/rad/herniation.)

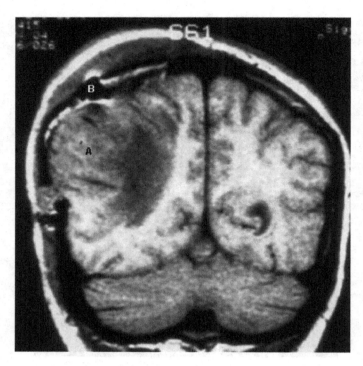

Figure 7.6. Extracranial herniation. Coronal T1-weighted magnetic resonance image of the brain showing an edematous right hemisphere **(A)** herniating through a craniotomy defect **(B)**. (Copyright H. Irvine and J.G. Smirniotopoulos, MD, rad.usuhs. mil/rad/herniation.)

Extracranial herniation occurs when there is a defect in the skull that allows expanding intracranial contents to herniate outward (Figure 7.6). This is most often seen as the intended consequence of a decompressive craniotomy performed for the relief of increased ICP.

Diagnostic Testing

Routine laboratory testing of a patient with coma of unknown etiology should include an immediate bedside test for serum glucose level, a complete blood count, and a complete metabolic profile that includes measurement of serum electrolytes, calcium, blood urea nitrogen, creatinine, liver transaminases, ammonia, and lactate levels. The blood count may demonstrate leukocytosis or leukopenia related to infection or hematologic malignancy, macrocytosis related to folate or cobalamin deficiency, or anemia caused by hemorrhage. Any suspicion for infection should lead to the collection of blood, urine, and CSF cultures. A complete metabolic profile may disclose the presence of an electrolyte imbalance, a disorder of osmolality, renal or hepatic dysfunction, or an inborn error of metabolism. If a blood gas is measured for respiratory management it may provide the first evidence of metabolic acidosis associated with hypotension, intoxication, or an inborn error of metabolism. If the clinical suspicion for an inborn error of metabolism is high, more specific tests can be performed, such as serum amino acids, urine organic acids, and serum carnitine and acylcarnitines, but the results of such tests are often unavailable for days or weeks. Testing of children in coma that remains unexplained despite a routine workup may expand to measures of thyroid function, cortisol, and urine porphyrins.

Toxic ingestions are best identified by history and by the recognition of specific clinical syndromes (toxidromes), but it is known that children are more likely than adults to present with unfamiliar or atypical clinical features [23,24]. Some laboratory tests can provide rapid results and are commonly ordered as a batch, including standard serum or urine tests for common drugs of abuse (barbiturates, benzodiazepines, opioids, amphetamines, cocaine metabolites, phencyclidine, and marijuana metabolites) and serum tests for acetaminophen, salicylates, ethanol, sympathomimetic amines, and tricyclic antidepressants. Broader drug screens, such as thin-layer chromatography and ultraviolet spectroscopy, can detect less common causes of intoxication but are not rapidly available and often require confirmatory tests [25].

Neuroimaging by computed tomography (CT) is most suited to the critically ill patient because of its fast scanning. Computed tomography is able to detect pathology in need of immediate surgical intervention, including hydrocephalus, herniation, and mass lesions caused by infection, neoplasia, hemorrhage, and edema. Magnetic resonance imaging (MRI) provides greater structural detail but may be uniquely able to show early evidence of infection, infarction, diffuse axonal injury, petechial hemorrhage, sinovenous thrombosis, and demyelination [26,27]. Some advanced but not universally available methods of MRI, such as proton spectroscopy, can also offer significant information regarding prognosis in patients with anoxic or traumatic coma. Magnetic resonance imaging is therefore preferred but may often be delayed until a child is stable enough to endure the long acquisition time within the scanner. It is recommended that some form of neuroimaging be considered before lumbar puncture in any patient with a decreased level of consciousness, given the perception of an increased risk of inducing herniation.

Additional neuroimaging studies may be suggested by the initial CT or MRI, such as magnetic resonance angiography or conventional angiography for cases of suspected vascular malformation, vasculitis, or venous thrombosis. Repeated scanning, usually with CT, is often undertaken on an emergent basis in patients with clinical deterioration and can demonstrate worsening edema, hemorrhage, herniation, and hydrocephalus. Patients without a surgically remediable lesion on initial 24 or 48 hr CT scans do not appear to benefit from continued routine imaging [28]. There is currently no role for the routine use of functional MRI, positron emission tomography, or single photon emission tomography in the evaluation of comatose patients.

An electroencephalogram (EEG) should be among the tests performed routinely in patients with coma of unknown etiology and is often the only means of recognizing nonconvulsive status epilepticus (NCSE), especially in patients who are paralyzed [29]. Periodic epileptiform discharges have been associated with NCSE [30]. In patients without epilepsy, these discharges are suggestive of underlying brain injury and, when lateralized, are suggestive of herpes encephalitis or infarction. Multifocal or generalized periodic discharges can also be seen with metabolic and infectious causes of widespread cerebral dysfunction and are characteristic of subacute sclerosing panencephalitis [31]. Nonepileptiform features of the EEG, such as slowing or asymmetry, are largely nonspecific but can sometimes provide diagnostic or prognostic information [32,33]. Continuous EEG is useful to assess and titrate the depth of sedation in patients placed under anesthesia for control of status epilepticus or increased ICP.

Other electrodiagnostic tests, such as somatosensory, auditory, and visual evoked potentials, are sometimes used in comatose patients for assessment of prognosis but do not have a well-defined diagnostic utility. Nerve conduction and needle electromyographic studies also have no place in the routine evaluation of coma, although they are essential for diagnosing the locked-in syndrome caused by peripheral nervous system disorders and are generally useful in the evaluation of paralysis in critically ill patients.

Management of Coma

After initial evaluation and stabilization, and reversal of the underlying cause if possible, the treatment of a comatose patient is focused on prevention of secondary brain injury caused by systemic hypotension, hypoxia, hypoglycemia, seizures, hyperthermia, infection, and herniation [34]. Our ability to recognize and treat these secondary factors has steadily gotten better, although parallel improvements in outcomes are difficult to demonstrate [35]. Children with severe traumatic injuries have been shown to have better outcomes when treated in pediatric trauma centers [36].

Our understanding of the pathophysiology of brain injury, regardless of etiology, has also improved. Cell death along necrotic and apoptotic pathways involves energy failure, loss of ion homeostasis, membrane depolarization, release of excitatory neurotransmitters, elevation of intracellular calcium, production of excessive free radicals, release of proinflammatory cytokines, activation of proapoptotic proteins, cleavage of DNA, lysis of proteins, and peroxidation of lipids [37]. Interventions to inhibit each of these biochemical derangements have been developed, and many have shown promise in animal and in vitro experiments; however, none has as yet been translated successfully into clinical practice.

Table 7.4 outlines steps in the management of coma. Tracheal intubation for airway protection and mechanical ventilation will be required in most instances. Stabilizing the circulation in patients with brain injury involves maintaining an adequate cerebral perfusion pressure (CPP), calculated as the difference between the mean arterial pressure and the ICP. A CPP of 50 mm Hg or more is correlated with improved survival after traumatic brain injury [38]. Steps to maintain the CPP, even in patients at risk for cerebral edema, lead to better outcomes than routine dehydration [39]. A bedside test of the serum glucose level allows early recognition and treatment of hypoglycemia. Hyperglycemia, on the other hand, is associated with increased morbidity and mortality in patients with traumatic and ischemic brain injuries. It is currently recommended that normoglycemia be maintained [40,41]. Reversal of known or suspected intoxication with opiates, anticholinergics, and benzodiazepines can be attempted using the specific antagonists naloxone, physostigmine, and flumazenil. These agents can induce

withdrawal symptoms and cause other potentially serious side effects. Adult patients with unexplained coma can often safely be treated with a *coma cocktail* that includes dextrose, thiamine, and sedative reversal agents [42]. Given evidence that children are even less likely to experience adverse reactions from flumazenil and naloxone, their empiric use has been suggested [43].

Patients suspected of having increased ICP need urgent neuroimaging and neurosurgical consultation. Urgent surgical management of increased ICP may require placement of an intracranial pressure monitor, decompression of a hematoma or other mass lesion, decompressive craniotomy, or cerebrospinal fluid shunting. Efforts to maintain an ICP at less than 20 mm Hg improve the outcomes of patients with severe traumatic brain injury [44]. Recent studies suggest a benefit from early decompressive craniotomy in these patients [45,46]. Lowering the ICPs of patients who have suffered a severe hypoxic insult, on the other hand, may only serve to improve the survival of profoundly impaired or vegetative patients [47]. Nonsurgical measures for lowering ICP include hyperventilation, head positioning, and the use of hyperosmolar fluids, corticosteroids, and sedatives. There are concerns that prolonged hyperventilation can decrease cerebral perfusion [48]. Osmolar diuretics such as mannitol carry a risk of dehydration, decreased cerebral perfusion, and rebound cerebral edema. The use of hypertonic saline has been established as safe and effective [49].

Early post-traumatic seizures, most of which occur in the first 24 hr, can elevate ICP and increase cerebral metabolic demand, potentially worsening secondary brain injury. Prophylactic anticonvulsants do improve neurologic outcomes in children after severe trauma [50] but do not lower the incidence of post-traumatic epilepsy, and their prolonged use may impair rehabilitation [51]. Status epilepticus necessitates urgent anticonvulsant therapy but may be clinically subtle or nonconvulsive. An epileptic etiology should be considered whenever neurologic deterioration or vital sign abnormalities are otherwise unexplained.

Infection is often suspected and treated on the basis of initial clinical signs and laboratory test results. Intracranial infections can be difficult to diagnose without cerebrospinal fluid analysis. Even when bacterial meningitis is strongly suspected it is acceptable and often prudent to treat empirically and defer lumbar puncture in patients at an increased risk of cerebral herniation on the basis of a known or suspected intracranial mass lesion [52]. Neurogenic fever, which may be related to impairment of the hypothalamus, occurs in up to 40% of patients with severe traumatic brain injury and in up to 50% of patients with severe hypoxic–ischemic injury [53]. Hyperthermia is clearly detrimental to the injured brain, and cooling measures should be used as needed to bring core temperatures into the normal range [54]. However, clinical trials of therapeutic hypothermia in brain-injured patients do not currently support its routine use [55].

Critically ill patients are at risk for malnutrition and electrolyte and acid–base imbalances. Appropriate nutrition maximizes neurologic recovery and resistance to infection [56]. Rapid changes in serum osmolarity can cause myelinolysis or cerebral edema. Hyponatremia is frequently seen in patients with brain injuries and can be caused by inappropriate antidiuretic hormone release, which is associated with decreased urine output, or cerebral salt wasting, which is associated with increased urine output [57].

The risk of deep venous thrombosis and consequent pulmonary embolism is lower in comatose patients treated with low-molecular-weight heparin, sequential compression stockings, and foot pumps [58].

TABLE 7.4. Steps in the management of coma.

1. Ensure a stable airway, adequate oxygenation and ventilation, and circulation
2. Recognize and treat hypoglycemia
3. Consider specific antidotes for medication overdoses
4. Monitor for, prevent, and treat increased intracranial pressure
5. Evaluate for and treat seizures
6. Treat suspected infection
7. Normalize body temperature
8. Optimize nutrition
9. Correct electrolyte and acid–base disturbances
10. Prevent deep venous thrombosis

TABLE 7.5. Glasgow Outcome Scale.

1. Death
2. Persistent vegetative state
3. Severe disability: conscious but dependent
4. Moderate disability: independent but disabled
5. Good recovery

Source: Tilford et al. [50].

Outcome of Coma

Despite efforts to prevent secondary brain injury, clinical outcomes are often frustratingly poor and largely depend on the etiology and severity of the initial injury. Trauma is consistently among the most common causes of mortality in childhood, and many survivors are left with severe neurologic handicaps [59]. Studies often report neurologic outcomes using one of several scales. The commonly used Glasgow Outcome Scale (GOS), outlined in Table 7.5, emphasizes functional independence [60]. The Pediatric Cerebral Performance Category Scale (PCPCS), outlined in Table 7.6, evaluates both the independence and age-appropriateness of a child's function [61]. These scales are easily applied and have good inter-rater reliabilities but do not take into account the effects of emotional and social impairments common among survivors of brain injury. Among the more broadly inclusive scales in use are the Functional Independence Measure (FIM) and its pediatric counterpart (WeeFIM), which assess 18 items in six categories, including self-care, sphincter control, mobility, locomotion, communication, and social/cognitive function [62,63]. When a patient is able to cooperate, testing by a clinical neuropsychologist provides the most comprehensive assessment of cognitive recovery [64].

Outcome Prediction

Families may be frustrated when recovery from coma proceeds slowly, perhaps conditioned to expect a sudden and dramatic awakening. Such recoveries do occur but are exceptional, as are recoveries from a severely disabled state lasting more than 6 months. Most children with traumatic brain injury reach their highest GOS score within that time frame, although independence can continue to subtly improve for months and years. Most children who survive traumatic coma (up to 90% of those with coma lasting less than 6 weeks) will eventually achieve a GOS score of moderately disabled or better, although cognitive and emotional problems may persist. Similar outcomes are seen with nontraumatic causes of pediatric coma, as in one population-based study of 278 children in which 46% died, 64% of the survivors were neurologically intact, 16% had

TABLE 7.6. Pediatric Cerebral Performance Category Scale (51).

1. Normal: able to perform all age-appropriate activities
2. Mild disability: conscious, alert, and able to interact at an age-appropriate level but may have a mild neurologic deficit
3. Moderate disability: conscious, sufficient cerebral function for most age-appropriate independent activities
4. Severe disability: conscious, dependent on others for daily support because of impaired brain function
5. Persistent vegetative state or coma
6. Death

Source: Beghi [50].

mild to moderate disability, and 14% were severely disabled or in a vegetative state [65]. The widespread use of the GOS, emphasizing motor independence, has contributed to a belief that brain injuries affect younger children less than they do adults. However, cognitive deficits may have a more profound influence on subjects with a lifetime of impaired learning ahead of them [66].

Families of children in coma are often presented with difficult decisions about the institution, continuation, or withdrawal of medical care. Early measures that predict eventual death or severe impairment allow some to decline what they perceive to be futile care, even though most measures are less than ideal. The accuracy of outcome predictions made using combined clinical, serologic, radiologic, and electrophysiologic measures is as high as 90%, but no measures have been able to avoid predicting bad outcomes for children who nevertheless make meaningful recoveries.

The clinical measure most commonly used for prediction is the presenting GCS score. Children whose injuries are severe but who present with a GCS from 4 to 8 are very unlikely to die, whereas those with the lowest score of 3 have a mortality rate of 50% to 60%, often dying within a few days of hospitalization [67]. Outcome from severe traumatic brain injury is also correlated with multiple trauma, hypoxia, hypotension, disseminated intravascular coagulation, hyperglycemia, and early post-traumatic seizures [68]. Outcome from nontraumatic coma is also worse for patients with lower presenting GCS scores, especially lower motor scores, and is negatively correlated with younger age, absent brain stem reflexes, and hypotension [69].

Electrophysiologic somatosensory evoked potentials (SSEPs) can add even more to outcome prediction. Pooled studies of adults and children have shown a more than 90% accuracy in using bilaterally intact SSEPs within 48 hr of resuscitation to predict good recovery and bilaterally absent SSEPs to predicts severe disability or death [69]. However, absent SSEPs are far more likely to be misleading in children and adolescents, who are more likely to awaken from coma and go on to recover significant independence [70]. Other electrophysiologic tests, including EEGs, brain stem auditory evoked responses (BAERs), and visual evoked potentials (VEPs), have limited value in outcome prediction [33]. Nevertheless, some EEG patterns, such as burst-suppression and isoelectricity, are highly predictive of a very poor prognosis. These patterns were seen only in children with a fatal outcome in one series of near-drownings [71].

Some clinical scenarios offer little hope for intact survival. Children who suffer cardiopulmonary arrest, especially those who remain pulseless on arrival to the emergency room after an out-of-hospital arrest, nearly always die or remain profoundly impaired. Some children, such as those who are found pulseless after an unwitnessed arrest, who require more than 25 min of cardiac resuscitation, or who suffer warm-water near-drowning and are pulseless on arrival to the emergency room, are so unlikely to survive or recover that any continuation of care may be futile [72–75]. On the other hand, intact recovery rates of up to 75% have been reported with other scenarios, including witnessed cardiopulmonary arrest, isolated respiratory arrest, and ice-water submersion. For submersion victims, other factors found to be associated with better recovery include preservation of pupillary reflexes, a GCS of greater than 5 in the emergency room, female gender, and initial blood glucose of less than 250 mg/dL [76].

Neuroimaging studies, particularly proton magnetic resonance spectroscopy (MRS), are of great value for outcome prediction. Lower N-acetyl aspartate to creatine (NAA/Cr) ratios and higher lactate levels on MRS are highly predictive of poorer outcomes in

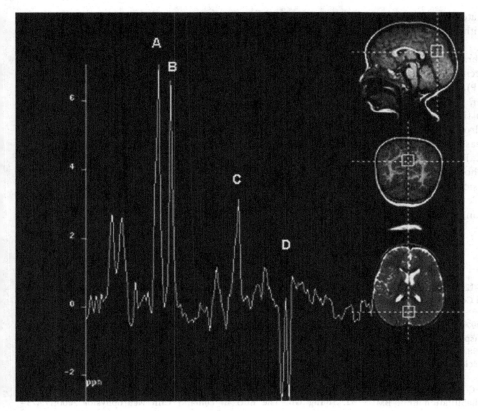

FIGURE 7.7. Proton magnetic resonance spectroscopy. Proton magnetic resonance spectroscopy of a voxel centered within the occipital gray matter of a 15-month-old child who suffered an axphyxial injury from a foreign body aspiration, showing an extremely depressed ratio between N-acetyl aspartate (C) and creatine (B), indicating neuronal loss or dysfunction. The ratio between choline (A) and creatine is elevated, suggesting membrane disruption or glial activation. The presence of a large lactate peak (D) is consistent with a severe anoxic injury. The patient has remained in a persistent vegetative state. (Courtesy of Barbara Holshouser, MD, Department of Neuroradiology, Loma Linda University School of Medicine.)

near-drowning patients (Figure 7.7) [77,78]. Even conventional MRI has a significant advantage over CT scanning for patients with traumatic brain injury: one series found that signal abnormalities in the brain stem, seen in 60% of cases, were 100% predictive of mortality [79]. Similarly, the extent of signal abnormality on MRI after hypoxic–ischemic injury, especially in watershed and basal ganglia areas, is strongly correlated with neurologic outcome [80]. Susceptibility weighted MRI is particularly helpful in demonstrating the presence and extent of intracranial hemorrhages in patients with diffuse axonal injury (Figure 7.8). Studies using higher reso-

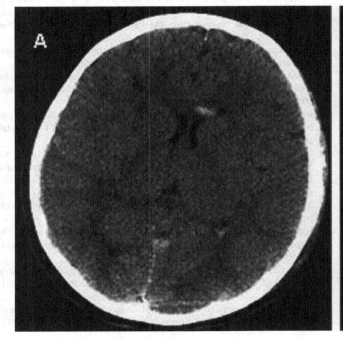

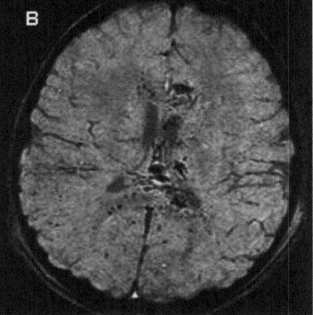

FIGURE 7.8. Magnetic resonance imaging of a 10-year-old pedestrian hit by an automobile. The axial computed tomography scan (A) shows bleeding within the anterior corpus callosum. Magnetic resonance imaging using susceptibility weighting (B) is able to demonstrate more extensive hemorrhage within the corpus callosum, thalamus, and ventricles. (Courtesy of Karen Tong, MD, Department of Neuroradiology, Loma Linda University School of Medicine.)

lution images may eventually show even greater precision, especially in correlating regional abnormalities with specific cognitive deficits among survivors.

Serum tests for markers of the severity of brain injury, such as the glial and neuronal proteins neuron-specific enolase (NSE), S100, and glial fibrillary acidic protein (GFAP), are also showing great promise in early studies [81]. However, the limitations of outcome prediction are such that caution in their application is warranted. Even victims of warm-water near-drowning who appear to have little chance of survival are given at least 48 hr of intensive support under current recommendations [82]. Furthermore, decisions to order tests for outcome prediction should be mindful of the family's desire for the information. A decision to continue care may seem futile to some families but reasonable to others, depending on many factors, including culture, religion, and education.

References

1. Zeman A. Consciousness. Brain 2001;124:1263–1289.
2. Plum F, Posner JB. The Diagnosis of Stupor and Coma, 3rd ed, revised. Philadelphia: FA Davis; 1982.
3. Zeman A. Persistent vegetative state. Lancet 1997;350:795–799.
4. The Multi-Society Task Force on PVS. Medical aspects of the persistent vegetative state. N Engl J Med 1994;330:1499–508.
5. Ashwal S. Medical aspects of the minimally conscious state in children. Brain Dev 2003;25:535–545.
6. Andrews K, Murphy L, Munday R, Littlewood C. Misdiagnosis of the vegetative state: retrospective study in a rehabilitation unit. BMJ 1996;313:13–16.
7. Laureys S. Functional neuroimaging in the vegetative state. NeuroRehabilitation 2004;19:335–341.
8. Landrieu P, Fromentin C, Tardieu M, Menget A, Laget P. Locked in syndrome with a favourable outcome. Eur J Pediatr 1984;142:144–145.
9. Masuzawa H, Sato J, Kamitani H, Kamikura T, Aoki N. Pontine gliomas causing locked-in syndrome. Childs Nerv Syst 1993;9:256–259.
10. Rosman NP, Adhami S, Mannheim GB, Katz NP, Klucznik RP, Muriello MA. Basilar artery occlusion in children: misleading presentations, "locked-in" state, and diagnostic importance of accompanying vertebral artery occlusion. J Child Neurol 2003;18:450–462.
11. Bakshi N, Maselli RA, Gospe SM Jr, Ellis WG, McDonald C, Mandler RN. Fulminant demyelinating neuropathy mimicking cerebral death. Muscle Nerve 1997;20:1595–1597.
12. Echenberg RJ. Permanently locked-in syndrome in the neurologically impaired neonate: report of a case of Werdnig-Hoffmann disease. J Clin Ethics 1992;3:206–208.
13. Golden GS, Leeds N, Kremenitzer MW, Russman BS. The "locked-in" syndrome in children. J Pediatr 1976;89:596–598.
14. van Mourik M, van Dongen HR, Catsman-Berrevoets CE. The many faces of acquired neurologic mutism in childhood. Pediatr Neurol 1996;15:352–357.
15. Abekura M. Akinetic mutism and magnetic resonance imaging in obstructive hydrocephalus. Case illustration. J Neurosurg 1998;88:161.
16. Mellon AF, Appleton RE, Gardner-Medwin D, Aynsley-Green A. Encephalitis lethargica–like illness in a five-year-old. Dev Med Child Neurol 1991;33:158–161.
17. Shinoda M, Tsugu A, Oda S, Masuko A, Yamaguchi T, Yamaguchi T, Tsugane R, Sato O. Development of akinetic mutism and hyperphagia after left thalamic and right hypothalamic lesions. Childs Nerv Syst 1993;9:243–245.
18. Kadota Y, Kondo T, Sato K. Akinetic mutism and involuntary movements following radical resection of hypothalamic glioma—case report. Neurol Med Chir 1996;36:447–450.
19. Wijdicks EF. The diagnosis of brain death. N Engl J Med 2001;344:1215–1221.
20. Wong CP, Forsyth RJ, Kelly TP, Eyre JA. Incidence, aetiology, and outcome of non-traumatic coma: a population based study. Arch Dis Child 2001;84:193–199.
21. Bates D. The management of medical coma. J Neurol Neurosurg Psychiatry 1993;56:589–598.
22. Carty H, Pierce A. Non-accidental injury: a retrospective analysis of a large cohort. Eur Radiol 2002;12:2919–2925.
23. Abbruzzi G, Stork CM. Pediatric toxicologic concerns. Emerg Med Clin North Am 2002;20:223–247.
24. Lifshitz M, Shahak E, Sofer S. Carbamate and organophosphate poisoning in young children. Pediatr Emerg Care 1999;15:102–103.
25. Hammett-Stabler CA, Pesce AJ, Cannon DJ. Urine drug screening in the medical setting. Clin Chim Acta 2002; 315:125–135.
26. Tong KA, Ashwal S, Holshouser BA, Shutter LA, Herigault G, Haacke EM, Kido DK. Hemorrhagic shearing lesions in children and adolescents with posttraumatic diffuse axonal injury: improved detection and initial results. Radiology 2003;227:332–339.
27. Sundgren PC, Reinstrup P, Romner B, Holtas S, Maly P. Value of conventional, and diffusion- and perfusion weighted MRI in the management of patients with unclear cerebral pathology, admitted to the intensive care unit. Neuroradiology 2002;4:674–680.
28. Figg RE, Burry TS, Vander Kolk WE. Clinical efficacy of serial computed tomographic scanning in severe closed head injury patients. J Trauma 2003;55:1061–1064.
29. Markand ON. Pearls, perils, and pitfalls in the use of the electroencephalogram. Semin Neurol 2003;23:7–46.
30. Brenner RP. Is it status? Epilepsia 2002;43:S103–S113.
31. Yemisci M, Gurer G, Saygi S, Ciger A. Generalised periodic epileptiform discharges: clinical features, neuroradiological evaluation and prognosis in 37 adult patients. Seizure 2003;12:465–472.
32. Young GB. The EEG in coma. J Clin Neurophysiol 2000;17:473–485.
33. Mewasingh LD, Christophe C, Fonteyne C, Dachy B, Ziereisen F, Christiaens F, Deltenre P, De Maertelaer V, Dan B. Predictive value of electrophysiology in children with hypoxic coma. Pediatr Neurol 2003;28:178–183.
34. Kochanek PM, Clark RS, Ruppel RA, Adelson PD, Bell MJ, Whalen MJ, Robertson CL, Satchell MA, Seidberg NA, Marion DW, Jenkins LW. Biochemical, cellular, and molecular mechanisms in the evolution of secondary damage after severe traumatic brain injury in infants and children: lessons learned from the bedside. Pediatr Crit Care Med 2000;1:4–19.
35. Pfenninger J, Santi A. Severe traumatic brain injury in children—are the results improving? Swiss Med Wkly 2002;132:116–120.
36. Potoka DA, Schall LC, Ford HR. Improved functional outcome for severely injured children treated at pediatric trauma centers. J Trauma 2001;51:824–832.
37. Bramlett HM, Dietrich WD. Pathophysiology of cerebral ischemia and brain trauma: similarities and differences. J Cereb Blood Flow Metab 2004;24:133–150.
38. Hackbarth RM, Rzeszutko KM, Sturm G, Donders J, Kuldanek AS, Sanfilippo DJ. Survival and functional outcome in pediatric traumatic brain injury: a retrospective review and analysis of predictive factors. Crit Care Med 2002;30:1630–1635.
39. Yu PL, Jin LM, Seaman H, Yang YJ, Tong HX. Fluid therapy of acute brain edema in children. Pediatr Neurol 2000;22:298–301.
40. Jeremitsky E, Omert LA, Dunham CM, Wilberger J, Rodriguez A. The impact of hyperglycemia on patients with severe brain injury. J Trauma 2005;58:47–50.
41. Wass CT, Lanier WL. Glucose modulation of ischemic brain injury: review and clinical recommendations. Mayo Clin Proc 1996;71:801–812.
42. Bartlett D. The coma cocktail: indications, contraindications, adverse effects, proper dose, and proper route. J Emerg Nurs 2004;30:572–574.
43. Perry HE, Shannon MW. Diagnosis and management of opioid- and benzodiazepine-induced comatose overdose in children. Curr Opin Pediatr 1996;8:243–247.

44. Wahlstrom MR, Olivecrona M, Koskinen LO, Rydenhag B, Naredi S. Severe traumatic brain injury in pediatric patients: treatment and outcome using an intracranial pressure targeted therapy—the Lund concept. Intensive Care Med 2005;31:832–839.

45. Ruf B, Heckmann M, Schroth I, Hugens-Penzel M, Reiss I, Borkhardt A, Gortner L, Jodicke A. Early decompressive craniectomy and duraplasty for refractory intracranial hypertension in children: results of a pilot study. Crit Care 2003;7:R133–R138.

46. Figaji AA, Fieggen AG, Peter JC. Early decompressive craniotomy in children with severe traumatic brain injury. Childs Nerv Syst 2003;19: 666–673.

47. Bohn DJ, Biggar WD, Smith CR, Conn AW, Barker GA. Influence of hypothermia, barbiturate therapy, and intracranial pressure monitoring on morbidity and mortality after near-drowning. Crit Care Med 1986;14:529–534.

48. Skippen PA, Seear M, Poskitt K, Kestle J, Cochrane D, Annich G, Handel J. Effect of hyperventilation on regional cerebral blood flow in head-injured children. Crit Care Med 1997;25:1402–1409.

49. Georgiadis AL, Suarez JI. Hypertonic saline for cerebral edema. Curr Neurol Neurosci Rep 2003;3:524–530.

50. Tilford JM, Simpson PM, Yeh TS, Lensing S, Aitken ME, Green JW, Harr J, Fiser DH. Variation in therapy and outcome for pediatric head trauma patients. Crit Care Med 2001;29:1056–1061.

51. Beghi E. Overview of studies to prevent posttraumatic epilepsy. Epilepsia 2003;44:S21–S26.

52. Oliver WJ, Shope TC, Kuhns LR. Fatal lumbar puncture: fact versus fiction—an approach to a clinical dilemma. Pediatrics 2003;112: e174–e176.

53. Thompson HJ, Pinto-Martin J, Bullock MR. Neurogenic fever after traumatic brain injury: an epidemiological study. J Neurol Neurosurg Psychiatry 2003;74:614–619.

54. Bernardo LM, Henker R, O'Connor J. Treatment of trauma-associated hypothermia in children: evidence-based practice. Am J Crit Care 2000;9:227–234.

55. Bernard SA, Buist M. Induced hypothermia in critical care medicine: a review. Crit Care Med 2003;31:2041–2051.

56. Taylor SJ, Fettes SB, Jewkes C, Nelson RJ. Prospective, randomized, controlled trial to determine the effect of early enhanced enteral nutrition on clinical outcome in mechanically ventilated patients suffering head injury. Crit Care Med 1999;27:2525–2531.

57. Berkenbosch JW, Lentz CW, Jimenez DF, Tobias JD. Cerebral salt wasting syndrome following brain injury in three pediatric patients: suggestions for rapid diagnosis and therapy. Pediatr Neurosurg 2002;36:75–79.

58. Spain DA, Bergamini TM, Hoffmann JF, Carrillo EH, Richardson JD. Comparison of sequential compression devices and foot pumps for prophylaxis of deep venous thrombosis in high-risk trauma patients. Am Surg 1998;64:522–525.

59. Arias E, MacDorman MF, Strobino DM, Guyer B. Annual summary of vital statistics—2002. Pediatrics 2003;112:1215–1230.

60. Jennett B, Bond M. Assessment of outcome after severe brain damage. Lancet 1975;1:480–484.

61. Fiser DH. Assessing the outcome of pediatric intensive care. J Pediatr 1992;121:68–74.

62. Keith RA, Granger CV, Hamilton BB, Sherwin FS. The functional independence measure: a new tool for rehabilitation. Adv Clin Rehabil 1987;1:6–18.

63. Msall ME, DiGaudio K, Rogers BT, LaForest S, Catanzaro NL, Campbell J, Wilczenski F, Duffy LC. The Functional Independence Measure for Children (WeeFIM). Conceptual basis and pilot use in children with developmental disabilities. Clin Pediatr 1994;33:421–430.

64. Hannay HJ, Sherer M. Assessment of outcome from head injury. In: Narayan RK, Wilberger JE Jr, Povlishock JT, eds. Neurotrauma. New York: McGraw-Hill; 1996.

65. Forsyth RJ, Wong CP, Kelly TP, Borrill H, Stilgoe D, Kendall S, Eyre JA. Cognitive and adaptive outcomes and age at insult effects after non-traumatic coma. Arch Dis Child 2001;84:200–204.

66. Fletcher JM, Ewing-Cobbs L, Francis DJ, Levin HS. Variability in outcomes after traumatic brain injury in children: a developmental perspective. In: Broman SH and Michel ME, eds. Traumatic Head Injury in Children. New York: Oxford; 1995:22–39.

67. Bruce DA. Outcome, does it work? In: Harris BH, ed. Progress in Pediatric Trauma. Boston: Nobb Hill Press; 1985.

68. Chiaretti A, Piastra M, Pulitano S, Pietrini D, De Rosa G, Barbaro R, Di Rocco C. Prognostic factors and outcome of children with severe head injury: an 8-year experience. Childs Nerv Syst 2002;18:129–136.

69. Johnston B, Seshia SS. Prediction of outcome in non-traumatic coma in childhood. Acta Neurol Scand 1984;69:417–427.

70. Beca J, Cox PN, Taylor MJ, Bohn D, Butt W, Logan WJ, Rutka JT, Barker G. Somatosensory evoked potentials for prediction of outcome in acute severe brain injury. J Pediatr 1995;126:44–49.

71. Robinson LR, Mickelsen PJ, Tirschwell DL, Lew HL. Predictive value of somatosensory evoked potentials for awakening from coma. Crit Care Med 2003;31:960–967.

72. Kruus S, Bergstrom L, Suutarinen T, Hyvonen R. The prognosis of near-drowned children. Acta Paediatr Scand 1979;68:315–322.

73. Goyco PG, Beckerman RC. Sudden infant death syndrome. Curr Probl Pediatr 1990;6:297–346.

74. Quan L, Wentz KR, Gore EJ, Copass MK. Outcome and predictors of outcome in pediatric submersion victims receiving prehospital care in King County Wash. Pediatrics 1990;86:586–593.

75. Spack L, Gedeit R, Splaingard M, Havens PL. Failure of aggressive therapy to alter outcome in pediatric near-drowning. Pediatr Emerg Care 1977;13:98–102.

76. Ibsen LM, Koch T. Submersion and asphyxial injury. Crit Care Med 2002;30:S402–S408.

77. Holshouser BA, Ashwal S, Luh GY, Shu S, Kahlon S, Auld KL, Tomasi LG, Perkin RM, Hinshaw DB Jr. Proton MR spectroscopy after acute central nervous system injury: outcome prediction in neonates, infants and children. Radiology 1997;202:487–496.

78. Dubowitz DJ, Bluml S, Arcinue E, Dietrich RB. MR of hypoxic encephalopathy in children after near drowning: correlation with quantitative proton MR spectroscopy and clinical outcome. Am J Neuroradiol 1998;19:1617–1627.

79. Woischneck D, Klein S, Reissberg S, Peters B, Avenarius S, Gunther G, Firsching R. Prognosis of brain stem lesion in children with head injury. Childs Nerv Syst 2003;19:174–178.

80. Christophe C, Fonteyne C, Ziereisen F, Christiaens F, Deltenre P, De Maertelaer V, Dan B. Value of MR imaging of the brain in children with hypoxic coma. AJNR Am J Neuroradiol 2002;23:716–723.

81. Vos PE. Glial and neuronal proteins in serum predict outcome after severe traumatic brain injury. Neurology 2004;62:1303–1310.

82. Christensen DW, Jansen P, Perkin RM. Outcome and acute care hospital costs after warm water near drowning in children. Pediatrics 1997;99:715–721.

83. Teasdale G, Jennett B. Assessment of coma and impaired consciousness: a practical scale. Lancet 1974;ii:81–84.

84. Simpson DA, Cockington RA, Hanieh A, Raftos J, Reilly PL. Head injuries in infants and young children: the value of the Paediatric Coma Scale. Review of literature and report on a study. Childs Nerv Syst. 1991 Aug;7(4):183–190.

8

Hypoxic Ischemic Encephalopathy After Cardiorespiratory Arrest

Dermot R. Doherty and James S. Hutchison

Introduction

This chapter focuses on the temporary cessation and subsequent restoration of cerebral blood flow, otherwise known as *transient global cerebral ischemia*. For the vast majority of patients, this is caused by cardiorespiratory arrest (CRA). Ischemic mechanisms also come into play in traumatic brain injury, stroke, acute hydrocephalus, and other encephalopathies complicated by severe intracranial hypertension [1–3]. Consequently, there is overlap in the metabolic and cellular processes of diseases of differing etiologies. A thorough review of the mechanisms of global cerebral ischemia therefore provides a basis for understanding the mechanisms of other brain injuries and encephalopathies.

There are four distinct phases relating to CRA in children: (1) pre-CRA physiologic deterioration, (2) the period of no flow, (3) the period of low flow during resuscitation, and (4) the return of circulation. The cardiopulmonary resuscitation (CPR) algorithms, and indeed much of resuscitation research, have focused on establishing the return of spontaneous circulation (ROSC). Effective resuscitation with the goal of early ROSC will have a profound impact on mortality and morbidity. This is being addressed by coordinated "code-blue" teams and training of first responders in basic cardiac life support, advanced cardiac life support, and pediatric advanced life support algorithms [4]. It is also possible that the identification of those children at risk for CRA would have a functional outcome and survival benefit, given that many children may have raised red flags of their impending deterioration in the hours before CRA. In this respect, the organization of hospital pediatric early warning systems or medical emergency teams may also have an important role [5,6].

More recently there has been a change in emphasis from merely achieving ROSC using advanced life support techniques to minimizing the impact of CRA and subsequent reperfusion injury in the brain [7]. Importantly, the term *cardiopulmonary cerebral resuscitation* (CPCR) is slowly beginning to enter medical consciousness. This is underscored by the fact that in both the adult and pediatric populations, there remains a large discrepancy between those patients who are successfully resuscitated from CRA and those patients who ultimately survive to leave the hospital without neurologic consequences. This discrepancy has been the focus of both basic and clinical research in recent times, but more research is needed to provide clinicians with the tools to treat the reperfusion injury effectively.

When ROSC is achieved after prolonged resuscitative attempts, there is significant insult to the brain, which often results in death or significant neurologic morbidity. Even with the availability of highly invasive techniques such as extracorporeal membrane oxygenation (ECMO), which can successfully restore circulation, clinicians must be aware that implementing neuroprotective strategies early in the resuscitative process is likely to improve patient outcomes.

Definitions

In 1995, a consensus paper was published describing the recommendations of a taskforce representing the American Academy of Pediatrics, The American Heart Association, and the European Resuscitation Council on the uniform reporting of pediatric advance life support [8]. It is known as the pediatric Utstein reporting style. It has standardized the way investigators record and report data from CRA studies. The essential components of the pediatric Utstein criteria are standardized descriptions of prehospital variables, hospital variables, arrest and event variables, and outcome variables. It is imperative that researchers in this field be familiar with this reporting style during the design of studies. This reporting style provides a tool to critically examine and compare studies of pediatric CRA. There have been many reports of pediatric CRA, but unfortunately the number of prospective studies to date reported using the pediatric Utstein style has been relatively small, making comparison difficult.

D.S. Wheeler et al. (eds.), *The Central Nervous System in Pediatric Critical Illness and Injury*,
DOI 10.1007/978-1-84800-993-6_8, © Springer-Verlag London Limited 2009

Epidemiology

It is difficult to know the true incidence of CRA in the pediatric population largely because of differences in how the data have been defined and collected [9,10]. An excellent review by Morris and Nadkarni summarizes much of the data from the pre-Utstein era [9]. The incidence of all inhospital CRAs is 1%–3% of the hospital population [11,12]. Approximately one third of children will have had their CRA in the community [13]. Within the pediatric intensive care unit (PICU) population, a 32-institution study reported an incidence of 1.8% of all PICU admissions [14]. Others have reported higher incidences, ranging from 6% to 14% [11,12]. Within the cardiac PICU population in a single center over 2 years, an incidence of 4% was reported [15], and the Pediatric Perioperative Cardiac Arrest Registry (POCA) reports an incidence of 1.4/10,000 related to anesthesia [16]. Not surprisingly, approximately 75% of inhospital CPR events occur in the intensive care unit [12,13].

Etiology

In recent prospective studies by Reis et al. [11] and Lopez-Herce et al. [13] most patients (71%) had chronic medical conditions before CRA. The chronic medical conditions were cardiac in 20%–21.6%, neurologic in 11%–16%, respiratory in 6%–13%, congenital malformations in 3%–11.7%, oncologic in 2.9%–13%, and other diseases in 13.8%–19% [11,13]. Of those patients having CRA in the community, the etiology was sudden infant death syndrome in 23%, trauma in 20%, sepsis in 12%, near-drowning in 9%, cardiac disease in 7%, and seizures in 7%, as reported by Schindler et al. in Toronto in 1996 [17].

Cardiac arrests are far more common than respiratory arrests, accounting for approximately three fourths versus one fourth of all CRA events [13]. However, the failing system that precipitates the CRA is predominantly the respiratory system (approximately 60%), with septic shock as the next leading cause, accounting for 18% of CRAs [11,13]. Not surprisingly, bradycardia and asystole are the predominant cardiac rhythms (88%) at the time of CRA [11,12]. Pulseless ventricular arrhythmias are less common, accounting for 10% of CRAs [13], which is in stark contrast to the adult population [13,18] where ventricular tachyarrhythmias account for the vast majority. An important exception to these etiologies is seen within the cardiac PICU population, where arrhythmia and shock account for 60%–70% of CRAs [12,15].

Pathophysiology of Global Cerebral Ischemia

Energy Failure

Following cardiac arrest there is complete cessation of blood flow, which deprives the brain of substrates for energy production (oxygen and glucose). The remaining glucose and glycogen are rapidly metabolized to lactate as cells switch from oxidative phosphorylation to anaerobic respiration. Lactate levels will rise exponentially and proportional to plasma glucose levels and will coincide with hydrolysis of adenosine triphosphate (ATP), causing $[H^+]$ to increase [19]. Hyperglycemia will worsen hypoxic brain damage [20].

During global ischemia the brain loses its ability to generate energy (Figure 8.1). The breakdown of ATP to adenosine and

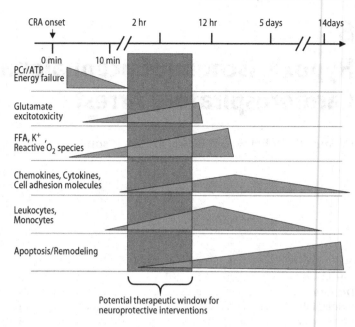

FIGURE 8.1. Pathophysiology of hypoxic–ischemic brain injury following cardiorespiratory arrest (CRA) and potential therapeutic window for neuroprotective strategies. ATP, adenosine triphosphate; FFA, free fatty acids; PCr, phosphocreatine.

organic phosphate is buffered initially by creatine phosphokinase, adenosine diphosphate (ADP), and adenosine monophosphate (AMP), but, if no phosphate bonds are being generated, the buffering capacity is rapidly exceeded [21]. During this early phase, the brain will conserve energy by inhibiting neural activity through membrane hyperpolarization, caused initially by the opening of voltage-dependent K^+ channels and later by ATP-dependent K^+ channels [22]. Clinically, we see this manifest as unconsciousness and quickly followed by isoelectric EEG within a minute of CRA. This "neural shutdown" is short lived, as it is followed by a failure to maintain membrane electrochemical gradients over the next few minutes. There is rapid uncoordinated depolarization caused by K^+ efflux and Na^+ and Ca^{2+} influx into the cell. This will result in two major events. First, there will be an osmotic shift and conformational change in the cell membrane, which will lead to dysfunction of transmembrane structures. Some cells may rapidly lyse or progress to necrosis. Second, the electrochemical threshold for excitation will be passed, and there is rapid uncontrolled synaptic activity known as *anoxic depolarization*. This will lead to excessive release of primarily excitatory neurotransmitters, which is known as *excitotoxicity* [22].

Excitotoxicity and Calcium

Neurotransmitters released initially by changes in electrochemical gradients and ionic flux will cause further release of predominantly excitatory compounds of which the most abundant and most studied is glutamate. Although not the only mediator in this synaptic maelstrom, glutamate acts in three main receptor types, N-methyl-D-aspartate (NMDA), alpha-amino-3-hydroxy-5-methyl-4-isoxazoleproprionate (AMPA), and kainate receptors, causing further ionic flux. Other substances, such as gamma-aminobutyric acid (GABA), adenosine, and serotonin, attenuate the effect of glutamate, but excitotoxic effects predominate.

N-methyl-D-aspartate receptor activation provides a major stimulus for the rapid influx of calcium, more so than AMPA or kainate receptor activation, and, because of this, NMDA receptor antagonism has been a primary therapeutic target for neuroprotective research [23]. A vicious circle of uncontrolled metabolic activity, neuronal body swelling, and further neurotransmitter release ensues.

The role of calcium as a second messenger is pivotal, as it promotes spreading depolarization and triggers a multitude of cytotoxic molecular cascades that will further deplete cell energy stores [24] and promote apoptosis or necrosis [25]. Calcium concentrations in the cell increase secondary to influx of interstitial calcium but also from the release of calcium from the endoplasmic reticulum. The plethora of Ca^{2+}-activated events includes the activation of proteases, DNAses, and lipases. Examples include mitogen activated protein kinases (MAP kinases), including c-Jun NH_2-terminal kinase, p38, and extracellular signal regulating kinases, that may trigger cell death pathways [26]. Calpains are Ca^{2+}-activated serine proteases that have been implicated in excitotoxic neuronal death [27]. Protein kinase C (PKC) activation will exacerbate excitotoxicity and neuronal excitability [28].

Membrane phospholipids are broken down during ischemia by the activation of phospholipase A_2 and phospholipase C [29]. The products of lipid breakdown such as free fatty acids (FFA), diacylglycerol (DAG), and platelet-activating factor (PAF) will behave as lipid messengers and activate important modulators of neuronal activity such as PKC [30]. Lipid membrane products generated by the lipase activation have further implications. The first relates to the loss of structural integrity within the cells or its organelles, and the second relates to the generation of metabolites of FFA, DAG, and PAF. The peroxidation of lipid membrane molecules by reactive oxygen species (ROS) can generate nitric oxide, superoxide, and hydroxyl radicals, which further damage membranes and DNA and can lead to cell death.

Reactive Oxygen Species and Reperfusion Injury

Under normal circumstances, the brain controls its regional/local blood flow in proportion to neuronal activity with important vasoregulatory compounds such as nitric oxide (NO). Nitric oxide is generated from NO synthase (NOS) in the endothelium, neuron, and interstitium from the amino acid L-arginine. In the presence of ROS, NOS combines with ROS to generate peroxynitrite at a rate outpacing the rate of its absorption by scavengers, such as superoxide dismutase. Peroxynitrite is an extremely volatile substance that damages DNA and other cellular components.

Mitochondrial Injury

The increase in cytosolic calcium can trigger the formation of membrane transport pores in the mitochondrial membrane [31]. These portals can allow free passage of cytosolic compounds into the mitochondrial lumen and interfere with the inner mitochondrial membranes and elements of the respiratory chain. The mitochondrion can lyse in this scenario, or its contents will leak out. Cytochrome c is one of the mitochondrial compounds that leaks into the cytosol and executes the intrinsic apoptotic cascade by activating caspases and poly(ADP)-ribose polymerase (PARP) cleavage [32]. Energy failure therefore precipitates mitochondrial disruption, which triggers programmed cell death (apoptosis) through cytochrome c release.

Inflammation

The inflammatory responses in the first few minutes of hypoxic–ischemic encephalopathies consist of both humeral and cellular components. Proinflammatory cytokines such as interleukin (IL)-1β, tumor necrosis factor (TNF)-α, and IL-8 are released from the cerebral microvascular endothelium and brain parenchyma. Chemotaxis and activation of leukocytes and microglia will occur, and upregulation of cell adhesion molecules will stimulate increased leukocyte trafficking in the cerebral microcirculation. Compared with thromboembolic stroke, where leukocytes are very prominent in the perinecrotic tissue, the role of leukocytes in transient global ischemia is not yet clear. There has been no temporal or mechanistic relationship demonstrated between inflammation and the fate of neural tissue in transient global ischemia [33]. It is, however, probable that leukocytes play some role in transient global ischemia, as they are seen to be adherent to the cerebral endothelium within minutes of reperfusion [34].

The blood–brain barrier (BBB) is intermittently disrupted after cerebral ischemia. Microstructural conformational changes mediated by inflammation lead to this loss of BBB integrity [35]. This creates another vicious cycle in which a combination of vasogenic edema from increased BBB permeability and cytogenic edema generated through multiple pathways leads to cerebral edema.

Apoptosis and Necrosis

Cell death occurs by both apoptotic and necrotic mechanisms following transient global ischemia. Many of the mediators reviewed earlier can trigger pathways leading to cell death. Some of the cardinal features of apoptosis are not always present following global ischemia because of overlap between some of the molecular and morphologic features of cell death [36,37]. In global ischemia, there is not an anatomically defined penumbra as there is in stroke, where apoptosis plays a clear role [38,39]. However, in various animal models of transient global ischemia cell death is attenuated by pharmacologic therapies that inhibit apoptotic cascades [40,41]. It is possible that there is a spectrum of neuronal death following global ischemia, with both necrosis and apoptosis playing a role. Molecules that trigger cell death, such as ROS, can lead to DNA damage and activation of caspases and PARP. The PARPs are an important group of enzymes, whose activation may not be adequate to repair the damaged DNA, in which case the damaged cells are removed by apoptosis. Excessive activation of PARPs leads to depletion of nicotinamide adenine dinucleotide and ATP, causing deterioration in the cell's energy potential leading to necrosis. Cell content leakage leads to promotion of transcription of proinflammatory genes by neighboring cells [42].

No Reflow and Delayed Hypoperfusion

The no-reflow phenomenon describes a situation in which there is no flow in some microvessels upon reperfusion following cerebral ischemia [43]. This has been attributed to adherent neutrophils, endothelial swelling, blood hyperviscosity, and platelet aggregates accumulating in microvessels in the no-flow period during CRA [44].

It has been understood for some time that, after global cerebral ischemia and reperfusion, there is a brief (several minute) period of relative hyperperfusion followed by a prolonged (several hour) period of low cerebral blood flow (delayed hypoperfusion [45,46].

The mechanism of delayed hypoperfusion is not clear, but there is evidence of vasoactive substances mediating vasoconstriction. For example endothelin-1 antagonism and L-arginine infusion have been shown to reduce delayed hypoperfusion [47,48]. It is important to note that during delayed hypoperfusion metabolic recovery is impaired by an inability to deliver adequate substrate to meet the metabolic demands.

Neuropathology

The pattern of selective vulnerability of neurons to hypoxia ischemia evolves with the developing brain. Infants tend to have selective neuronal loss in the diencephalons, olives, and hippocampus, with relative sparing of the cerebral cortex and cerebellum. In contrast, older children and adults have selective neuronal loss in layers III and V of the cortex (especially in the watershed zones between the anterior-middle and posterior cerebral arteries), the CA1 and CA3 regions of the hippocampus, and the Purkinje layers of the cerebellum [49,50]. This type of damage is usually delayed and is preceded by a maturation period, which tends to be inversely proportional to the length of the precipitating ischemic event [51]. Krep et al. reported a timeline of metabolic recovery using diffusion and perfusion weighted magnetic resonance imaging (MRI) studies of animals resuscitated from CRA [52]. The rate and topographic pattern of recovery reflects those areas that show histologic evidence of ischemic injury in other models.

Outcomes

Historically, the outcome of CRA in children has been dismal. The mechanism of the arrest is also important, with a better survival outcome from respiratory arrest than from cardiac arrest (approximately 70% vs. 33%) [9,13]. Out-of-hospital CRA has the worst prognosis, with an ROSC rate of approximately 14%, hospital survival rate of approximately 7%, and an intact neurologic survival rate of approximately 3% [9,17,53]. In hospital CRA has a better outcome, with approximately 60% achieving ROSC; however, the survival rate drops to 30% at 24hr and 15% at 1 year [11,12,15,54]. It is clear from this discrepancy between short- and long-term survival rates following ROSC that other factors play a major role in the mortality and functional outcome.

Neurologic Injury After Cardiorespiratory Arrest

The outcome of CRA is related to many different factors, with many children dying of the disease that precipitated the CRA. Survival is inversely proportional to the duration of the cardiac arrest [13], which reflects the duration of cerebral ischemia. A diagnosis of brain death accounted for 15% of those children who died between days 1 and 7 after ROSC, but this represents the severest of neurologic injuries. Approximately one half of the children who could be neurologically assessed (i.e., not sedated or muscle relaxed) demonstrated neurologic injury, which was reflected with significantly increased mortality (56.8%) compared with those who could not be assessed or respond to tactile stimulus (18.7%) [13]. Interestingly, of those children who are alive at 1 year (10%–18%), the vast majority (73%–84%) return to baseline function and have a good neurologic outcome (pediatric cerebral performance category [PCPC] grade 1–2) [11,15,55]. Children with the most severe neurologic injury have a

high mortality rate. In addition, many of those patients who remain comatose will ultimately have their life support withdrawn [13].

Therapy

At this time, there are no specific therapies aimed at neuroprotection recommended for children. This situation is likely to change as translational research emerges from the basic science models and the results of current research are analyzed. The clinician can, however, use existing knowledge of pathophysiology and make use of monitoring modalities available to intensivists to optimize care aimed specifically at the brain after ROSC or commencement of ECMO flow (Table 8.1). The restoration of an adequate cerebral blood flow and oxygen delivery on the one hand, with the minimization of metabolic activity on the other hand, should be the main principles of post-ROSC brain care.

TABLE 8.1. Suggested algorithm after return of spontaneous circulation (ROSC).

Established Care Standard
Normal oxygen
Normocarbia
Normotension
Normothermia
Normoglycaemia
Normal hematocrit
Treat seizures
Determine Risk of CNS Injury

Short CRA Duration 1–5 min	Moderate CRA Duration 5–20 min	Prolonged CRA Duration >20 min

Balanced Clinical Decision Given Factors Determined by:
1. Pre-morbid physiological deterioration severity
2. Chronic medical condition
3. Duration of resuscitation and interventions
4. Expressed wishes of patient, parent(s) or guardians
5. Likelihood of meaningful recovery

Continue conventional care	Consider experimental therapies	Limiting/withdrawing life support if prognosis grave
• Early neurologic assessments.	• Mild hypothermia up to 48 hr (32°–34°C)	• Clinical prognostic examination
• Attention to normal physiologic parameters	• Post-ROSC hypertension	• Electrophysiology
• Option to broaden scope of neuroprotection	• Targeted sedation	• MRI
	• Hyperosmolar therapy	• Biochemical tests

Prognostic Tools
Neurological examination
• Good: Conjugate eye movements, extensor motor response at 24 hr
• Bad: Absent pupillary response, disconjugate eye movement, flexor motor response or worse (24 hr)

Somatosensory evoked potential
• Bad: Absent N20 Median SSEPs at 24 hr
• Good: Long-latency SSEPs less than 120 msec

Electroencephalograph
• Good: Return of EEG slowing and sleep pattern preservation
• Bad: Isoelectric, burst suppression, low amplitude, alpha rhythm

MRI scanning
• Good: MRI scan score ≤2
• Bad: MRI scan score >2

Note: CNS, central nervous system; CRA, cardiorespiratory arrest; MRI, magnetic resonance imaging; SSEP, somatosensory evoked potential.

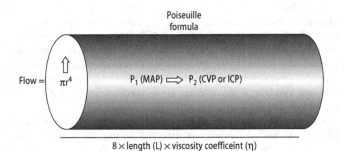

FIGURE 8.2. The Poiseuille equation. CVP, central venous pressure; ICP, intracranial pressure; MAP, mean arterial pressure.

Optimizing Perfusion

Using the Poiseuille-Hagan formula (which describes flow in a tube), one can conceptualize the perfusion variables with regard to the brain (Figure 8.2). For blood to flow, there must be an arteriovenous pressure gradient (P_1–P_2), and in the brain the upstream pressure is mean arterial pressure (MAP). Under normal circumstances the downstream pressure is intracerebral pressure (ICP) or cerebral/central venous pressure. However, in pathologic circumstances, the ICP is the effective downstream pressure. In this context, cerebral perfusion pressure (CCP) is MAP – ICP.

The other major contribution of the Poiseuille-Hagan formula is that flow is a function of πr^4, where r = the radius of the tube. This formula clearly demonstrates that flow and substrate delivery are far more dependent on the radius of a blood vessel than the arterial to venous pressure gradient. Within the brain, carbon dioxide tension is a major contributor to vascular diameter. In the recent past, control of ICP was achieved through hyperventilation promoting cerebral vasoconstriction and lowering total brain blood volume. Hyperventilation clearly reduces flow to the brain, leading to poorer outcomes following CRA, and should not be used [56].

The final variable from the Poiseuille-Hagan formula is viscosity. Because viscosity (η) is a denominator in the equation, a lower value of η would result in a higher value for Q, or flow [57]. However, this needs to be balanced by the fact that there must be adequate hematocrit for oxygen delivery, and the effect of higher viscosity must be balanced by the need to decrease microvascular flow disturbance [58]. The balance of cerebral oxygen supply and demand can be monitored by measuring the surrogate of cerebral venous blood oxygenation (jugular venous oxygen saturation).

The roles of delayed hypoperfusion and the no-reflow phenomenon in the pathophysiology of hypoxic–ischemic brain injury have been addressed using several models [44]. In the 1970s, the late Peter Safer of Pittsburgh, who was a luminary in the field of resuscitation research, demonstrated in dogs that high perfusion pressure after ROSC overcame the no-reflow problem and was associated with better outcome. He recommended a "hypertensive bout" after ROSC that would act as a hydrodynamic rescue for hypoperfusion [59].

Metabolic Supply and Demand

Administration of 100% oxygen is recommended during CPCR. Some have questioned this recommendation, as higher PaO_2 levels may provide a ready source of ROS. There are some animal and human data to support resuscitation using room air to decrease ROS. However, a recent Cochrane review concludes that there is insufficient evidence to recommend this [60]. There is little rationale or evidence to use hypoxic mixtures to prevent reperfusion injury, so normal physiologic oxygen tension is a reasonable goal. Indeed, it may be that the recovering brain has a higher oxygen extraction ratio. Clues to this come from intraparenchymal oxygen sensors in brain that reflect lower brain tissue oxygen tensions than those measured systemically [61].

As mentioned previously, $PaCO_2$ has an enormous role in control of cerebral blood volume and ICP. For reasons mentioned earlier, hypocarbia is not recommended following cardiac arrest. There is a suggestion that in other models of organ dysfunction higher CO_2 has cytoprotective functions [62]. However, the current recommendation is to maintain normocarbia following global cerebral ischemia.

As mentioned previously, the ability to regenerate the energy potential of the brain is key to reestablishment of homeostasis. There is, however, evidence that oversupply of glucose leads to generation of excessive lactate or H^+, which is injurious after hypoxic brain injury. The avoidance of hypoglycemia and the pursuit of normoglycemia are reasonable therapeutic goals after ROSC.

Hypothermia Therapy

Hypothermia therapy remains the basis of neuroprotection for circulatory arrest or low-flow cardiopulmonary bypass in complex cardiac surgery and also in certain neurosurgical procedures [63,64]. It was also used in the 1980s to treat cerebral edema in children following cardiac arrest caused by near-drowning [65,66]. Interest in this therapy has increased again recently after the simultaneous publication of two studies that demonstrated a tangible improvement in survival and neurologic outcome when hypothermia therapy was used following cardiac arrest caused by acute ventricular fibrillation in adults [67,68]. Indeed, current recommendations for resuscitation are that adults resuscitated after cardiac arrest because of ventricular dysrhythmia should undergo hypothermia therapy [7]. Recent studies of hypothermia therapy in newborns with hypoxic–ischemic encephalopathy also demonstrate an improved survival rate and neurologic outcome [69]. The effect of hypothermia therapy in children following cardiac arrest is unknown, but it is clear from research that we have carried out that hypothermia therapy is being used in children. At this time, there is clinical equipoise among pediatric intensivists regarding the use of therapeutic hypothermia, so an appropriately powered randomized controlled trial needs to be done in this patient population.

Recently, research in rodent models of global cerebral ischemia demonstrated that if mild hypothermia was implemented within 1–6 hr following the ischemia for durations of 12–48 hr, both histologic and functional outcomes were improved [70–72]. It may be that the use of hypothermia may be more pronounced in younger animals [73]. Mild hypothermia protects against neuronal loss in the hippocampus (CA1) and improves neurobehavioral outcome following 5 min of global (two-vessel occlusion) cerebral ischemia in the gerbil [36,70,71,73]. The protection against loss of CA1 neurons and memory deficits is sustained for at least 6 months following the injury [71]. Mild hypothermia is most beneficial when applied immediately following the ischemic insult [36] and for longer durations (i.e., 48 hr). Mild hypothermia of 48 hr duration is effective even when the onset of hypothermia is delayed 6 hr after 10 min of severe forebrain ischemia in the rat [72].

Proposed mechanisms of action of postischemic hypothermia therapy include decreased cerebral metabolism [74], antiinflammatory effects [75,76], decreased glutamate concentrations [2,77], decreased generation of free radicals and lipid peroxidation [78], decreased heat shock protein response [79], and kinase activation [80]. We have also demonstrated that hypothermia has selective antiinflammatory effects decreasing the expression of nuclear factor kappa B (NFκB) and secretion of IL-8 by cerebral endothelial cells, thereby limiting leukocyte recruitment to the cerebral microcirculation [76]. In summary, the results of animal studies and studies of adult and newborn humans support further study of therapeutic hypothermia after CRA for children.

Pharmacotherapy

Anesthesia and Sedation

Sedation therapy is ubiquitous in intensive care units, aimed primarily at the facilitation of mechanical ventilation, invasive procedures, and anxiolysis. Anesthetic agents and sedatives have the added benefit of decreasing the cerebral metabolic rate of oxygen ($CMRO_2$) in a dose-dependent manner. The degree to which they do this is variable depending on the compound, and both intravenous and gaseous aesthetics have been extensively investigated in this role. Most neuro-intensive care unit sedation studies focus on control of neurophysiology as an outcome, without the power to detect a survival difference related to the choice of agent [81].

Inhalation Anesthetics

Isoflurane produces an isoelectric EEG and dramatically decreases $CMRO_2$ at clinically relevant doses, and it has been shown to produce less necrosis than a fentanyl–nitrous oxide combination after global ischemia in mice [82]. A similar study of complete and incomplete forebrain ischemia showed significant neuroprotection in terms of selectively vulnerable neurons and functional outcome compared with fentanyl and ketamine [83]. Isoflurane has a neuroprotective effect through upregulation of the antiapoptotic protein kinase B (Akt) [84]. However, another study showed that isoflurane exerted a proapoptotic effect by endoplasmic reticulum calcium depletion in a neuronal cell model (in vitro) [85]. Traditionally, isoflurane has been called the neuroanesthetic of choice, but because, of its impracticality in terms of machinery, scavenging, and manpower, routine use in the intensive care unit has never occurred.

Barbiturates

Reports in the 1980s of the use of barbiturate-induced coma and hypothermia therapy for children following near-drowning described adverse outcomes, and both of these therapies fell out of favor for some time [66]. Studies previous to this cast doubt on the efficacy of high-dose barbiturate in complete cerebral ischemia in dogs [86,87]. Thiopental produces EEG burst suppression at clinically relevant doses, but, compared with hypothermia therapy, the time to reach anoxic depolarization is reached earlier with thiopental [88]. More recent data suggest a synergistic neuroprotective effect of hypothermia and thiopental after CRA [89]. While intuitively it makes sense to lower $CMRO_2$, adverse outcomes with barbiturates may reflect the side effects of the barbiturate rather than the central nervous system effect.

Propofol has been used in neuro-intensive care because of its titratable pharmacokinetic profile. It provides metabolic suppression, which can result in a fall in ICP [90], and it has potential neuroprotective properties [91]. Recently there has been some animal data showing the upregulation of antiapoptotic proteins by propofol after cerebral ischemia [92]. Given the reports of propofol infusion syndrome in children, prolonged use in the PICU is not recommended [93].

Sedation therapy is used in most cases after PICU admission after CRA, and the reader is directed to the relevant literature [81,94]. The choice of agents varies among PICUs. The clinician should be familiar with each agent and understand and prescribe based on the goals to be achieved by a given agent and the risk/benefit ratio and cost of the sedative for a specific patient. When the prognosis is grave, sedative agents should be withheld in order to assess the neurologic status of the patient.

Suppressing Excitotoxicity and Calcium Flux

The rationale for the use of GABA agonists is that they will raise the threshold for uncontrolled depolarization by their action on the chloride channel. Chlormethiazole, GABA, gamma-hydroxybutyrate, and tiagabine have been examined in mainly rodent models. There was protection against neuronal death when animals were treated with these agents; however, promising early studies did not translate into a long-term functional outcome benefit [95–98]. Similarly, the NMDA antagonist properties of ketamine did not result in significant improvement in neurohistologic outcome [83]. Indeed, ketamine may be proapoptotic in the developing brain [99].

Calcium channel blockers in many forms have been studied in stroke studies. In a review by Horn and Limburg, an analysis of 47 trials of calcium antagonists failed to show a clinically important effect [100]. While acknowledging that stroke and transient global ischemia are different entities, the role of calcium certainly overlaps. Nimodipine is used in neuro-intensive care for prophylaxis against cerebral vasospasm following subarachnoid haemorrhage. It does not provide a neuroprotective effect in rodent models of CRA, especially at high doses [101], but lower doses may offer some albeit marginal benefit [102]. In the same study, the author reports that flunarizine provided more substantial neurohistologic protection at a lower dose range [102], which has also been seen in a fetal brain injury model in sheep [103]. Dantrolene, which stabilizes the release of calcium from the endoplasmic reticulum, has been shown to attenuate glutamate release and improve neurohistologic outcome in a rodent model [104]. Recently a report in *Cell* suggests that calcium flux may be mediated by the effect of acidosis on sensitive transmembrane ion channels, which would offer a new therapeutic approach for modulating calcium in hypoxia ischemia [105]. As more is learned about the role of calcium channels in reperfusion injury, there will be future investigation into targeted calcium channel manipulation following global cerebral ischemia (Aarts, 2002).

No Reflow and Delayed Reperfusion

Recently, investigators have studied mechanisms of improving flow by addressing some of the causes of no reflow and delayed hypoperfusion. Osmotic therapies using starches and hypertonic saline have had mixed results. The rationale behind their use is twofold: to increase the circulating volume and to reduce brain edema volume (and hence ICP). Hypertonic saline is of particular interest, as it may have an antiinflammatory mechanism in that it sheds adhesion molecules and hence may reduce the leukocyte–endothelial interaction [106]. Other attempts have been reported addressing platelet plugging specifically as a cause of no reflow using heparin and tissue plasminogen activator [52]. These have failed to produce sustained improvements in delayed hypoperfusion.

Antiinflammatory Therapies and Immunomodulation

Given that the inflammatory response is significant after reperfusion, and the inducible cyclooxygenase (COX) synthase plays a key role, it is not surprising that numesulide, a COX-2 inhibitor, had a beneficial effect in a gerbil global ischemia model, as did a COX-2 knockout model [107,108]. Similarly, ibuprofen has been shown to be neuroprotective in vitro and in vivo by an antiinflammatory mechanism [109]. Immunosuppressants have neuroprotective effects, albeit specific to their mechanisms of action.

Adhesion molecules may play an important role after CRA in terms of their effects on the cellular inflammatory response and cerebral blood flow/no reflow. Antiadhesion antibodies (CD11b/CD18, intercellular adhesion molecule [ICAM]-1, vascular cell adhesion molecule [VCAM]) hold promise in stroke [34,110]. The rationale for their use is that first there have been reports that neutrophil depletion or adhesion antagonism improves microvascular flow and second that antiinflammatory effects may attenuate cell death pathways. Clinical trials of anticellular adhesion molecule antibodies in stroke have not been successful [111]. Although there is upregulation of adhesion molecules after transient global ischemia, there is not a strong leukocyte response in this type of injury [33]. Intercellular adhesion molecule-1–deficient mice failed to demonstrate neuroprotection after global ischemia [112]. We have demonstrated that hypothermia therapy significantly attenuates cerebral endothelial adhesion receptor expression and leukocyte adhesion to the endothelium following global ischemia [113], and this is associated with neuroprotection. However, we are currently investigating whether this effect is an important therapeutic mechanism of hypothermia therapy.

Other pharmacologic therapies have been approached and reported in this immense field of neuroprotection research. Some of the notable reports are with hormones, especially progesterone and estrogens. For a concise review of pharmacotherapeutic approaches, the reader is directed to a review by Weigl et al. [114].

Monitoring of Parameters That Affect the Brain After Return of Spontaneous Circulation

With data emerging from neuromonitoring studies, it is clear that secondary hypoxic–ischemic injury can occur following ROSC. The concept of anoxic depolarization describes waves of synaptic activity after injury [115]. This depolarization can increase metabolic demand at a time when cerebral blood flow is low (delayed hypoperfusion) [116]. This poses a challenge for the intensivist in that further evolution of the injury may be taking place, and we are not routinely monitoring for or able to prevent it.

Standard cardiorespiratory monitoring is essential for the acute phase of ischemic encephalopathy to create the correct physiologic substrate for brain recovery after CRA. Blood pressure, central venous oxygen saturations as a surrogate measure of cardiac output, and respiratory gas tensions should be monitored and maintained in the normal range. Temperature should also be recorded and normothermia maintained. We monitor lower esophageal temperature as a surrogate of brain temperature (Bissonnette, 2000). Even though tight parameters are being achieved and recorded, occult hypoxic events in the brain are common [117].

Jugular venous bulb oximetry ($SjvO_2$) measures the venous oxygen saturation in the jugular venous bulb (which is consider the venous outflow tract from the brain), using a similar principle to the pulse oximeter. Modern fiberoptic sensor probes provide continuous monitoring of the percentage saturation of jugular bulb venous blood, which is around 55%–71%. A value of <50% may represent ischemia, but it must be taken in the context of the cerebral DO_2. Isolated from the PaO_2 and lactate, a low or normal $SjvO_2$ may be erroneous as there is the potential for technical error caused by catheter misplacement or displacement. For example, a catheter too low will mix with extracranial venous blood, and a catheter placed too high may measure a nondominant hemisphere. A normal $SjvO_2$ may also reflect decreased oxygen extraction because of shunting or a shift in the O_2 dissociation curve to the left. Management of $SjvO_2$ is concisely reviewed by Feldman and Robertson [118], and further study is needed it can be recommended for general use in children after CRA.

Near-infrared spectroscopy (NIRS) is a noninvasive method of measuring regional cerebral oxygenation saturation ($StcrO_2$). Near-infrared spectroscopy works on the principle that the cranium is transparent to near-infrared wavelengths, and there is differential absorption of near-infrared light by substances relevant to oxygenation. The peak absorbance of deoxygenated hemoglobin is 760 nm and that of oxygenated hemoglobin is 900 nm, with the absorbance of total hemoglobin peaking at approximately 800 nm. Oxidized cytochrome oxidase has an absorbance spectrum of approximately 800–900 nm, and, when this substance becomes reduced during anoxia, this absorbance spectrum will disappear from the blood. This ratio of deoxyhemoglobin to O_2 hemoglobin and cytochrome oxidase is reported as a percentage of saturated blood or as an absolute value, reflecting the metabolic status of the tissue under the probe. However, there are sources of error caused by nonspecific absorbance from other chromophores and, depending on the patient, a variable optical path length for light. Modern monitors will compensate for these sources of error. However, three problems recur. First, there is interpatient variability because of bone and/or soft tissue density differences, which makes comparison or definition of relative values difficult. Second, despite one probe measuring the oxygenation of the cerebral tissue compartment and the second measuring the oxygenation of the noncerebral tissue compartment, there is contamination between the two compartments. Third, NIRS will measure the metabolic status of the venous compartment, the arterial compartment, and the cerebral microcirculation. The proportion to which any one of these compartments contributes to the absorbance of near-infrared light at any one time varies particularly in pathologic conditions. It is generally accepted that the $StcrO_2$ is a mixture of arterial and venous saturations.

As the technology was initially thought to be more accurate for neonates and children, most of the experience with NIRS is reported in the pediatric literature, particularly in cardiopulmonary bypass for congenital heart disease. Considering the potential problems with accuracy, this technology does correlate well with metabolic status [119]. When compared with $SjvO_2$, in pediatric cardiac surgical patients, $NIRS/TcrO_2$ generally correlates well, with the proviso that it overestimates low $SjvO_2$ and underestimates high $SjvO_2$

values [120]. A recent study in adults with traumatic brain injury reported that TcrO$_2$ <60% correlated with CPP, severity of injury, and outcome [116]. Unfortunately, there are no data relating to children resuscitated from CRA to our knowledge. Given the improvement in this technology, and the fact it is noninvasive and portable, its utility should be investigated for children after CRA.

Invasive ICP monitoring has been used in the past, but treatment of ICP was not associated with improved outcome so the practice has been abandoned. Transcranial cerebral Doppler measurement, similar to other sonographic vascular assessments, can give the user real-time information on the volume, velocity, and characteristics of flow, usually measured in the middle cerebral artery [121]. The clinician can see the effects of raised ICP on the volume of blood and judge therapeutic maneuvers in real time [90]. The presence of diastolic flow reversal may indicate severe ICP elevation where there is little or no antegrade cerebral blood flow. Given the emerging technologies available, we recommend that the use of one or a combination of these neuromonitoring techniques to assess the adequacy of cerebral oxygen delivery should be further investigated [122].

Prognosis

Many patients resuscitated after CRA remain comatose for a variable period of time, and even experienced clinicians cannot reliably predict prognosis in terms of functional outcome or survival early after CRA [123] using standard clinical criteria. There are clinical, radiologic, biochemical, and electrophysiologic tests described, but the physician must balance the entire clinical picture with an eye to determine what is useful, practical, and available to help predict outcome.

History and Physical Examination

As mentioned earlier, the duration of cardiac arrest and the location (out-of-hospital or inhospital) of CRA have an impact on survival. Confounders to this are hypoxic preconditioning because of the child's chronic medical condition and hypothermic near-drowning. Anecdotally, chronically hypoxic children seem to be able to tolerate CRA better than previously healthy children, and there may be sound metabolic reasons for this.

Levy et al. [124] determined that absent pupillary reflexes at initial examination universally predicted poor outcome. The presence of a pupillary response with spontaneous conjugate albeit roving eye movements and the presence of motor extensor response or better was associated with favorable outcome. At 24 hr, the absence of conjugate eye movements and motor responses that were flexor or worse predicted adverse outcome [124]. The loss of other brain stem reflexes is usually a sinister sign, as it would be unlikely that higher cortical function would remain normal in the presence of a compromised brain stem. The development of seizures and myoclonus evolving to status myoclonus or epilepticus is significant [125].

Biochemical Markers

Three markers have been reported to have prognostic value after CRA; neuron-specific enolase (NSE), S100β protein, and neurofilament protein. However, there are few pediatric data for CRA. In a prospective adult study, NSE demonstrated a wide range (1.8–250 μg/L) in those patients who did not recover consciousness after CRA, predicting 64% of poor neurologic outcomes [126]. Similar reports have been made for the protein S100β. Most reports use these neurobiologic markers along with clinical and electrophysiologic investigations. Zingler et al. reported NSE and S100β on days 1,3, and 7, combined with somatosensory evoked potentials (SSEPs) had a 100% specificity [127], whereas clinical and biochemical examinations at 72 hr have been recommended by others [128]. There is variation in the literature as to the level of NSE or S100β that is the cut-off for prediction of poor outcome, but a serum concentration >25 μg/L should raise concerns of unfavorable outcome. Importantly, high levels of these proteins were predictive of poor outcome measured using the Glasgow Outcome Scale but were not predictive of the secondary outcomes of the activity of daily living index and the mini-mental state examination [129].

Electroencephalography

The EEG has been extensively studied following CRA in adults and in birth asphyxia in neonates, but there are few studies with children [130]. There have been attempts to provide prognostic criteria with the EEG, but unfortunately they have not gained wide acceptance [131]. As a general principle, patients with isoelectric EEGs, burst suppression, invariant and unreactive low-amplitude recordings, and alpha rhythms usually have poor outcomes [131,132]. Patients with mild slowing of the EEG and the return of sleep patterns tend to have better outcomes [133]. Electroencephalographic findings should be taken in context with the whole clinical picture. Further investigation is needed for children with CRA.

Somatosensory Evoked Potentials

Using the median nerve bilaterally, two types of SSEPs have been used to predict outcome in hypoxic–ischemic brain injury; short-latency and long-latency peaks. Short-latency peaks (N20) SSEPs reflect the thalamocortical region or the cervicomedullary region to the sensory cortex. Long-latency SSEP (N70) peaks reflect corticocortical activity. A bilaterally absent N20 peak at 24 hr is uniformly fatal; however, preservation of the N20 does not predict favorable or undesirable outcome [123]. Early appearance (less than 110 msec) of long-latency (N70) peaks is usually a good sign; however, when the long-latency N70 peak appears with increasing delay or is absent, it correlates with adverse outcome [134]. Madl et al. [134] demonstrated that an N70 peak measured after 130 msec is a sensitive measurement of poor outcome. A range of outcomes is seen in patients whose N70 peaks are seen between 111 and 127 msec.

A systematic review by Zandbergen et al. [130] demonstrated that absent pupillary reflexes, absent motor responses on day 3, isoelectric EEG, and burst suppression were 100% specific, albeit with sometimes wide confidence intervals. They concluded that short cortical SSEPs had the lowest pooled false-positive rates and narrowest confidence intervals and as such was the most useful method to predict outcome [130].

Imaging Modalities

Standard CT scanning is probably the most available imaging modality. However, it lacks sensitivity or specificity to address prognosis. An MRI score has a high sensitivity (96%) for predicting poor outcome in children with hypoxic–ischemic brain injury

[135]. Diffusion weighted MRI, which is sensitive to cellular water shifts, may also be a sensitive tool for prognostication after CRA [136].

Conclusion

Following a significant CRA and ROSC, children need to be monitored and treated in a PICU to prevent a secondary brain injury from hypoxia, hypotension, hypo- or hyperglycemia, seizures, and hyperthermia. Recognizing children at risk of CRA is very important for those who have their CRA on the hospital wards, and for this early warning mechanisms will clearly have a role. Given that 70% of patients have their CRA in the intensive care unit, they have been identified as already being at high risk. The use of prophylactic interventions such as appropriate use of ECMO might be indicated in specific cases. Further studies of neuromonitoring techniques for cerebral oxygenation and electrical and metabolic activities are needed. Further studies of hypothermia therapy are also needed for this patient population. There is increasing knowledge of the molecular pathways that lead to cell death in the brain during the reperfusion injury, and hopefully this research will lead to novel therapies. Prognosis can be determined clinically in patients with prolonged arrest who remain comatose following ROSC. For some patients, EEG, SSEPs, and MRI will help the clinician to determine prognosis.

References

1. Czosnyka M, Pickard JD. Monitoring and interpretation of intracranial pressure. J Neurol Neurosurg Psychiatry 2004;75(6):813–821.
2. Marion DW, Penrod LE, Kelsey SF, Obrist WD, Kochanek PM, Palmer AM, Wisniewski SR, DeKosky ST. Treatment of traumatic brain injury with moderate hypothermia. N Engl J Med 1997;336(8):540–546.
3. Teasdale GM, Graham DI. Craniocerebral trauma: protection and retrieval of the neuronal population after injury. Neurosurgery 1998; 43(4):723–737.
4. Lopez-Herce J, Carrillo A, Sancho L, Moral R, Bustinza A, Serina C. Pediatric basic and advanced life support courses: first experiences in Spain. Resuscitation 1996;33(1):43–48.
5. Duncan H, Hutchison J, Parshuram CS. The Pediatric Early Warning System score: a severity of illness score to predict urgent medical need in hospitalized children. J Crit Care 2006;21(3):271–278.
6. Tibballs J, Kinney S, Duke T, Oakley E, Hennessy M. Reduction of paediatric in-patient cardiac arrest and death with a medical emergency team: preliminary results. Arch Dis Child 2005;90:1148–1152.
7. Nolan JP, Morley PT, Vanden Hoek TL, Hickey RW, Kloeck WG, Billi J, Bottiger BW, Morley PT, Nolan JP, Okada K, Reyes C, Shuster M, Steen PA, Weil MH, Wenzel V, Hickey RW, Carli P, Vanden Hoek TL, Atkins D. International Liaison Committee on Resuscitation. Therapeutic hypothermia after cardiac arrest. An advisory statement by the Advanced Life Support for the International Committee on Resuscitation. Circulation 2003;108:118–121.
8. Zaritsky A, Nadkarni V, Hazinski MF, Foltin G, Quan L, Wright J, Fiser D, Zideman D, O'Malley P, Chameides L. Recommended guidelines for uniform reporting of pediatric advanced life support: the pediatric Utstein style. A statement from a task force of the American Academy of Pediatrics, the American Heart Association, and the European Resuscitation Council. Circulation 1995;92(7):2006–2020.
9. Morris MC, Nadkarni VM. Pediatric cardiopulmonary-cerebral resuscitation: an overview and future directions. Crit Care Clin 2003; 19:337–364.
10. Whitelaw CC, Goldsmith LJ. Comparison of two techniques for determining the presence of a pulse in an infant. Acad Emerg Med 1997;4: 153–154.
11. Reis AG, Nadkarni V, Perundi MB, Grisi S, Berg RA. A prospective investigation into the epidemiology of in-hospital pediatric cardiopulmonary resuscitation using the international Utstein reporting style. Pediatrics 2002;109(2):200–209.
12. Suominen P, Olkkola KT, Voipio V, Korpela R, Palo R, Rasanen J. Utstein style reporting of in-hospital cardiopulmonary resuscitation. Resuscitation 2000;46:17–25.
13. Lopez-Herce J, Garcia C, Dominguez P, Carrillo A, Rodriguez-Nunez A, Calvo C, Delgado MA; Spanish Study Group of Cardiopulmonary Arrest in Children. Characteristics and outcome of cardiorespiratory arrest in children. Resuscitation 2004;63(3):311–320.
14. Slonim AD, Patel KM, Ruttimann UE, Pollack MM. Cardiopulmonary resuscitation in pediatric intensive care units. Crit Care Med 1997; 25(12):1951–1955.
15. Parra DA, Totapally BR, Zahn E, Jacobs J, Aldousany A, Burke RP, Chang AC. Outcome of cardiopulmonary resuscitation in a pediatric cardiac intensive care unit. Crit Care Med 2000;28:3296–3000.
16. Morray JP, Geiduschek JM, Ramamoorthy C, Haberkern CM, Hackel A, Caplan RA, Domino KB, Posner K, Cheney FW. Anesthesia-related cardiac arrest in children: initial findings of the Pediatric Perioperative Cardiac Arrest (POCA) Registry. Anesthesiology 2000; 93(1):6–14.
17. Schindler MB, Bohn D, Cox PN, McCrindle BW, Jarvis A, Edmonds J, Barker G. Outcome of out of hospital cardiac or respiratory arrest in children. N Engl J Med 1996;335(20):1473–1479.
18. Waalewijn RA, de Vos R, Koster RW. Out-of-hospital cardiac arrest in Amsterdam and its surrounding areas: results form the Amsterdam resuscitation study (ARREST) in Utstein style. Resuscitation 1998; 38(3):157–167.
19. Katsura K, Asplund B, Ekholm A, Siesjo BK. Extra- and intracellular pH in the brain during ischaemia, related to tissue lactate content in normo- and hypercapnic rats. Eur J Neurosci 1992;4(2):166–176.
20. Park WS, Chang YS, Lee M. Effects of hyperglycemia or hypoglycemia on brain cell membrane function and energy metabolism during the immediate reoxygenation–reperfusion period after acute transient global hypoxia–ischemia in the newborn piglet. Brain Res 2001; 901(1–2):102–108.
21. Ekholm A, Katsura K, Seisjo BK. Ion fluxes in ischemia: relationship to excitatory amino acids. Drug Res Rel Neuroactive Amino Acids 1992;4:351–361.
22. Lee JM, Grabb MC, Zipfel GJ, Choi DW. Brain tissue responses to ischemia. J Clin Invest 2000;106(6):723–731.
23. Katsura K, Siesjo BK, Bazan NG. Excitotoxicity, free radicals, and cell membrane changes. Ann Neurol 1989;35(Suppl):S17–S21.
24. Nicotera P. Molecular switches deciding death of injured neurons. Toxicol Sci 2003:744–749.
25. Ankarcrona M, Dypbukt JM, Bonfoco E, Zhivotovsky B, Orrenius S, Lipton SA, Nicotera P. Glutamate-induced neuronal death: a succession of necrosis or apoptosis depending on mitochondrial function. Neuron 1995;14(4):961–973.
26. Cohen P. The search for physiological substrates of MAP and SAP kinases in mammalian cells. Trends Cell Biol 1997;7:353–361.
27. Siman R, Noszek JC. Excitatory amino acids activate calpain-1 and induce structural protein breakdown in vivo. Neuron 1988;1:279–287.
28. Kaczmarek L. The role of Protein Kinase C in the regulation of ion channels and neurotransmitter release. Trends Neurosci 1987;10: 30–34.
29. Aveldano MI, Bazan NG. Rapid production of diacylglycerols enriched in arachidonate and stearate during early brain ischemia. J Neurochem 1975;25(6):919–920.
30. Katsura K, Rodriguez de Turco EB, Siesjo BK, Bazan NG. Effects of hyperglycemia and hypercapnia on lipid metabolism during complete brain ischemia. Brain Res 2005;1030(1):133–140.

31. Smaili SS, Russell JT. Permeability transition pore regulates both mitochondrial membrane potential and agonist evoked Ca^{2+} signals in oligodendrocyte progenitors. Cell Calcium 1999;26(3–4):121–130.

32. MacManus JP, Linnik MD. Gene expression induced by cerebral ischemia: an apoptotic perspective. J Cereb Blood Flow Metab 1997; 17(8):815–832.

33. Emerich DF, Dean RL 3rd, Bartus RT. The role of leukocytes following cerebral ischaemia: pathogenic variable or bystander reaction to emerging infarct. Exp Neurology 2002;173:168–181.

34. Gidday JM, Park TS, Gonzales ER, Beetsch JW. CD-18 dependent leukocyte adherence and vascular injury in pig cerebral circulation after ischemia. Am J Physiol 1997;272(6 Pt 2):H2622–H2629.

35. Mayhan W. Cellular mechanisms by which tumor necrosis factor-α produces disruption of the blood brain barrier. Brain Res 2002;927: 144–152.

36. Colbourne F, Sutherland GR, Auer RN. Electron microscopic evidence against apoptosis as the mechanism of neuronal death in global ischemia. J Neurosci 1999;19(11):4200–4210.

37. Martin LJ, Al-Abdulla NA, Brambrink AM, Kirsch JR, Sieber FE, Portera-Cailliau C. Neurodegeneration in excitotoxicity, global cerebral ischemia, and target deprivation: a perspective on the contributions of apoptosis and necrosis. Brain Res Bull 1998;46(4):281–309.

38. Mergenthaler P, Dirnagl U, Meisel A. Pathophysiology of stroke: lessons from animal models. Metab Brain Dis 2004;19:151–157.

39. Manabat C, Han BH, Wendland M, Derugin N, Fox CK, Choi J, Holtzman DM, Ferriero DM, Vexler ZS. Reperfusion differentially induces caspase-3 activation in ischemic core and penumbra after stroke in immature brain. Stroke 2003;34:207–213.

40. Zhan RZ, Wu C, Fujihara H, Taga K, Qi S, Naito M, Shimoji K. Both caspase-dependent and caspase-independent pathways may be involved in hippocampal CA1 neuronal death because of loss of cytochrome c from mitochondria in a rat forebrain ischemia model. J Cereb Blood Flow Metab 2001;21:529–540.

41. Chan P. Mitochondria and neuronal death/survival signaling pathways in cerebral ischemia. Neurochem Res 2004;29:1943–1949.

42. Jagtap P, Szabo C. Poly(ADP-ribose) polymerase and the therapeutic effects of its inhibitors. Nature Rev Drug Discovery 2005;4(5):421–440.

43. Ames A 3rd, Wright RL, Kowada M, Thurston JM, Majno G. Cerebral ischemia II. The no-reflow phenomenon. Am J Pathol 1968;52(2): 437–453.

44. Safer P, Kochanek P. Cerebral blood flow promotion after prolonged cardiac arrest. Crit Care Med 2000;28(8):3104–3106.

45. Tsuchidate R, He QP, Smith ML, Siesjo BK. Regional cerebral blood flow after 2 hours of middle cerebral artery occlusion. J Cereb Blood Flow Metab 1997;17(10):1066–1073.

46. Siesjo B. Cerebral blood flow. In: Pinsky M, ed. Mechanisms of Ischemia, Diagnosis and Therapy. [Update in Intensive Care Medicine.] Berlin: Springer-Verlag; 2002:45–60.

47. Krep HB, et al. Endothelin type A-antagonist improves long term neurological recovery after cardiac arrest in rats. Crit Care Med 2000;28(8):2873–2880.

48. DeWitt DS, Smith TG, Deyo DJ, Miller KR, Uchida T, Prough DS. L-arginine and superoxide dismutase prevent or reverse cerebral hypoperfusion after fluid percussion traumatic brain injury. J Neurotrauma 1997;269:H23–H29.

49. Auer RN. Sutherland GR. Hypoxia and related conditions. In: Greenfield's Neuropathology. London: Hodder Headline Group; 2002:233–280.

50. Ellison D, Love S. Adult hypoxic and ischemic lesions. In: Neuropathology: A Reference Text of Central Nervous System Pathology. 1998.

51. Ito U, Spatz M, Walker JT Jr, Klatzo I. Experimental ischemia in the Mongolian gerbil. 1. Light microscope observations. Acta Neuropathol 1975;32:209–223.

52. Krep H, Bottiger BW, Bock C, Kerskens CM, Radermacher B, Fischer M, Hoehn M, Hossmann KA. Time course of circulatory and meta-

bolic recovery of cat brain after cardiac arrest assessed by perfusion and diffusion weighted imaging and MR-spectroscopy. Resuscitation 2003;58(3):337–348.

53. Sirbaugh PE, Pepe PE, Shook JE, Kimball KT, Goldman MJ, Ward MA, Mann DM. A prospective population-based study of the demographics, epidemiology, management and outcome of out of hospital pediatric cardiopulmonary arrest. Ann Emerg Med 1999;33(2): 174–184.

54. Torres A, Pickert CB, Firestone J, Walker WM, Fiser DH. Long-term functional outcome of inpatient cardiopulmonary resuscitation. Pediatr Emerg Care 1997;13(6):369–373.

55. Lopez-Herce J, Garcia C, Rodriguez-Nunez A, Dominguez P, Carrillo A, Calvo C, Delgado MA; Spanish Study Group of Cardiopulmonary Arrest in Children. Long-term outcome of pediatric cardiorespiratory arrest in Spain. Resuscitation 2005;64:79–85.

56. Clausen T, Scharf A, Menzel M, Soukup J, Holz C, Rieger A, Hanisch F, Brath E, Nemeth N, Miko I, Vajkoczy P, Radke J, Henze D. Influence of moderate and profound hyperventilation on cerebral blood flow, oxygenation and metabolism. Brain Res 2004;1019(1–2):113–123.

57. Gruber EM, Jonas RA, Newburger JW, Zurakowski D, Hansen DD, Laussen PC. The effect of hematocrit on cerebral blood flow velocity in neonates and infants undergoing deep hypothermic cardiopulmonary bypass. Anesth Analg 1999;89(2):322–327.

58. Duebener L, Sakamoto T, Hatsuoka S, Stamm C, Zurakowski D, Vollmar B, Menger MD, Schafers HJ, Jonas RA. Effects of hematocrit on cerebral microcirculation and tissue oxygenation during deep hypothermic bypass. Circulation 2001;104(12 Suppl):I260–I264.

59. Safar P, Behringer W, Bottiger BW, Sterz F. Cerebral resuscitation potentials for cardiac arrest. Crit Care Med 2002;30(4):S140–S144.

60. Tan A, Schulze A, O'Donnell CP, Davis PG. Air versus oxygen for resuscitation of infants at birth. Cochrane Database Syst Rev 2005;18(2):CD002273.

61. Reinert M, Barth A, Rothen HU, Schaller B, Takala J, Seiler RW. Effects of cerebral perfusion pressure and increased fraction of inspired oxygen on the brain tissue oxygen, lactate and glucose in patients with severe head injury. Acta Neurochir 2003;145(5):341–350.

62. Laffey JG, O'Croinin D, McLoughlin P, Kavanagh BP. Permissive hypercapnia-role in protective lung ventilation strategies. Intensive Care Med 2004;30(3):347–356.

63. Bellinger DC, Wypij D, Kuban KC, Rappaport LA, Hickey PR, Wernovsky G, Jonas RA, Newburger JW. Developmental and neurological status of children at 4 years of age after heart surgery with hypothermic circulatory arrest or low-flow cardiopulmonary bypass. Circulation 1999;100(5):526–532.

64. Pemberton PL, Dinsmore J. The use of hypothermia as a method of neuroprotection during neurosurgical procedures and after traumatic brain injury: a survey of clinical practice in Great Britain and Ireland. Anaesthesia 2003;58(4):370–373.

65. Biggart M, Bohn DJ. Effect of hypothermia and cardiac arrest on outcome of near drowning accidents in children. J Pediatr 1990; 117:179–183.

66. Bohn DJ, Biggar WD, Smith CR, Conn AW, Barker GA. The influence of hypothermia, barbiturate therapy, and intracranial pressure monitoring on morbidity and mortality after near-drowning. Crit Care Med 1986;(14):529–534.

67. The Hypothermia after Cardiac Arrest Study Group. Mild therapeutic hypothermia to improve neurologic outcome after cardiac arrest. N Engl J Med 2002;346:549–556.

68. Bernard SA, Gray TW, Buist MD, Jones BM, Silvester W, Gutteridge G, Smith K. Treatment of comatose survivors of out of hospital cardiac arrest with induced hypothermia. N Engl J Med 2002;346(8): 557–563.

69. Shankaran S, Laptook AR, Ehrenkranz RA, Tyson JE, McDonald SA, Donovan EF, Fanaroff AA, Poole WK, Wright LL, Higgins RD, Finer NN, Carlo WA, Duara S, Oh W, Cotten CM, Stevenson DK, Stoll BJ, Lemons JA, Guillet R, Jobe AH; National Institute of Child Health and Human Development Neonatal Research Network. Whole body

hypothermia for neonates with hypoxic-ischemic encephalopathy. N Engl J Med 2005;353:1574–1584.

70. Colbourne F, Corbett D. Delayed and prolonged post-ischemic hypothermia is neuroprotective in the gerbil. Brain Res 1994;654(2): 265–272.

71. Colbourne F, Corbett D. Delayed post ischemic hypothermia: a six month survival study using behavioral and histological assessments of neuroprotection. J Neurosci 1995;15(11):7250–7260.

72. Colbourne F, Li H. Buchan AM. Indefatigable CA1 sector neuroprotection with mild hypothermia induced 6 hours after severe forebrain ischemia in rats. J Cereb Blood Flow Metab 1999;19(7):742–749.

73. Corbett D, Nurse S, Colbourne F. Hypothermic neuroprotection. A global ischemia study using 18- to 20-month-old gerbils. Stroke 1997; 28(11):2238–2242.

74. Kaibara T, Sutherland GR, Colbourne F, Tyson RL, Hypothermia: depression of tricarboxylic acid cycle flux and evidence for pentose phosphate shunt upregulation. J Neurosurg 1999;90(2):339–347.

75. Smith SL, Hall E. Mild pre- and posttraumatic hypothermia attenuates blood–brain barrier damage following controlled cortical impact injury in the rat. J Neurotrauma 1997;13(1):1–9.

76. Sutcliffe IT, Smith HA, Staninimirovic D, Hutchison, JS. Effects of moderate hypothermia on IL1B induced leukocyte rolling and adhesion in pial microcirculation of mice and on proinflammatory gene expression in human cerebral endothelial cells. J Cereb Blood Flow Metab 2001;21:1310–1319.

77. Globus MY, Alonso O, Dietrich WD, Busto R, Ginsberg MD. Glutamate release and free radical production following brain injury: effects of posttraumatic hypothermia. J Neurochem 1997;65(4):1704–1711.

78. Lei B, Tan X, Cai H, Xu Q, Guo Q. Effect of moderate hypothermia on lipid peroxidation in canine brain tissue after cardiac arrest and resuscitation. Stroke 1994;25(1):147–152.

79. Hicks SD, DeFranco D, Callaway CW. Hypothermia during reperfusion after asphyxial cardiac arrest improves functional recovery and selectively alters stress-induced protein expression. J Cereb Blood Flow Metabolism 2000;20(2):520–530.

80. Hicks SD, Parmele KT, DeFranco DB, Klann E, Callaway CW. Hypothermia differentially increases extracellular signal-regulated kinase and stress-activated protein kinase/c-Jun terminal kinase activation in the hippocampus during reperfusion after asphyxial cardiac arrest. Neuroscience 2000;98(4):677–685.

81. Rhoney DH, Parker D Jr. Use of sedative and analgesic agents in neurotrauma patients: effects on cerebral physiology. Neurol Res 2001;23: 237–259.

82. Homi HM, Mixco JM, Sheng H, Grocott HP, Pearlstein RD, Warner DS. Severe hypotension is not essential for forebrain isoflurane neuroprotection in mice. Anesthesiology 2003;99:1145–1151.

83. Miura Y, Mackensen GB, Nellgard B, Pearlstein RD, Bart RD, Dexter F, Warner DS. Differential effects of anesthetic agents on outcome from near complete but not incomplete global ischemia in the rat. Anesthesiology 1998;89:391–400.

84. Gray JJ, Bickler PE, Fahlman CS, Zhan X, Schuyler JA. Isoflurane neuroprotection in hypoxic hippocampal slice cultures involves increases in intracellular Ca^{2+} an mitogen activated kinases. Anesthesiology 2005;102(3):606–615.

85. Wei H, Kang B, Wei W, Liang G, Meng QC, Li Y, Eckenhoff RG. Isoflurane and sevoflurane affect cell survival and BCL-2/BAX ratio differently. Brain Res 2005;1037(1–2):139–147.

86. Steen PA, Newberg L, Milde JH, Michenfelder JD. Hypothermia and barbiturates: individual and combined effects on canine oxygen consumption. Anesthesiology 1983;58:527–532.

87. Steen P, Milde JH, Michenfelder JD. No barbiturate protection in a dog model of complete cerebral ischemia. Ann Neurol 1979;5: 343–349.

88. Nakashima K, Todd MM, Warner DS. The relation between cerebral metabolic rate and ischemic depolarization. A comparison of the effects of hypothermia, pentobarbital, and isoflurane. Anesthesiology 1995;82:1199–1208.

89. Ebmeyer U, Safar P, Radovsky A, Xiao F, Capone A, Tanigawa K, Stezoski SW. Thiopental combination treatments for cerebral resuscitation after prolonged cardiac arrest in dogs. Explanatory outcome study. Resuscitation 2000;45(2):119–131.

90. Oertel M, Kelly DF, Lee JH, McArthur DL, Glenn TC, Vespa P, Boscardin WJ, Hovda DA, Martin NA. Efficacy of hyperventilation, blood pressure elevation, and metabolic suppression therapy in controlling intracranial pressure after head injury. J Neurosurg 2002;97(5): 1045–1053.

91. Grasshoff C. Gillessen T. The effect of propofol on increased superoxide concentration in cultured rat cerebrocortical neurons after stimulation with N-methyl-d-aspartate receptors. Anesth Analg 2002;95(4): 920–922.

92. Engelhard K, Werner C, Eberspacher E, Pape M, Stegemann U, Kellermann K, Hollweck R, Hutzler P, Kochs E. Influence of propofol on neuronal damage and apoptotic factors after incomplete ischemia and preperfusion in rats: a long term observation. Anesthesiology 2004; 101(4):912–917.

93. Wooltorton E. Propofol: contraindicated for sedation of pediatric intensive care patients. CMAJ 2002;167(5):507.

94. Citerio, G. Cormio M. Sedation in neurointensive care: advances in understanding and practice. Curr Opin Crit Care 2003;9(2):120–126.

95. Shuaib A, Murabit MA, Kanthan R, Howlett W, Wishart T. The neuroprotective effects of gamma-vinyl GABA in transient global ischemia: a morphological study with early and delayed evaluations. Neurosci Lett 1996;204(1–2):1–4.

96. Thaminy S, Reymann JM, Heresbach N, Allain H, Lechat P, Bentue-Ferrer D. Is chlormethiazole neuroprotective in experimental global ischemia. A microdialysis and behavioral study. Pharmacol Biochem Behav 1997;56(4):737–745.

97. Vergoni AV, Ottani A, Botticelli AR, Zaffe D, Guano L, Loche A, Genedani S, Gessa GL, Bertolini A. Neuroprotective effect of gamma-hydroxybutyrate in transient global cerebral ischemia in the rat. Eur J Pharmacol 2000;397:75–84.

98. Iqbal S, Baziany A, Gordon S, Wright S, Hussain M, Miyashita H, Shuaib A, Rajput AH. Neuroprotective effect of tiagabine in transient forebrain global ischemia: an in vivo microdialysis, behavioral, and histological study. Brain Res 2002;946:162–170.

99. Wang C, Sadovova N, Fu X, Schmued L, Scallet A, Hanig J, Slikker W. The role of the N-methyl-d-aspartate receptor in ketamine-induced apoptosis in rat forebrain culture. Neuroscience 2005;132(4): 967–977.

100. Horn J, Limburg M. Calcium antagonists for ischemic stroke: a systematic review. Stroke 2000;32:570–576.

101. Calle PA, Paridaens K, De Ridder LI, Buylaert WA. Failure of nimodipine to prevent brain damage in global cerebral ischemia in the rat. Resuscitation 1993;25(1):57–71.

102. Zapater P, Moreno J, Horga JF. Neuroprotection by novel calcium antagonist PCA50938, nimodipine and flunarizine, in gerbil global brain ischemia. Brain Res 1997;772(1–2):57–62.

103. Berger R, Lehmann T, Karcher J, Garnier Y, Jensen A. Low dose flunarizine protects the fetal brain from ischemic injury. Pediatr Res 1998;44(3):277–282.

104. Hayashi T, Kagaya A, Motohashi N, Yamawaki S. Possible mechanism of dantrolene stabilization of cultured neuroblastoma cell plasma membranes. J Neurochem 1994;63(5):1849–1854.

105. Xiong ZG, Zhu XM, Chu XP, Minami M, Hey J, Wei WL, MacDonald JF, Wemmie JA, Price MP, Welsh MJ, Simon RP. Neuroprotection in ischemia: blocking calcium permeable acid sensing ion channels. Cell 2004;118(6):687–698.

106. Oreopoulos GD, Hamilton J, Rizoli SB, Fan J, Lu Z, Li YH, Marshall JC, Kapus A, Rotstein OD. In vivo and in vitro modulation of intercellular adhesion molecule (ICAM)-1 expression by hypertonicity. Shock 2000;14(3):409–414.

107. Sasaki T, Kitagawa K, Yamagata K, Takemiya T, Tanaka S, Omura-Matsuoka E, Sugiura S, Matsumoto M, Hori M. Amelioration of hippocampal neuronal damage after transient forebrain ischemia in

cyclooxygenase deficient mice. J Cereb Blood Flow Metab 2004;24(1): 107–113.

108. Candelario-Jalil E, Gonzalez-Falcon A, Garcia-Cabrera M, Alverez D, Al-Dalain S, Martinez G, Leon OS, Springer JE. Assessment of the relative contributions of COX-1 and COX-2 in ischemia induced oxidative damage and neurodegeneration following transient global ischemia. J Neurochem 2003;86(3):345–355.

109. Park EM Cho BP, Volpe BT, Cruz MO, Joh TH, Cho S. Ibuprofen protects ischemia-induced neuronal injury via up-regulating interleukin-1 antagonist expression. Neuroscience 2005;132(3):625–631.

110. Zhang ZG, Chopp M, Tang WX, Ning J, Zhang RL. Post ischemic treatment (2–4h) with anti-CD11b and anti-CD18 monoclonal antibodies are neuroprotective after transient (2h) focal ischemia in the rat. Brain Res 1995;698(1–2):79–85.

111. Degraba T. The role of inflammation after acute stroke. Utility of perusing anti-adhesion molecule therapy. Neurology 1998;51(3 Suppl 3):S62–S68.

112. Kitagawa K, Matsumoto M, Ohtsuki T, Kuwabara K, Mabuchi T, Yagita Y, Hori M, Yanagihara T. Deficiency of intercellular adhesion molecule 1 fails to mitigate selective neuronal death after transient global ischemia. Brain Res 1999;847(2):166–174.

113. Hutchison JS, Sutcliffe IT, Cui H, Zhang W, Stanimirovic DB. Hypothermia inhibits leukocyte adhesion and gene expression in cerebral endothelial cells following hypoxia/ischaemia. Intensive Care Med 2003 (MMDICM Symposium).

114. Weigl M, Tenze G, Steinlechner B, Skhirtladze K, Reining G, Bernardo M, Pedicelli E, Dworschak M. A systematic review of currently available pharmacological neuroprotective agents as a sole intervention before anticipated or induced cardiac arrest. Resuscitation 2005;65: 21–39.

115. Anderson TR, Jarvis CR, Biederman AJ, Molnar C, Andrew RD. Blocking the anoxic depolarization protects without functional compromise following simulated stroke in cortical brain slices. J Neurophysiol 2005;93(2):963–979.

116. Dunham CR, et al. Cerebral hypoxia in severely brain injured patients is associated with admission Glasgow Coma Score, computed tomography severity, cerebral perfusion pressure and survival. J Trauma 2004;56(3):482–491.

117. Gracias VH, Guillamondegui OD, Stiefel MF, Wilensky EM, Bloom S, Gupta R, Pryor JP, Reilly PM, Leroux PD, Schwab CW. Cerebral oxygenation, a pilot study. J Trauma 2004;56(3):469–474.

118. Feldman Z, Robertson CS. Monitoring of cerebral hemodynamics with jugular venous bulb catheters. Crit Care Clin 1997;13(1):51–77.

119. Nollert G, Jonas RA Reichart B. Optimizing cerebral oxygenation during cardiac surgery: a review of experimental and clinical investigations with near infrared spectrophotometry. Thorac Cardiovasc Surg 2000;48(4):247–253.

120. Daubeney PE, Pilkington SN, Janke E, Charlton GA, Smith DC, Webber SA. Cerebral oxygenation measured by near-infrared spectroscopy: comparison with jugular bulb oximetry. Ann Thorac Surg 1996;61(3): 930–934.

121. Asil T, Uzunca I, Utku U, Berberoglu U. Monitoring of increased intracranial pressure resulting from cerebral edema with transcranial Doppler sonography in patients with middle cerebral artery infarction. J Ultrasound Med 2003;22(10):1049–1053.

122. Edmonds HL, Zhang YP, Shields CB. New neurophysiology and central nervous system dysfunction. Curr Opin Crit Care 2003;9(2):98–105.

123. Madl C, Kramer L, Domanovits H, Wollard RH, Gervais H, Gendo A, Eisenhuber E, Grimm G, Sterz F. Improved outcome prediction in unconscious cardiac arrest survivors with sensory evoked potentials compared with clinical assessment. Crit Care Med 2000;28(3):721–726.

124. Levy DE, Caronna JJ, Singer BH, Lapinski RH, Frydman H, Plum F. Predicting outcome from hypoxic–ischemic coma. JAMA 1985;253(10): 1420–1426.

125. Krumholz A, Stern BJ, Weiss HD. Outcome from coma after cardiopulmonary resuscitation: relation to seizures and myoclonus. Neurology 1988;38(3):401–405.

126. Meynaar IA, Oudemans-van Straaten HM, van der Wetering J, Verlooy P, Slaats EH, Bosman RJ, van der Spoel JI, Zandstra DF. Serum neuron specific enolase predicts outcome in post-anoxic coma: a prospective cohort study. Intensive Care Med 2003;29(2):189–195.

127. Zingler VC, Krumm B, Bertsch T, Fassbender K, Pohlmann-Eden B. Early prediction of neurological outcome after cardiopulmonary resuscitation: a multimodal approach combining neurobiological and electrophysiological investigations may provide high prognostic certainty in patients after cardiac arrest. Eur Neurol 2003;49(2):79–84.

128. Pfeiffer R, Borner A, Krack A, Sigusch HH, Surber R, Figull HR. Outcome after cardiac arrest: predictive values and limitations of the neuroproteins neuron-specific enolase and protein S-100 and the Glasgow Coma Scale. Resuscitation 2005;65(1):49–55.

129. Rosen H, Sunnerhagen KS, Helitz J, Blomstrand C, Rosengren L. Serum levels of the brain derived proteins S-100 and NSE predict long-term outcome after cardiac arrest. Resuscitation 2001;49(2): 183–191.

130. Zandbergen EG, de Haan R, Stoutenbeek CP, Koelman JH, Hijdra A. Systematic review of early prediction of poor outcome in anoxic–ischaemic coma. Lancet 1998;352(9143):1808–1812.

131. Shewmon A. Coma prognosis in children. J Clin Neurophysiol 2000;15(5):467–742.

132. Hulihan JS, Syna DR. Electroencephalographic sleep pattern in post anoxic stupor and coma. Neurology 1994;44(4):758–760.

133. Evans BM, Bartlett JR. Prediction of outcome in severe head injury based on recognition of sleep related activity in the polygraphic electroencephalogram. J Neurol Neurosurg Psychiatry 1995;59(1):17–25.

134. Madl C, Grimm G, Kramer L, Yeganehfar W, Sterz F, Schneider B, Kranz A, Schneeweiss B, Lenz K. Early prediction of individual outcome after cardiopulmonary resuscitation. Lancet 1993;341(8849): 855–858.

135. Christophe C, Fonteyne C, Ziereisen F, Christiaens F, Deltenre P, De Maertelaer V, Dan B. Value of MR imaging of the brain in children with hypoxic coma. Am J Neuroradiol 2002;23(4):716–723.

136. Els T, Kassubek J, Kubalek R, Klisch J. Diffusion weighted MRI during early global cerebral hypoxia: a predictor for clinical outcome. Acta Neurol Scand 2004;110:361–367.

9

Toxic and Metabolic Encephalopathies

Ashok P. Sarnaik and Kathleen L. Meert

Central nervous system (CNS) dysfunction can result from a variety of metabolic derangements or endogenous/exogenous toxins. The outcome from a diverse group of neurologic insults has improved considerably in recent years due to a better understanding of the CNS response to injurious agents and aggressive neurointensive care. Threat to neuronal integrity is posed by the primary injury (e.g. trauma, infection, toxin etc) as well as by the secondary injury resulting from the altered CNS metabolism and intracranial milieu. Although the management of the primary injury is of major importance, it is the secondary injury that often determines the outcome. Manifestations of secondary injury may occur within minutes, hours or days after the primary insult. It should be recognized that secondary injury may occur in the absence of, in spite of, or sometimes even because of therapeutic interventions. The window of opportunity to prevent or treat secondary injury may be extremely narrow over a few minutes or ongoing over several days.

Pathophysiologic Considerations

The Central Nervous System and Its Osmolar Environment

The tight junctions between the CNS capillary endothelial cells, fortified by astrocytic end-feet processes and the thick neuronal cell membrane constitute the blood brain barrier (BBB). Recent advances have shed light on the complex molecular basis for the unique properties of the BBB [1]. Solutes, including crystalloids, take several hours to equilibrate across this barrier, whereas water moves rapidly in either direction. An osmolar gradient therefore would have a significant and unique effect on total brain size which is not seen in other organs (Figures 9-1A and 9-1B). In muscle tissue for example, an increase in serum osmolarity is rapidly shared by the interstitium as the osmols readily pass across the capillary endothelium. Since these osmols cannot easily pass across the cell membrane, intracellular water moves into the interstitial space to attain osmotic equilibrium. Diminished cell size is thus compensated for by an increased interstitial fluid with little or no change in the overall tissue size. Because of the BBB however, in the CNS the osmolar dysequilibrium occurs at the level of the capillary endothelium, resulting in movement of water from both the intracellular and interstitial fluid spaces into the vascular space. Therefore, in the face of acute hyperosmolarity, there is an overall decrease in brain volume (Figure 9-1A). Conversely, when serum osmolarity rapidly decreases, the brain intracellular and interstitial osmols cannot easily enter the vascular space. The brain acts as an "osmolar trap", imbibing water, increasing its size as it equilibrates with a hypo-osmolar environment and reaches osmotic equilibrium (Figure 9-1B).

The CNS also has unique adaptive mechanisms to defend its tissue volume in response to a sustained change in serum osmolarity. In chronic hyperosmolar states, the brain water content returns to normal as different solutes (idiogenic osmoles) appear inside the brain cells [2]. These osmoles, better characterized as organic osmolytes, have been identified as various amino acids, polyols, and methylamines [3]. They are transported into the brain when faced with hyperosmolarity and allow for normalization of brain water content. Organic osmolytes are transported into the brain in response to a sustained exposure to a variety of serum osmoles including sodium, glucose, and urea. It is of interest that the rapidity with which brain water content is normalized may be different with different osmoles. For example, the brain water content is normalized much more rapidly (few hours) in hyperglycemia compared to hypernatremia (several days) [4]. Rapid correction of hyperosmolarity before the brain can normalize its osmolar content results in cerebral edema as an increased amount of brain solute draws water into the intracellular and interstitial spaces. The brain also has the ability to lose osmoles and minimize the gain in water when hypo-osmolarity is sustained. This occurs because of an initial decrease in sodium and potassium with subsequent depletion of non-electrolyte solute. Thus the gain in brain water after an acute decrease in osmolarity is followed by return to normalcy as hypo-osmolarity persists [5]. Whereas acute hyponatremia can cause life-threatening cerebral edema, patients with chronic hyponatremia are often asymptomatic.

Cerebral Edema

Cerebral edema is conventionally classified into vasogenic, cytotoxic and interstitial edema according to its underlying pathogenesis [6]. Disruption of the BBB is the hallmark of vasogenic cerebral edema. The increased capillary permeability allows intravascular

D.S. Wheeler et al. (eds.), *The Central Nervous System in Pediatric Critical Illness and Injury,*
DOI 10.1007/978-1-84800-993-6_9, © Springer-Verlag London Limited 2009

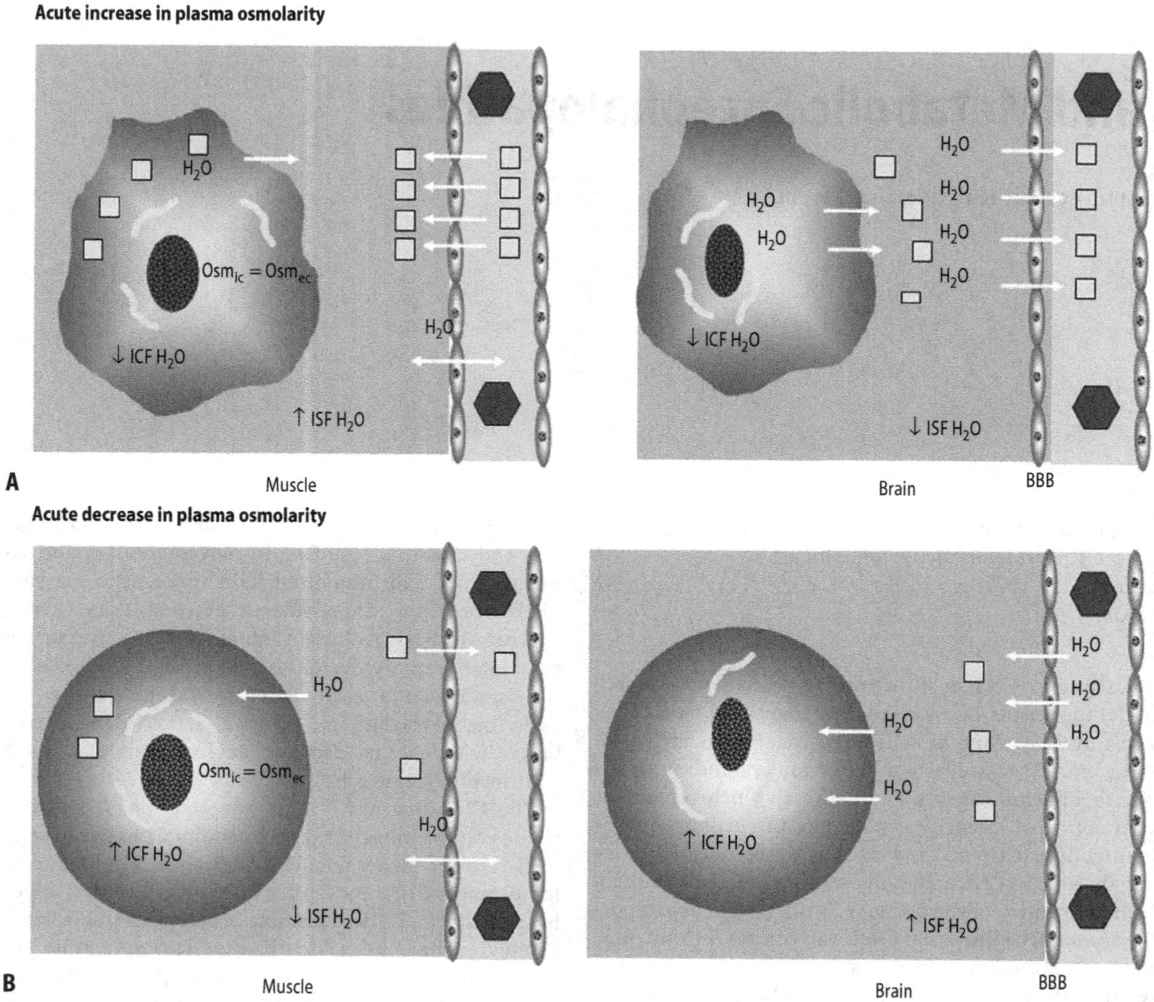

Acute increase in plasma osmolarity

Acute decrease in plasma osmolarity

FIGURES 9.1 (A and B) Effects of acute changes in plasma osmolarity on brain size compared to muscle. See text for explanation.

fluid and solutes to enter brain interstitial fluid, causing its expansion. It should be recognized that the disruption of the BBB is not absolute, and therapeutic agents such as mannitol can still be effective in producing an osmotic gradient across the brain capillaries, thus drawing water from interstitial fluid into the vascular space. Clinically, vasogenic edema is encountered in head trauma, bacterial meningitis, brain abscess, tumor, hypertensive encephalopathy, and lead poisoning. In cytotoxic edema, there is a relatively higher amount of intracellular solute compared to that in the extracellular fluid space drawing water into the cells to maintain osmotic equilibrium. Disease states with impaired cellular metabolism (hypoglycemia, Reye's syndrome, trauma, infection, and hypoxia) are associated with accumulation of abnormal quantities of intracellular osmoles resulting in movement of water into the cells. Intracellular cerebral osmolar content is also increased in response to sustained hyperosmolarity, e.g. in hypernatremia, hyperglycemia, and uremia [2–4]. Rapid lowering of serum osmolarity, before the intracerebral osmoles are normalized, results in increased brain water content. Similarly acute hypo-osmolar states such as water intoxication and the syndrome of inappropriate antidiuretic hormone (SIADH) result in neuronal swelling in the face of normal intracellular osmolar content. Interstitial edema occurs when an increased hydrostatic pressure gradient exists between the ventricular system and the brain interstitium, resulting in transependymal movement of cerebrospinal fluid (CSF) into periventricular white matter.

A consideration of pathophysiologic mechanisms in cerebral edema has important therapeutic significance. Osmotherapy is more effective in cytotoxic cerebral edema, whereas relief of CSF obstruction is necessary to treat interstitial cerebral edema. It is important to realize however, that vasogenic, cytotoxic and interstitial edema may occur concurrently in the same patient.

Intracranial Contents and Pressure-Volume Relationship

The skull with fused sutures is a relatively rigid container filled with non-compressible fluid and solid tissues. Intracranial contents include fluid, brain parenchyma, and meninges. Intracranial fluid is partitioned into four compartments: intravascular space, brain interstitial fluid, intracellular fluid and cerebrospinal fluid (CSF). Even open sutures and fontanels offer only a limited capacity for expansion. Thus, for intracranial pressure (ICP) to remain

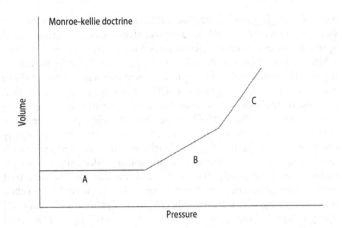

Monroe-kellie doctrine

FIGURE 9.2. Intracranial pressure-volume relationship. Initial increase in volume in one of the intracranial compartments is associated with little or no increase in ICP (A). Subsequent increases in volume result in exponential rise in ICP (B and C).

constant, any increase in the brain water content must be accompanied by a displacement of an equal volume of blood or CSF into extracranial spaces (Monroe-Kellie doctrine, Figure 9-2). When this spatial compensation is exhausted, ICP begins to rise. There are several implications of this doctrine. First, in the early phase, accumulation of abnormal fluid in the intracranial space may be associated with little or no increase in ICP as intracranial CSF gets displaced in the distensible spinal subarachnoid space. Second, ICP begins to rise when equivalent volume cannot be displaced to compensate for the pathologic increase in one of the intracranial compartments. Third, life-threatening intracranial hypertension and distortion/displacement of brain tissue (herniation syndromes) may occur with relatively small increases in intracranial volume after a critical capacity is exceeded. Finally, a relatively small decrease in intracranial volume may rapidly lower ICP to a safer level and reverse encephalopathy if appropriate therapy is instituted before irreversible brain injury occurs [7].

Brain Metabolism

In an adult, the brain comprises 2% of body weight and accounts for 20% of whole body glucose and oxygen consumption [8]. Under normal conditions, glucose is the sole source of energy for the brain. Although ketone bodies and amino acids can serve as an alternate fuel, they cannot completely replace glucose to meet cerebral metabolic demands [9]. The brain is thus exquisitely susceptible to hypoglycemia. Glucose uptake occurs through a glucose transporter in cerebral capillaries [10].

Many nutrients and vitamins are also important for cerebral metabolism. Among these, thiamine deficiency is perhaps the most relevant as a cause of encephalopathy in the critical care setting. Thiamine plays a crucial role in carbohydrate metabolism. Patients with chronic debilitating diseases dependent on total parenteral nutrition (TPN), on hemodialysis or peritoneal dialysis and those with diabetes mellitus and poor nutrition may be at risk for severe thiamine deficiency. Three important enzymes, essential for glucose metabolism, are dependent on thiamine pyrophosphate: transketolase (TK), pyruvate dehydrogenase (PDH) and α ketoglutarate dehydrogenase [11–13]. TK is necessary for glucose metabolism through the pentose phosphate pathway, which is the sole source of ribose for the synthesis of nucleic acid precursors and the major source of NADPH. PDH and α ketogluterate dehydrogenase are necessary for processing pyruvate through the Krebs cycle and generation of ATP. NADPH and NADP are crucial in catalyzing oxidation/reduction reactions in the Krebs cycle. Thiamine deficiency results in severe impairment of glucose metabolism, elevated pyruvate and lactate levels, and encephalopathy.

Diseases such as Reye's syndrome are characterized by severe mitochondrial dysfunction and are associated with severe metabolic derangements, cytotoxic cerebral edema and encephalopathy [14,15]. Similarly, inborn errors of metabolism such as organic acidemias, urea cycle disorders and aminoacidurias can manifest with varying levels of encephalopathy. Either endogenous (ammonia, urea, sepsis etc) or exogenous toxins (drugs, carbon monoxide, alcohols etc) causing alteration of cerebral metabolism are frequently encountered in pediatric critical care settings.

When to Suspect Toxic/Metabolic Encephalopathy?

History and clinical features often provide important clues to the presence of toxic/metabolic encephalopathy. A careful social history and chronology of events leading to discovery of CNS dysfunction might point the clinician in the direction of exogenous toxin as being the culprit. Similarly, recognition of an underlying clinical disorder such as hepatic failure, uremia, sepsis etc is of obvious importance. Inborn errors of metabolism may present acutely with rapidly progressing encephalopathy or subacutely after varying periods of subtle symptoms such as vomiting and poor weight gain. In general, toxic/metabolic encephalopathies should be suspected when history, clinical examination and imaging studies (when indicated) cannot explain cerebral dysfunction on the basis of structural abnormalities of the brain. Secondary structural damage may be present in such cases as a consequence of metabolic derangements.

Clinical Features

Although certain clinical features are unique to an individual disease entity, certain manifestations are common to all toxic/metabolic encephalopathies [16]. Alteration in level of consciousness is a hallmark of such disorders. This can manifest as either a depressed state such as lethargy, stupor, confusion, obtundation, and lack of arousal; or an excited state such as agitation, delirium, and seizures. As a general rule, manifestations of CNS dysfunction show rostrocaudal progression from cerebral cortex to brain stem. Abnormalities of respirations are quite common. Global CNS depression may manifest as slow and shallow respirations with resultant hypoventilation and respiratory acidosis. Bihemispheric and diancephalic pathology can lead to Cheyne-Stokes respirations. Injuries within the rostral brain stem or tegmentum can lead to central neurogenic hyperventilation and respiratory alkalosis. Mid to caudal pontine lesions can result in an apneustic breathing pattern characterized by a prolonged inspiratory pause. Medullary lesions result in ataxic, irregular breathing or apnea.

Laboratory evaluation should be directed at individual toxic/metabolic disease entities as suspected by history, clinical examination and circumstantial evidence. Imaging studies have a limited role unless a structural lesion is a possibility. They should not delay institution of supportive and specific therapy.

Specific Disorders

Reye's Syndrome

Association of acute encephalopathy and fatty degeneration of viscera was described independently by Reye et al. and Johnson et al. in 1963 [17,18]. Reye's syndrome (RS) is a prototypical metabolic encephalopathy which is characterized by mitochondrial dysfunction. Brain and liver are the two most consistently affected organs. CNS dysfunction, the only threat to survival, is independent of hepatic involvement. In other words, RS is distinct from hepatic encephalopathy which results from endogenous toxic metabolites accumulating because of liver dysfunction.

The classic clinical scenario is presented in Figure 9-3. Most cases occur in the fall and winter, with a peak age incidence between 5 and 15 years. A strong association with influenza A and B, and varicella is observed. Although the exact causative mechanism has remained elusive, many meticulous, independent epidemiologic studies have shown strong association between the use of salicylates during the antecedent viral illness and the development of RS [19–22]. The Surgeon General's recommendation against the use of salicylates for children with influenza and chickenpox and a decreasing use of aspirin in the community has coincided with a sharp decline in the incidence of RS in the United States since the early 1980s [21,22]. However, RS is by no means an extinct disease entity [23].

The disease is often biphasic in nature with the first phase consisting of a trivial viral infection from which the patient is seemingly recovering. Four commonly observed antecedent clinical illnesses are: upper respiratory infection, chickenpox, gastroenteritis and influenza-like ailment. The second phase, encephalopathy, is highly stereotypic and heralded by persistent, unrelenting vomiting lasting from several hours to a day. Progressive disturbance in the level of consciousness soon follows and reaches varying degrees of severity in a typical rostrocaudal fashion. The extent of cerebral dysfunction is the basis for clinical staging. Recognition of RS in

early stages is important. The earliest signs of encephalopathy (stage I) can be subtle such as excessive sleepiness, decreased verbal spontaneity, behavior and personality changes, confusion, and irritability. Stage II encephalopathy is a hyperexcitable state manifesting as disorientation and violent maniacal behavior. Some of these patients may be misdiagnosed as CNS excitatory drug intoxication because of their delirious state. Signs of sympathetic overactivity such as tachycardia, systolic hypertension, wide pulse pressure, dilated pupils, sweating, tachypnea and fever are commonly encountered. Stage III encephalopathy is characterized by central neurogenic hyperventilation and respiratory alkalosis. The respirations are increasingly deep and rapid. Muscle tone is increased with dystonic decorticate posturing. The oculocephalic reflex becomes sluggish, indicating brain stem dysfunction. Stage IV encephalopathy represents further brain stem impairment with decerebrate posturing, inconsistent or absent oculocephalic reflex, and dilated, sluggishly reacting pupils. If encephalopathy progresses to stage V, the patient becomes flaccid, apneic, areflexic and hypotensive. When prolonged, stage V represents brain death. The progression of one stage to another is variable between patients. In patients with severe encephalopathy the patient can progress to decerebrate coma within hours of the onset of vomiting.

Cytotoxic cerebral edema from mitochondrial dysfunction is the hallmark of RS [15]. In early stages, cerebral edema is not associated with intracranial hypertension because of the spatial compensation described earlier. Life-threatening intracranial hypertension however is the most important mechanism of brain herniation and death as encephalopathy progresses. Despite this, papilledema is uncommon unless ICP remains elevated for several days. The CNS dysfunction characteristically lasts for several days depending upon the severity. With adequate control of ICP and cerebral perfusion pressure (CPP), patients have potential for recovery with little or no sequelae.

There is no single laboratory test that can in and of itself be considered diagnostic of RS. The diagnosis is based on the clinical picture, evidence of hepatic dysfunction, <10 WBC/mm³ and normal protein in CSF and no reasonable explanation for encephalopathy. Serum AST and ALT are elevated more than two times normal in all patients. Because of easy availability and reliability, serum transaminase determination is an ideal screening test. The extent of transaminase elevation is of no clinical significance. Blood ammonia concentration is elevated in most cases and the extent of elevation (>300 μg/dl) is of poor prognostic significance. However, tt should be noted that RS is not due to ammonia intoxication. Severe encephalopathy may persist despite normalization of blood ammonia. Prothrombin time is often prolonged. Significant elevation (>5 mg/dl) in serum bilirubin level is uncommon. Acid base abnormalities are very common. The most consistent abnormality is that of respiratory alkalosis. Lactic acidemia is also commonly encountered although overt acidosis is rare. Histopathologic examination of the liver tissue shows characteristic diffuse microvesicular fatty infiltration of hepatocytes. Electron microscopic examination demonstrates mitochondrial swelling and disruption.

Management of RS is based on the premise that the generalized mitochondrial injury, including in the brain and the liver, is potentially completely reversible even in patients with severe disease. The challenge to the physician therefore is to protect the brain from irreversible injury until sufficient time is provided for spontaneous recovery. RS encephalopathy can progress rapidly and unexpectedly. Patients suspected of RS therefore should be transferred to a

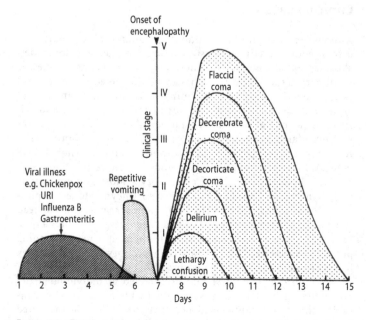

Figure 9.3. Clinical course of Reye's syndrome and rostrocaudal progression of encephalopathy.

hospital with a fully equipped pediatric intensive care unit. Sedatives should not be given to counteract agitation unless ventilation is controlled. Infusion of 10% to 15% dextrose in 0.2% saline at a rate of 1,500 ml/m^2/24 h, and maintaining normoglycemia are sufficient to manage stage I encephalopathy. Thirty mEq of potassium per liter as chloride and phosphate should be added to the infusion fluid. Insulin has been used to decrease fatty acidemia and protein catabolism. For this purpose 1 unit of insulin can be added to 5 g glucose in the intravenous (IV) fluid. Coagulation abnormalities can be corrected by administration of 1 to 5 mg of vitamin K and fresh frozen plasma.

Neurologic deterioration evidenced by inability to respond to verbal stimuli and lack of purposeful response to pain indicates worsening cerebral edema. Management is aimed at monitoring and treating intracranial hypertension and maintaining adequate CPP. Mannitol osmotherapy is extremely effective in treating RS encephalopathy because of the cytotoxic nature of the cerebral edema and intactness of the BBB. Mannitol in a dose of 0.25 to 0.5 g per kg should be infused over 15–20 minutes for stage II or more severe encephalopathy. Mannitol should be used every 4 to 6 hours until the patient regains consciousness and then tapered over 24 to 48 hours. Additional doses may be needed during the acute episodes of neurologic deterioration or elevations of ICP. Adequacy of renal function must be ensured for osmotherapy to be effective. Mannitol should be withheld if serum osmolarity exceeds 320 mOsm/kg H$_2$O. By acting as an osmotic diuretic, mannitol may also cause hypovolemia. Maintenance of adequate vascular volume as determined by central venous pressure around 5 mm Hg with appropriate volume expansion is necessary. Patients reaching stage III encephalopathy are best managed by elective tracheal intubation and mechanical ventilation to maintain PaCO$_2$ in mid 30 s. ICP monitoring is important in all such patients. The emphasis of management is to maintain euvolemia, serum osmolarity <310 mm Hg, ICP <20 mm Hg and CPP >50 mm Hg. Barbiturates are effective in reducing ICP. Pentobarbital is used as an adjunct to mechanical ventilation and mannitol for control of ICP. A loading dose of 2–3 mg/kg followed by a continuous infusion of 1–3 mg/kg/hour is a reasonable initial therapy. Additional boluses and adjustment of infusion rate is based upon the clinical state and ICP. At levels above 15–20 μg/ml, pentobarbital therapy is associated with myocardial depression. Inotropic support with dopamine or dobutamine should be instituted to maintain adequate perfusion. Additional strategies to control ICP such as ventricular drainage may be necessary.

Prognosis depends upon successful maintenance of ICP and CPP control. Some patients are resistant to therapy and develop lethal intracranial hypertension and brain herniation. However, if secondary injury from intracranial hypertension and cerebral ischemia is prevented, the underlying mitochondrial dysfunction is potentially reversible and excellent neurologic outcome can be expected even in patients with severe encephalopathy. Advances in neurointensive care have led to improvement in survival in patients with RS.

Hyponatremic Encephalopathy

Clinical settings in which significant hyponatremia is encountered are numerous [24–27]. Excessive ingestion of water (water intoxication) is the most common cause of hyponatremic encephalopathy in infants. Because of their lower glomerular filtration rate, infants have diminished capacity to excrete free water compared to older children and adults. Administration of free water in patients with SIADH is also an important cause of symptomatic hyponatremia in hospitalized patients. Other causes include gastrointestinal losses, diuretic therapy, adrenal insufficiency, renal salt wasting, cystic fibrosis, and drug therapy such as with oxcarbazepine (Trileptal) and cisplatin. The most important clinical consequences of hyponatremia and its treatment involve the CNS. In this context, the rapidity with which hyponatremia develops is crucial in terms of pathophysiologic consequences. Seizures, cerebral edema, brain stem herniation, permanent brain damage, respiratory arrest, and death can result from severe untreated hyponatremia of rapid onset [24,25]. Conversely, gradual development of hyponatremia may not result in neurologic dysfunction even at serum sodium levels <110 mmol/L [28]. The apparent discrepancy in clinical observations and management recommendations among various studies can be explained by the response of the CNS to its changing osmolar environment. An acute decrease in serum sodium is associated with an increase in brain water content. Autopsy findings in fatal cases of acute water intoxication have shown cerebral edema with uncal and brain stem herniation [29]. Consequently, rapid correction of serum sodium level in acutely hyponatremic patients would be expected to decrease brain water content and restore CNS function [24,30]. However, with chronic hyponatremia, brain water content tends to normalize with time. In such patients rapid correction of hyponatremia with hypertonic saline carries the risk of osmotic desiccation, central pontine and extrapontine myelinolysis and severe neurologic abnormalities [31,32]. In clinical practice, the exact duration over which hyponatremia has developed is often unknown. Hyponatremic patients with CNS symptoms such as lethargy, seizures and coma should be considered acute and treated promptly, whereas the asymptomatic ones should be considered chronic and should be corrected gradually.

Acute symptomatic hyponatremia is a medical emergency. A rapid IV bolus of 4 to 6 mL/kg body weight of 3% saline is suitable for this purpose [24]. With apparent volume of distribution of 0.6 L/kg body weight for sodium, one could anticipate an immediate increase of 3 to 5 mmol/L serum sodium concentration with such treatment. This relatively small but rapid elevation in serum sodium is a safe and effective means of managing hyponatremic encephalopathy. After this acute increase, further restoration of serum sodium occurs mainly by water diuresis, especially in infantile water intoxication. Patients with SIADH and symptomatic hyponatremia should be first treated with furosemide (1 mg/kg IV) to increase free water clearance followed by administration of 3% saline and fluid restriction.

Diabetic Encephalopathy

Cerebral edema is by far the most feared complication of type I diabetic ketoacidosis (DKA). Although cerebral edema has been described at presentation, it is most frequently encountered during treatment. Several risk factors have been identified. These include younger age, new-onset, greater degree of dehydration and a lower PaCO$_2$ [33]. Despite a great deal of controversy, excessive fluid administration during the period when the brain has increased osmolar content appears to be the most important factor [33–35]. There are several reasons why children with type I DKA have a potential to receive more fluids than they actually need. The dry mouth and lips resulting from Kussmaul breathing and poor perfusion secondary to acidosis make them appear more dehydrated than they really are. Additionally, the traditional method of estimation of 5%, 10% and 15% for mild, moderate and severe degrees of dehydration respectively, although reasonable in infants, is inappropriate at a later age. Older children have less total body water to start with, and therefore, their fluid deficits are less for the same clinical severity of dehydration compared with infants. Organic osmolytes accumulate rapidly in the brain during hyperglycemia [4]. Administration of a large amount of hypotonic fluids from overestimating fluid deficits, at a time when the brain is most vulnerable to osmotic shifts, poses a significant risk of cerebral edema [34,36]. An increase in brain water was observed during treatment of DKA even in asymptomatic patients who were receiving hypotonic fluid for rehydration [37]. This increase in brain water content was not observed when hypotonic fluids were avoided [36]. In some patients, this increase in brain water may reach catastrophic proportions, resulting in severe intracranial hypertension, brain stem herniation, and death. Increasing lethargy in the face of biochemical improvement should be considered a manifestation of brain swelling unless proven otherwise. Early manifestations such as headache, drowsiness, and agitation may rapidly progress to seizures, brain stem herniation, and irreversible brain damage in a matter of 1 to 2 hours. Early recognition and prompt therapy can potentially reverse this encephalopathy. After shock and circulatory insufficiency are treated with isotonic fluid expansion, subsequent fluid administration should be at maintenance plus estimated deficit which should not exceed 5% of body weight per day. Potassium as chloride and phosphate should be added to the rehydration fluids as soon as urine output and a fall in serum potassium level are established. We prefer isotonic saline as the initial rehydration solution. Glucose should be added after serum glucose falls to <300 mg/dL at which time 0.45% saline along with potassium salts could be used as the rehydration fluid. Occurrence of cerebral edema has not been conclusively shown to be associated with the rate of fall in serum glucose concentrations. Most clinicians consider a decline of serum glucose level of approximately 100 mg/dL/h as reasonable. In most cases this can be accomplished by a continuous infusion of 0.1 U/kg/h insulin. An initial infusion rate of 0.05 U/kg/h is advisable for patients with new-onset DKA. The role of bicarbonate administration in causing cerebral edema in DKA has received considerable attention recently. A retrospective, case controlled, multicenter study showed that treatment with bicarbonate was associated with an increased risk of cerebral edema [38]. However in this study, patients who developed cerebral edema also had a lower PCO_2 and higher BUN. The role of bicarbonate therapy in the pathogenesis of cerebral edema has not been established in prospective controlled studies. Nonetheless, bicarbonate administration is unnecessary in the vast majority of cases and should be reserved for life-threatening acidosis and hyperkalemia. Recent studies have suggested that cerebral edema in DKA is vasogenic in nature with impaired BBB [39]. However, this may be a manifestation earlier in the course, while the brain remains susceptible to osmotic shifts later leading to symptomatic cerebral dysfunction and intracranial hypertension [40].

All children receiving treatment for DKA should be monitored with frequent neurologic examination. Early manifestations of cerebral edema can be effectively treated with mannitol (0.5 g/kg) or 3% saline (4–6 ml/kg). In the presence of persistent obtundation, unresponsiveness, and inadequate ventilatory response to acidosis, tracheal intubation and hyperventilation are necessary. Decreasing the rate of rehydration and fall in serum glucose concentration are also indicated in such patients.

Hepatic Encephalopathy

Hepatic encephalopathy is a potentially reversible form of cerebral dysfunction that occurs with both acute and chronic liver disease [41–45]. Acute liver failure (ALF) often leads to an encephalopathy that progresses from altered mental status to stupor and coma over a period of days. Progressive cerebral edema and raised ICP result in mortality rates as high as 50–90% [46]. Hepatic encephalopathy is graded based on the severity of neurological symptoms (Table 9-1).

The pathogenesis of cerebral edema and intracranial hypertension is multifactorial. It is to be recognized that symptomatic brain edema can occur without an increase in ICP. In ALF, intracranial hypertension is a result of increased brain water content and increased cerebral blood flow [47]. Both acute and chronic hepatic failure results in the accumulation of ammonia in the brain, and alterations in astrocyte structure and function with preservation of neurons. Astrocytes are crucial for normal brain function since they regulate the composition of extracellular fluid surrounding neurons. Astrocyte swelling is a common finding in the brains of patients dying of ALF [48]. Hyperammonemia appears to play a crucial role in the pathogenesis of cerebral edema in ALF. Cerebral herniation is closely associated with plasma ammonia levels >150 μmol/L [49]. Ammonia is detoxified in the brain by formation of glutamine mainly in the astrocytes. The osmotic effect of intracellular accumulation of glutamine in astrocytes is proposed to be one of the mechanisms of cytotoxic cerebral edema in ALF. Alterations of BBB, also described in ALF, could aggravate cerebral edema that is predominantly cytotoxic in nature. Cerebral blood flow autoregulation is impaired in hepatic encephalopathy [47,50,51]. Cerebral hyperemia has been associated with severity of encephalopathy, brain edema and adverse outcome [52]. Altered neurotransmission also has been implicated in the pathogenesis of hepatic encephalopathy. Glutamate is the major excitatory neurotransmitter in the brain involved in more than 80% of synapses [43,47]. In ALF, decreased reuptake by astrocytes results in increased extracellular glutamate concentrations. Abnormal trafficking of glutamate between neurons and astrocytes may contribute to the neurological manifestations of ALF. Similarly, monoamines [53,54], peripheral-type benzodiazepine receptors [43,55] and nitric oxide [56] have been proposed as important contributing factors for hepatic encephalopathy. Other stressors such as hypoglycemia, hyponatremia, hypokalemia and infections can precipitate the onset of hepatic encephalopathy in a patient with previously compensated liver failure.

Management of hepatic encephalopathy involves strategies to lower blood ammonia concentrations and manage elevated ICP. Judicious protein intake is advocated. While excessive protein intake increases ammonia load, negative nitrogen balance is detrimental to liver regeneration and preservation of skeletal muscle mass. Protein intake of 1–2 g/kg/d is often needed to prevent muscle wasting. A recent meta-anaysis concluded that branched chain

TABLE 9.1. Grades of hepatic encephalopathy.

Grade I	Mild confusion, irritability, depression, euphoria, abnormal sleep patterns
Grade II	Moderate confusion, lethargy, decreased ability to perform mental tasks, personality changes
Grade III	Severe confusion, disorientation, unable to perform mental tasks, somnolent, incomprehensible speech
Grade IV	Coma

amino acid supplementation has no beneficial effect on patients with hepatic encephalopathy [57]. Maintenance of normoglycemia is critically important. Lactulose is a commonly recommended agent to reduce ammonia production and absorption from the gut [42,58]. The dose of lactulose is adjusted to achieve 2–3 bowel movements per day. Oral neomycin has been used to reduce ammonia-producing bacteria in the gut when lactulose is not tolerated [42]. Neomycin has been associated with significant side effects such as renal and ototoxicity.

Cytotoxic cerebral edema associated with ALF is best managed with osmotherapy such as mannitol and hypertonic saline. Care must be taken to avoid hypovolemia, hypokalemia, and hyperosmolarity. Moderate hypothermia with core temperature of 32–33°C may be useful in decreasing ICP and reducing transfer of ammonia across the BBB [59]. Barbiturate therapy and moderate hyperventilation are useful adjuncts in decreasing ICP. The benefit of invasive ICP monitoring must be weighed against the risk of bleeding associated with the often accompanying coagulopathy. Vitamin K, fresh frozen plasma and in some cases, factor VII concentrates are necessary to reverse coagulopathy. Epidural monitors may be preferable to subdural ones for ICP monitoring. Maximum International Normalized Ratio (INR) >4, young age (<2 yrs), and presence of radiologic evidence of cerebral edema are of poor prognostic significance [46,60,61].

Short-term extracorporeal support as a bridge to liver transplantation has not been shown to be more effective than standard supportive care [60]. Liver transplantation offers the best chance of survival in a select group of patients with ALF. The important consideration is the probability of survival with supportive management versus liver transplantation. Patient selection and timing of the liver transplantation play a major role in outcome. Presence of cerebral edema greatly decreases chances of successful liver transplantation. On the other hand, cerebral edema may develop during or shortly after transplantation making survival unlikely [46].

Encephalopathy of Inborn Errors of Metabolism

A variety of inborn errors of carbohydrate, fat and protein metabolism result in accumulation of endogenous toxins such as ammonia, organic acids, and amino acids. Also, hypoglycemia may be a presenting feature. While such patients often present in early infancy, some inborn errors of metabolism may manifest at a later age. Unexplained encephalopathy accompanied by hypoglycemia and acid/base abnormalities should raise concern about the presence of inborn errors of metabolism. Such patients should have serum and urine measurements of amino acids and organic acids. Blood ammonia and lactate/pyruvate determination may also provide useful diagnostic clues. Treatment depends upon the individual disease entity. Peritoneal dialysis or hemodialysis may be required for severe hyperammonemia.

Nutritional Encephalopathy

Severe thiamine deficiency is potentially fatal if it is unrecognized and untreated. Patients with chronic debilitating diseases with unique nutritional needs may be at risk of developing thiamine deficiency. These include patients who are dependent on TPN, hemodialysis, and peritoneal dialysis. Patients with long-term metabolic derangements such as diabetes mellitus and renal failure, and those with poor nutritional habits are also at risk for developing severe thiamine deficiency. Thiamine is a water soluble vitamin with limited body stores. Severe thiamine deficiency may develop in as little as 5–7 days of deprivation [62,63]. Thiamine deficiency carries the risk of especially catastrophic and life-threatening consequences when associated with glucose loading such as in patients receiving TPN [64], and those treated with insulin for DKA. Incomplete combustion of products of glycolysis due to decreased activities of thiamine dependent transketolase, pyruvate dehydrogenase, and α-ketoglutarate dehydrogenase results in accumulation of pyruvate and Krebs cycle intermediates, and decreased synthesis of nucleic acids. The end result is energy failure, high anion gap metabolic acidosis, and multiorgan dysfunction. Clinically, a patient with acute thiamine deficiency manifests varying levels of encephalopathy progressing to unconsciousness. Myocardial insufficiency resulting in cardiogenic shock is also an important manifestation. Impairment of myocardial contractility and shock are often resistant to intravascular volume expansion and inotropic support. Both pyruvate and lactate concentrations are increased. The lactate/pyruvate ratio is often <20 because the major effect of thiamine deficiency is an inability to convert pyruvate to acetyl CoA. Pyruvate is then converted to lactate as an alternate albeit inferior source of energy.

Diagnosis of thiamine deficiency is mainly a clinical one. Critically ill patients with unexplained encephalopathy, myocardial dysfunction, and high anion gap metabolic acidosis in clinically relevant situations should raise suspicion of thiamine deficiency. Although the diagnosis could be supported by measurement of erythrocyte transketolase activity and biological assay for whole blood thiamine level, the treatment should not be delayed pending the results of these tests. The clinical response to IV administration of thiamine is dramatic as well as diagnostic in patients with thiamine deficiency. Immediate improvement occurs within minutes while complete resolution of symptomatology takes several hours. Thiamine is administered in a dose of 100 mg IV over 30 minutes and repeated in 4 hours as indicated clinically. Other vitamin and nutritional deficiencies such as that of niacin may also cause encephalopathy, however these are usually not encountered in the acute setting.

Miscellaneous Toxic/Metabolic Encephalopathies

A variety of illnesses encountered in intensive care units such as sepsis, renal failure etc, are associated with encephalopathy. The pathogenesis involves various endogenous toxins and cytokines according to individual conditions. Management is that of the underlying disorder. Improvement in encephalopathy coincides with resolution of the primary pathophysiology.

References

1. Drewes LR. What is the blood-brain barrier? A molecular perspective. Cerebral vascular biology. Adv Exp Med Biol 1999;474:111–122.

2. Fraser CL, Arieff AI. Metabolic encephalopathy. In: Arieff AI, DeFronzo RA, eds. *Fluid, Electrolyte and Acid-Base Disorders.* 2nd ed. New York: Churchill-Livingstone, 1995:685–740.

3. Lien YH, Shapiro JI, Chan L. Effects of hypernatremia on organic brain osmoles. J Clin Invest 1990;85:1427–1435.

4. Arieff AI, Schmidt RW. Fluid and electrolyte disorders and the central nervous system. In: Maxwell MH, Kleeman CR, eds. *Clinical Disorders of Fluid and Electrolyte Metabolism.* 3nd ed. New York: McGraw-Hill Book Company, 1980:1409–1480.

5. Sterns RH, Thomas DH. Brain dehydration and neurologic deterioration after rapid correction of hyponatremia. Kidney Int 1989;35:69–75.

6. Fishman RA. Brain edema. N Engl J Med 1975;293:706–711.
7. Preston G, Sarnaik AP, Nigro M. Transient intellectual and psychosocial regression during recovery phase of stage V Reye's syndrome. Dev Behav Pediatr 1982;3:206–208.
8. Magistretti PJ. Brain energy metabolism. In: Zigmond MJ, Bloom FE, Landis SC, Roberts JL, Squire LR, eds. *Fundamental Neuroscience*. San Diego, CA: Academic Press, 1999:389–413.
9. DeVivo DC. The effects of ketone bodies on glucose utilization. In: Passonneau JV, Hawkins RA, Lust WD, Welsh FA, eds. *Cerebral Metabolism and Neural Function*. Baltimore, MD: Williams and Wilkins, 1980:243–254.
10. Bachelard HS. Glucose transport to the brain in vivo and in vitro. In: Passonneau JV, Hawkins RA, Lust WD, Welsh FA, eds. *Cerebral Metabolism and Neural Function*. Baltimore, MD: Williams and Wilkins, 1980:106–119.
11. Wilson JD. Vitamin deficiency and excess. In: Isselbacher KJ, Braunwald E, Wilson JD, Martin JB, Fauci AS, Kasper DL, eds. *Harrison's Principles of Internal Medicine*. 13th ed. New York: McGraw-Hill, 1994:472–480.
12. Guyton AC. Dietary balances; regulation of feeding; obesity and starvation; vitamins and minerals. In: Guyton AC, Hall JE, eds. *Textbook of Medical Physiology*. 9th ed. Philadelphia: WB Saunders, 1996:889–901.
13. Tanphaichitr V. Thiamin. In: Shils ME, Olson JA, Shike M, eds. *Modern Nutrition in Health and Disease*. 8th ed. Philadelphia: Lea and Febiger, 1994:359–364.
14. Partin JC, Schubert WK, Partin JS. Mitochondrial ultrastructure in Reye's syndrome (Encephalopathy and fatty degeneration of the viscera). N Engl J Med 1971;285:1339–1343.
15. Partin JC, Partin JS, Schubert WK, et al. Brain ultrastructure in Reye's syndrome. J Neuropathol Exp Neurol 1975;34:425–444.
16. Chen R, Young GB. Metabolic encephalopathies. Baillieres Clin Neurol 1996;5:577–598.
17. Reye RDK, Morgan G, Baral J. Encephalopathy and fatty degeneration of the viscera. A disease entity in childhood. Lancet 1963;2:749–752.
18. Johnson GM, Scurletis TD, Carrol NB. A study of sixteen fatal cases of encephalitis-like disease in North Carolina children. N C Med J 1963;24:464–473.
19. Hall SM, Plaster PA, Glasgow JFT, et al. Preadmission antipyretics in Reye's syndrome. Arch Dis Child 1988;63:857–866.
20. Hurwitz ES, Barrett MJ, Bregman D, et al. Public Health Service study of Reye's syndrome and medications: Report of the main study. JAMA 1987;257:1905–1911.
21. Hurwitz ES. The changing epidemiology of Reye's syndrome in the United States: Further evidence for a public health success. JAMA 1988;260:3178–3180.
22. Centers for Disease Control and Prevention: Reye syndrome surveillance-United States, 1989. MMWR Morb Mortal Wkly Rep 1991;40:88–90.
23. Sarnaik AP. Reye's syndrome: Hold the obituary. Crit Care Med 1999;27:1674–1676.
24. Sarnaik AP, Meert K, Hackbarth R, et al. Management of hyponatremic seizures in children with hypertonic saline: A safe and effective strategy. Crit Care Med 1991;19:758–762.
25. Arieff AI. Hyponatremia, coma, convulsion, respiratory arrest, and permanent brain damage after elective brain surgery in healthy women. N Engl J Med 1986;314:1529–1535.
26. Corneli HM, Gormley CJ, Baker RC. Hyponatremia and seizures presenting in the first two years of life. Pediatr Emerg Care 1985;1:190–193.
27. Keating JP, Schears GJ, Dodge PR. Oral water intoxication in infants. An American epidemic. AJDC 1991;145:985–990.
28. Sterns RH. Severe symptomatic hyponatremia: treatment and outcome. A study of 64 cases. Ann Intern Med 1987;107:656–664.
29. Raskind M. Psychosis, polydipsia, and water intoxication: Report of a fatal case. Arch Gen Psychiatry 1974;30:112–114.
30. Arieff AI. Treatment of symptomatic hyponatremia: Neither haste nor waste. Crit Care Med 1991;19:748–751.
31. Sterns RH, Riggs JE, Schochet SS. Osmotic demylination syndrome following correction of hyponatremia. N Engl J Med 1986;314:1535–1542.
32. Laureno R, Karp BI. Pontine and extrapontine myelinolysis following rapid correction of hyponatremia. Lancet 1988;1:1439–1441.
33. Muir A. Do doctors cause or prevent cerebral edema in children with diabetic ketoacidosis? Pediatr Diabetes 2000;1:209–216.
34. Harris GD, Fiordalisi L, Harris WL, et al. Minimizing the risk of brain herniation during treatment of diabetic ketoacidemia: A retrospective and prospective trial. J Pediatr 1990;117:22–31.
35. Mahoney CP, Vlcek BW, DelAguila MA. Risk factors for developing brain herniation during diabetic ketoacidosis. Pediatr Neurol 1999;21:721–727.
36. Smedman L, Escobar R, Hesser U, et al. Subclinical cerebral oedema does not occur regularly during treatment of diabetic ketoacidosis. Acta Paediatr 1997;86:1172–1176.
37. Krane EJ, Rockoff MA, Waliman JK, et al. Subclinical brain swelling in children during treatment of diabetic ketoacidosis. N Engl J Med 1985;312:1147–1151.
38. Glaser N, Barnett P, McCaslin I, et al. Risk factors for cerebral edema in children with diabetic ketoacidosis. N Engl J Med 2001;344:264–269.
39. Glaser NS, Wootton-Gorges SL, Marcin JP, et al. Mechanism of cerebral edema in children with diabetic ketoacidosis. J Pediatr 2004;145:164–171.
40. Levitsky LL. Symptomatic cerebral edema in diabetic ketoacidosis: the mechanism is clarified but still far from clear. J Pediatr 2004;145:149–150.
41. Ferenci P, Lockwood A, Mullen K, et al. and the members of the working party. Hepatic encephalopathy—definition, nomenclature, diagnosis, and quantification: Final report of the working party at the 11th World Congress of Gastroenterology, Vienna, 1998. Hepatology 2002;35:716–721.
42. Lizardi-Cervera J, Almeda P, Guevara L, et al. Hepatic encephalopathy: A review. Ann Hepatol 2003;2:122–130.
43. Hazell AS, Butterworth RF. Hepatic encephalopathy. An update of pathophysiologic mechanisms. Pro Soc Exp Biol Med 1999;222:99–112.
44. Butterworth RF. Hepatic encephalopathy. Alcohol Res Health 2003;27:240–246.
45. Butterworth RF. Complications of cirrhosis. III. Hepatic encephalopathy. J Hepatol 2000;32 (suppl. 1):171–180.
46. Alper G, Jarjour IT, Reyes JD, et al. Outcome of children with cerebral edema caused by fulminant hepatic failure. Pediatr Neurol 1998;18:299–304.
47. Vaquero J, Chung C, Blei AT. Brain edema in acute liver failure. A window to the pathogenesis of hepatic encephalopathy. Ann Hepatol 2003;2:12–22.
48. Kato M, Hughes RD, Keays RT, et al. Electron microscopic study of brain capillaries in cerebral edema from fulminant hepatic failure. Hepatology 1992;15:1060–1066.
49. Clemmensen JO, Larsen FS, Kondrup J, et al. Cerebral herniation in patients with acute liver failure is correlated with arterial ammonia concentration. Hepatology 1999;29:648–653.
50. Larsen FS, Ejlersen E, Hansen BA, et al. Functional loss of cerebral blood flow autoregulation in patients with fulminant hepatic failure. J Hepatol 1995;23:212–217.
51. Strauss G, Hansen BA, Kirkegaard P, et al. Liver function, cerebral blood flow autoregulation, and hepatic encephalopathy in fulminant hepatic failure. Hepatology 1997;25:837–839.
52. Aggarwal S, Yonas H, Kang Y, et al. Relationship of cerebral blood flow, and cerebral swelling to outcome in patients with acute fulminant hepatic failure. Transplant Proc 1991;23:1978–1979.
53. Bergeron M, Reader TA, Layrargues GP, et al. Monoamines and metabolites in autopsied brain tissue from cirrhotic patients with hepatic encephalopathy. Neurochem Res 1989;14:853–859.

54. Bengtsson F, Bugge M, Johansen KH, et al. Brain tryptophan hydroxylation in the portacaval shunted rat: A hypothesis for the regulation of serotonin turnover in vivo. J Neurochem 1991;56:1069–1074.

55. Giguere JF, Hamel E, Butterworth RF. Increased densities of binding sites for the 'peripheral-type' benzodiazepine receptor ligand ^{3}H-PK11195 in rat brain following portacaval anastomosis. Brain Res 1992;585:295–298.

56. Rao VL, Giguere JF, Layrargues GP, et al. Increased activities of MAO_A and MAO_B in autopsied brain tissue from cirrhotic patients with hepatic encephalopathy. Brain Res 1993;621:349–352.

57. Als-Nielsen B, Koretz RL, Kjaergard LL, et al. Branched-chain amino acids for hepatic encephalopathy. The Cochrane Database of Systematic Reviews 2003;(2):CD001939.

58. Als-Nielsen B, Gluud LL, Gluud C. Non-absorbable disaccharides for hepatic encephalopathy: Systematic review of randomized trials. BMJ 2004;328:1046.

59. Jalan R, Olde Damink SW, Lee A, Hayes PC. Moderate hypothermia for uncontrolled intracranial hypertension in acute liver failure. Lancet 1999;354:1164–1168.

60. Marrero J, Martinez FJ, Hyzy R. Advances in critical care hepatology. Am J Respir Crit Care Med 2003;168:1421–1426.

61. Bhaduri BR, Mieli-Vergani G. Fulminant hepatic failure: Pediatric aspects. Semin Liver Dis 1996;16:349–355.

62. Kitamura K, Takahashi T, Tanaka H, et al. Two cases of thiamine deficiency-induced lactic acidosis during total parenteral nutrition. Tohoku J Exp Med 1993;171:129–133.

63. Valez R, Myers B, Guber MS. Severe acute metabolic acidosis (acute beriberi): an avoidable complication of total parenteral nutrition. JPEN J Parenter Enteral Nutr 1985;9:216–219.

64. Witkowski AA, Sarnaik AP, Heidemann SM, et al. Thiamine-responsive lactic acidosis, encephalopathy, and shock. J Pharm Technol 1998;14:240–242.

10
Infections of the Central Nervous System

Simon Nadel

Introduction

Infections affecting the central nervous system (CNS) in children have a varied and unpredictable outcome, often with a high morbidity and mortality, despite advances in available antimicrobial therapy and other adjunctive modes of treatment. Death or permanent disability is a common occurrence. There are many different organisms that initiate a variety of pathologic processes leading to the resulting clinical patterns. The subsequent conditions include meningitis, encephalitis, intracerebral abscesses, transverse myelitis, and noninfectious complications of systemic infection such as human immunodeficiency virus (HIV). The offending organism varies with age, immune function, and immunization status of the child. Although much of the focus in the management of these conditions is on eradication of a pathogen, many of these patients require organ-specific supportive care, including mechanical ventilation, and neuroprotective strategies where there is intracranial hypertension. This chapter reviews intracranial infections, their epidemiology, the nature of the infecting organism, and management of the clinical patterns that occur.

Meningitis

Although the spectrum between meningitis and encephalitis is broad, it is important to understand the pathophysiologic processes that take place that lead to meningitis and encephalitis. Meningitis is an inflammation of the pia and arachnoid meninges that surround the brain and spinal cord. In contrast, encephalitis is an inflammation of the brain parenchyma itself that typically presents with either diffuse or focal neuropsychological dysfunction.

Bacterial Meningitis

The definitive diagnosis of bacterial meningitis requires the isolation of the pathogen from cerebrospinal fluid (CSF). If for clinical reasons obtaining CSF is not possible, a clinical diagnosis of meningitis can be made by the finding of clinical signs of meningeal irritation (neck stiffness, positive Kernig's or Brudzinski's sign), together with positive blood culture, latex agglutination test for bacterial polysaccharide in blood or urine, or positive polymerase chain reaction for bacterial DNA in blood. Definitions of CNS infection have been recently proposed and for meningitis are divided into definite, probable, or possible bacterial meningitis (Table 10.1) [1].

Following bacterial meningitis, a poor outcome is common, with death or handicap occurring in up to 50% of patients depending on age, causative organism, and clinical status at presentation [2]. In the developed world, bacterial meningitis occurs at a frequency of approximately 3–5 patients per 100,000 population per year [3–5], apart from clusters or outbreaks. In the developing world, particularly during pandemics of meningococcal meningitis in sub-Saharan Africa, this figure may increase to over 500 patients per 100,000 population [6].

In neonates, pathogens causing meningitis are usually acquired from the maternal genital tract during delivery and include *Streptococcus agalactiae* (group B streptococci), *Escherichia coli*, and other organisms that colonize the perineal area [7]. Neonates are also at risk of infection from *Listeria monocytogenes*, acquired transplacentally. In older children, bacterial meningitis is usually acquired via hematogenous spread, and the most common infecting organisms are *Neisseria meningitidis*, *Streptococcus pneumoniae*, and *Haemophilus influenzae* (type b) (Hib) [8]. Routine vaccination programs have practically eradicated bacterial meningitis caused by Hib. Meningitis caused by *L. monocytogenes* may also occur in immunocompromised children. In addition, direct invasion by skin or respiratory pathogens and nosocomial infection may occur following trauma and neurosurgical interventions [9]. The organisms that predominate under these circumstances include *Pseudomonas aeruginosa*, enterococci, *Staphylococcus aureus*, and the coagulase-negative staphylococci. Table 10.2 lists the pathogens associated with acute bacterial meningitis according to age.

Pathophysiology

Bacterial invasion of the CSF causes a host inflammatory response, and ultimately it is this response that results in neuronal cell damage and death and the subsequent morbidity and mortality.

D.S. Wheeler et al. (eds.), *The Central Nervous System in Pediatric Critical Illness and Injury*,
DOI 10.1007/978-1-84800-993-6_10, © Springer-Verlag London Limited 2009

TABLE 10.1. Bacterial meningitis in children and infants >8 weeks old.

Definite bacterial meningitis
Compatible clinical syndrome +
  All ages: fever, 94%
  1–5 months: irritability, 85%
  6–11 months: impaired consciousness, 79%
  >12 months: vomiting, 82%, neck rigidity, 78%
  + positive culture of cerebrospinal fluid (CSF) or positive CSF Gram stain or bacterial
    antigen

Probable bacterial meningitis
Compatible clinical syndrome +
Positive blood culture + one of the following CSF changes:
>5 leukocytes, glucose <0.5 CSF/serum ratio, protein >1 g/L

Possible bacterial meningitis
Compatible clinical syndrome +
One of the following CSF changes:
>100 leukocytes, CSF/serum glucose ratio <0.5, protein >1 g/L +
Negative cultures or antigen for bacteria, virus, fungus, or mycobacteria

Neonatal meningitis <8 weeks old
Compatible clinical syndrome +
Isolation of likely pathogenic organism from CSF or positive bacterial antigen
Or abnormal CSF consistent with bacterial infection (see above)

Infecting pathogens reach CSF by hematogenous spread following colonization of the skin, the mucosal surface of the nasopharynx [10], or the respiratory or gastrointestinal tract; the organisms then translocate across the endothelial cells of the blood–brain barrier (BBB) in order to reach the CSF. Once in the CSF, bacterial products (e.g., peptidoglycan, lipoteichoic acid, endotoxin) stimulate the production of proinflammatory cytokines [11–13] (e.g., tumor necrosis factor [TNF]-α, interleukin [IL]-1β, and IL-6) and other mediators (e.g., nitric oxide and reactive oxygen species), leading to an influx of leukocytes into the subarachnoid space [14]. This is further enhanced following the induction of endothelial-derived adhesion molecules on the cerebral endothelium [15]. These blood-derived leukocytes, proinflammatory cytokines, and other inflammatory mediators cause an increase in BBB permeability, resulting in the leakage of plasma proteins into the CSF, further contributing to the development of cerebral edema and subsequent neuronal damage [16,17]. Diffuse cerebral endothelial damage leads to vasospasm and thrombosis, resulting in abnormal cerebral vascular autoregulation and a reduction in cerebral perfusion, and therefore to further neuronal damage [18]. The inflammatory effects of cytokines are regulated by the antiinflammatory cytokines: IL-10 and transforming growth factor (TGF)-β. It is the inflammatory response to an invading organism rather than direct effects of the pathogen itself that appears to cause most of the damage leading to morbidity and mortality in acute bacterial meningitis [19].

Clinical Manifestations

The classic signs of meningitis include fever, headache, photophobia, vomiting, neck stiffness, and an altered level of consciousness or mental status, including seizure activity [20]. In young children and infants, the signs may be nonspecific, and fever may be absent [21]; however, whenever a child has fever with an altered level of consciousness, meningitis must be considered high in the differential diagnosis.

Diagnosis

Obtaining CSF for culture is the gold standard investigation for the diagnosis of bacterial meningitis. When performing a lumbar puncture (LP) it is essential to measure and document the CSF opening pressure (normally <15 cm H_2O), appearance, cell count and differential count, glucose, protein, Gram stain, microbiological culture (including for viruses and fungi), viral and bacterial polymerase chain reaction, and stain for acid-fast bacilli, if indicated. Prompt diagnosis is essential, as a delay in commencing antibacterial therapy may be associated with an increased likelihood of morbidity, although the clinical evidence to support this assumption is surprisingly lacking [22].

Purulent meningitis is associated with intracranial hypertension, and brain stem or tentorial herniation may occur even in the absence of LP (approximately 5% of cases). Taking an accurate history, with appropriate recognition of the early systemic and neurologic signs of meningitis, allows an informed decision about whether an LP can be performed safely [23]. Performing an LP in the presence of intracranial hypertension may cause cerebral herniation. Therefore, if signs of raised intracranial pressure (ICP) are present, it is not safe to undertake an LP even in the presence of normal brain imaging [24]. Lumbar puncture is contraindicated (1) when there is significant respiratory and/or hemodynamic compromise, (2) when there is a bleeding diathesis, and (3) when focal neurologic signs and a fluctuating or significantly reduced (Glasgow Coma Score [GCS] ≤13) level of consciousness are present, usually indicating raised ICP. If there will be a delay in performing an LP, because of concerns about clinical status, it is important to start appropriate antimicrobial therapy as soon as possible, targeted toward the most likely offending agent based on age and immunologic status (see Table 10.2).

Up to 50% of children with meningitis receive oral antibiotics before a definitive diagnosis is made generally because of a nonspecific presentation [25]. This partial treatment often leads to a delay in presentation to the hospital and may cause diagnostic confusion [26]. Cerebral spinal fluid cultures may be rapidly sterilized, although cellular and biochemical changes will persist. The only bacterium whose growth is likely to be significantly affected following oral antibiotic administration is *Meningococcus*, and this is

TABLE 10.2. Pathogens by clinically important factors.

Age	Organisms
<1 month	*Streptococcus agalactiae* (group B streptococci), enteric bacilli (*Escherichia coli*, *Klebsiella pneumoniae*, *Proteus* spp.), *Listeria monocytogenes*
1–3 months	*S. agalactiae* (group B streptococci), enteric bacilli (*E. coli, K. pneumoniae, Proteus* spp.), *L. monocytogenes*, *Streptococcus pneumoniae*, *Neisseria meningitidis*, *Haemophilus influenzae* type b (Hib)
3 months to 5 years	*S. pneumoniae*, *N. meningitidis*, Hib
>5 years	*S. pneumoniae*, *N. meningitidis*
Immunocompromised	*S. pneumoniae*, *N. meningitidis*, Hib, *L. monocytogenes*, Gram-negative bacilli, *Salmonella* spp, enteric bacteria, *Pseudomonas aeruginosa*, *Cryptococcus neoformans*, other fungi, *Nocardia* spp
Postneurosurgery, postneurotrauma, CSF shunt	*S. pneumoniae*, *N. meningitidis*, Hib, *Staphylococcus aureus*, coagulase-negative staphylococci, Gram-negative bacilli, *Streptococcus pyogenes*, enterococci

Source: Williams and Nadel [9].

thought to be caused by the high sensitivity of the organism to low concentrations of antibiotics [27]. It is essential that CSF is sent for polymerase chain reaction and bacterial antigen detection as these will not usually be affected by the low CSF antibiotic concentrations found following oral administration.

A recent study suggested that CNS imaging played little part in the diagnosis and clinical management of children admitted to the hospital with an acute febrile encephalopathy, in the absence of focal neurologic signs [28,29]. In addition, cranial computed tomography (CT) scans have a poor positive predictive value for the detection of intracranial hypertension [30]. In various case series of children with meningitis, abnormal CT findings include subdural effusion, focal infarction, mild ventricular widening, contrast enhancing basal meninges, cerebral edema and pus, and widening in the basal cisterns [31–33]. Focal infarction and pus in the basal cisterns are associated with long-term neurologic sequelae. Transient dilatation of the subarachnoid space, however, is a relatively common finding and is not necessarily associated with long-term sequelae [32]. In another small series, parenchymal changes were found in nine children with bacterial meningitis. All children had neurologic impairment at the time of CT, and, during follow up, those with mild or moderate changes recovered without neurologic sequelae, whereas those with severe changes suffered severe neurologic sequelae [33]. Performing imaging for prognostication therefore appears to be of benefit.

Therapy

The management of bacterial meningitis requires specific antimicrobial agents (see below) as well as organ-specific supportive treatment targeted at reducing raised ICP with neuroprotective strategies. Bacterial multiplication within the CSF occurs quickly owing to a poor host immune response at this relatively immune-isolated site [34]. The CSF contains relatively low levels of specific antibody and complement, resulting in poor opsonization and phagocytosis [35].

Supportive Care

Some children may require tracheal intubation and mechanical ventilatory support. Indications for tracheal intubation and mechanical ventilatory support include (1) treatment of intracranial hypertension; (2) seizure management, including respiratory depression secondary to anticonvulsant medication; (3) coma; and (4) shock. A high Pediatric Risk of Mortality (PRISM) score upon admission and the presence of hypotension and tachycardia within the first 24 hr are typically associated with poor outcome [36].

All patients with bacterial meningitis will have evidence of increased ICP [37]. Increased ICP together with cerebral vasculitis and cerebral dysfunction are responsible for acute neurologic complications, including depression of conscious level, focal neurologic signs, and, potentially, cerebral herniation in the acute phase, all of which are associated with longer term neurologic sequelae. Initial resuscitation and management should be directed towards securing the airway (A = airway) and maintaining adequate oxygenation/ventilation (B = breathing) and hemodynamic stability (C = circulation) [38]. Early tracheal intubation and mechanical ventilatory support should be considered for children with a rapidly deteriorating GCS (>3 points in an hour), those with a GCS ≤8, those with a fluctuating level of consciousness, and those with any associated respiratory or cardiovascular organ failure. Mechanical ventilatory support should be tailored to maintain normal oxygen-ation and ventilation, with the goal of limiting ventilator-induced lung injury. Ventilation must be tailored to achieve arterial pCO_2 in the normal range [39], which avoids the dynamic complications associated with hyper- or hypocarbia. There is no evidence that the use of positive end-expiratory pressure (PEEP) exacerbates raised ICP, and its use is associated with a reduction in the risk of atelectasis [40]. Patients should be positioned appropriately to prevent obstruction to cerebral venous drainage, with elevation of the head of the bed by 20°–30° and head position maintained in the midline. Placement of internal jugular venous catheters should be avoided if possible, as they may obstruct venous drainage from the brain.

It is important to achieve a blood pressure that will achieve adequate cerebral perfusion pressure (CPP). Cerebral perfusion pressure is the equal to the mean arterial blood pressure (MAP) minus the ICP. It has been shown that a CPP of ≤40 mm Hg is associated with a poor outcome as determined by mortality and long-term disability in children with nontraumatic coma [41]. Recent studies have confirmed that maintenance of MAP with vasoconstrictive agents such as norepinephrine offer better protection of cerebral cellular oxygenation than other methods to support blood pressure in the presence of adequate intravascular volume [42,43].

Hyperthermia must be avoided [44] and when necessary active cooling measures instituted. In addition, tight control of serum electrolytes and blood glucose is required. There is some evidence that moderate hypothermia may be protective [45,46]; however, there are no data regarding its use in acute infectious encephalopathy.

Fluid management for bacterial meningitis is controversial. The guidelines recommending fluid restriction have been based on the frequent development of hyponatremia seen in children with bacterial meningitis, often found in conjunction with an increase in circulating concentration of antidiuretic hormone (ADH), as part of the syndrome of inappropriate ADH secretion (SIADH) [47]. The SIADH is associated with total body water overload and thus contributes to cerebral swelling. By restricting intravenous fluid administration in the presence of SIADH, the risk of developing cerebral edema is likely to be diminished. Some groups have found that children with bacterial meningitis who received maintenance fluid, as well as replacement of any deficits, had normal levels of ADH, whereas those who received restricted fluids had elevated ADH levels, suggesting that the increased ADH noted in meningitis was an appropriate response to dehydration. The explanation is that children who present to the hospital with bacterial meningitis have often had several days of fever and may have had vomiting, diarrhea, and inadequate fluid intake. In children with bacterial meningitis who were randomized to fluid restriction, when there was a reduction of >10 mL/kg in extracellular water, there was an increase in mortality and long-term neurologic morbidity [48]. When there is hyponatremia and normal ADH levels, it is thought that cerebral salt wasting contributes to the hyponatremia, the mechanism of which is unclear. Overall, although there are not enough data to firmly recommend fluid restriction, the main consideration should be avoidance of overzealous fluid administration.

In the face of an acute neurologic deterioration with signs of impending brain stem herniation, emergency management includes the administration of hyperosmolar therapy with mannitol or 3% saline [49]. There is no good evidence for one modality over another. In addition, in tracheally intubated and mechanically ventilated patients, short-term hyperventilation may prevent herniation [50].

Antibiotic Therapy

Empiric antibiotic therapy should be commenced based on the most likely causative organism for the individual patient, taking into account the patient's age, vaccination status, immune competence, and local patterns of antimicrobial resistance. In developed countries most authorities recommend a third-generation cephalosporin such as ceftriaxone or cefotaxime, which have good CSF penetration and are active against most pathogens causing bacterial meningitis [51,52].

Listeria monocytogenes, more common in infants under 3 months and adults over 50 years, is not sensitive to the cephalosporins; therefore, addition of a penicillin to this regimen is recommended [8]. However, antimicrobial resistance, among the common causes of acute bacterial meningitis, is of increasing clinical importance worldwide. The increasing emergence of resistant bacteria, particularly *Strep. pneumoniae*, methicillin-resistant *Staph. aureus* (MRSA), vancomycin-resistant enterococci (VRE), and the extended spectrum β-lactamase–producing Gram-negative organisms has presented enormous difficulties in the selection of adequate empiric antimicrobial therapy, before results of bacteriologic testing are available.

Factors to be taken into consideration when selecting the appropriate antibiotic for the therapy of bacterial meningitis include activity against the likely causative pathogen and its ability to penetrate and attain effective bactericidal concentrations in the CSF. The integrity of the BBB is compromised during meningitis, resulting in increased permeability to most antibiotics [53]. β-Lactam antibiotics achieve levels of 5%–20% of concomitant serum concentrations. Highly lipid-soluble antibiotics (e.g., rifampin, chloramphenicol, and the fluoroquinolones) achieve 30%–50% of their serum concentrations in CSF, even in the absence of BBB dysfunction. In contrast, the concentration of vancomycin is less than 5% of its serum concentration. Experimental models of bacterial meningitis in animals suggest that prompt bacteriologic cure is associated with antibiotic concentrations in CSF that are 10–30 times the minimal bactericidal concentration (MBC) for a specific microorganism [54].

The pharmacodynamic properties of different antimicrobials also affect their efficacy. Aminoglycosides and fluoroquinolones exhibit concentration-dependent activity. Their effectiveness is determined by the ratio between the peak concentration, or area under the concentration curve of the antibiotic, and the MBC of the infecting pathogen. In contrast, the β-lactams and vancomycin show concentration-independent activity. The time over the MBC during which the drug concentration exceeds the minimum inhibitory concentration (MIC) appears to be important in determining drug effectiveness. These drugs should therefore be administered at frequent dosing intervals.

For patients with a possible nosocomial infection, other broad-spectrum agents such as vancomycin and ceftazidime may be considered. Meropenem has been shown to be an excellent single agent for patients in whom resistant bacteria are likely or for those who have failed to respond to the primary choice [55]. However, there have been reports of treatment failures in patients with resistant pneumococcal meningitis and other resistant organisms [56,57].

The fluoroquinolones have been increasingly recognized as an important therapeutic option in both Gram-negative and Gram-positive meningitis, where their excellent CSF penetration and the potential for synergistic activity in combination with the cephalosporins and the carbapenems may indicate that they may play an important future role in the management of resistant pneumococcal and nosocomial meningitis [58].

Linezolid is the first agent of a new class of antibiotics called the oxazolidinones. Linezolid possesses excellent microbial activity against a wide variety of Gram-positive pathogens, including those resistant to methicillin and vancomycin. There have been several reports of its successful use in the management of resistant Gram-positive meningitis [59,60]. Table 10.3 lists the most common antibacterial agents used in the treatment of bacterial meningitis.

Antimicrobial resistance of organisms causing bacterial meningitis is becoming increasingly problematic in all parts of the world, with different resistance patterns emerging for different organisms in different places. Penicillin-resistant *Strep. pneumoniae* was first reported in 1967 [61] and has subsequently spread worldwide. Strains highly resistant to the penicillins, defined by the U.S. National Committee for Clinical Laboratory Standards [62] as an MIC of >2 μg/mL, are more likely to be resistant to other β-lactam and non-β-lactam antibacterials. The proportion of pneumococci causing invasive disease that are resistant to penicillin are reported to be as high as 59% in Hungary [63], 55% in Spain (pediatric patients) [64], 25% in Atlanta, Georgia [65], and 3.6% in the United Kingdom [66]. A Spanish study in 1999 found that 38% of all CSF isolates of pneumococci were resistant to penicillin [67]. More recently, pneumococcal strains resistant to the cephalosporins have been described [68]. In pneumococcal meningitis, strains are considered resistant to cefotaxime and ceftriaxone if the MIC is >0.5 μg/mL and highly resistant if the MIC is >2.0 μg/mL. There are several reports of treatment failure with third-generation cephalosporins [69,70], but there is some evidence to suggest that intermediate resistance (MIC = 1.0 μg/mL) is not associated with an altered clinical outcome when the third-generation cephalosporins are used for treatment [71].

Therapeutic modifications in light of increasing bacterial resistance to current antimicrobials have included the addition of vancomycin or rifampicin to a third-generation cephalosporin [72]. However, penetration of vancomycin into CSF is variable, particularly when concomitant corticosteroids are given, and there are recent reports of vancomycin-tolerant strains of pneumococci causing meningitis and of treatment failure in adults receiving vancomycin 30 mg/kg/24 hr [73]. Experimental evidence in animal models lends support to the possibility of delayed CSF sterilization when vancomycin is given with dexamethasone, as steroids reduce BBB permeability [74]. Rifampicin is a lipophilic compound with good CSF penetration [75] and is unaffected by the concomitant use of dexamethasone [76]. Its use has been recommended for adults receiving adjunctive steroid therapy and for children failing therapy on a combination of a cephalosporin and vancomycin.

TABLE 10.3. Empiric choice of antimicrobial by age.

Age	Empiric choice of antibacterial
<month	Penicillin or ampicillin and gentamicin
	Second line, ceftriaxone or cefotaxime
1–3 months	Ceftriaxone or cefotaxime and ampicillin
>3 months	Ceftriaxone or cefotaxime
Immunocompromised	Ceftriaxone and ampicillin and gentamicin
	Second line, meropenem and gentamicin
Postneurosurgery, postneurotrauma, CSF shunt	Ceftazidime and gentamicin and vancomycin
	Second line, meropenem and gentamicin and vancomycin

Unfortunately, along with penicillin resistance there has also been an increase in development of resistance to cephalosporins. To reduce the risk of treatment failure in meningitis because of resistant pneumococci, higher doses of cephalosporins have been assessed to increase CSF concentration of antibiotic. However, this has not been associated with reduction in treatment failure. More recently, recommendations have suggested antibacterial regimens that included vancomycin or rifampicin in combination with the cephalosporin [77]. In the United States, combination therapy of a cephalosporin and vancomycin is recommended for children with suspected pneumococcal meningitis, as adequate CSF concentrations of vancomycin have been demonstrated in children. However, because of concerns about CSF vancomycin concentrations in adults, rifampicin is recommended when pneumococcal meningitis is suspected.

Widespread penicillin resistance in *N. meningitidis* has also been reported [78], mainly caused by reduced affinity of penicillin for the penicillin binding proteins (PBP) 2 and 3 [79]. In addition, there are extremely rare, but worrying, reports of β-lactamase–producing meningococci [80]. A recent Spanish report suggests that penicillin-resistant meningococcal strains may be associated with a poorer clinical outcome [81], but there is no evidence of treatment failure with the third-generation cephalosporins or the newer fluoroquinolones. However, the emergence of rifampicin-resistant meningococci has important public health implications for chemoprophylaxis of close contacts of the index case [82].

β-Lactamase–producing strains of Hib are common, and chloramphenicol resistance is well described [83]. In countries where Hib conjugate vaccine is not in routine use, Hib meningitis because of resistant strains continues to be a clinical problem [84]; however, these strains are usually sensitive to the third-generation cephalosporins. In the postvaccine era, Hib meningitis or other non-Hib encapsulated *Haemophilus* (especially type f *Haemophilus*), accounted for 10% of all *Haemophilus* isolates from a recent epidemiologic study from Spain [85]. Most of these infections occurred in children <14 years of age, and 62% were ampicillin resistant, as well as resistant to tetracycline and chloramphenicol.

Most recommendations for duration of therapy are based on historical data with antimicrobials that are either no longer used or have become obsolete. There are few data on adequacy of length of therapy with the more commonly used modern antimicrobials. Table 10.4 provides additional information and recommendations on the duration of antimicrobial therapy in meningitis.

Antiinflammatory Agents

Cell wall–derived bacterial products, including endotoxin and peptidoglycan, lead to the activation of host inflammatory pathways, which further contribute to brain inflammation and edema. The release of proinflammatory cytokines, including the interleukins

TABLE 10.4. Recommended Duration of therapy by organism.

Infecting organism	Duration of therapy
Streptococcus pneumoniae	14 days
Streptococcus agalactiae (group B streptococci)	14–21 days
Listeria monocytogenes	14–21 days
Neisseria meningitidis	7 days
Haemophilus influenzae type b	7 days
Gram-negative organisms	21 days

Source: Data are from Gold [8].

(IL-1β, IL-6) and TNFα, leads to stimulation of the inflammatory cascade with the release of platelet activating factor (PAF), IL-8, and interferon-γ (IFN-γ). The activation of the inflammatory cascade results in the upregulation of cellular adhesion molecules in the vascular endothelium and blood leukocytes and the release of toxic products from activated neutrophils, which mediates meningeal inflammation, disruption of the BBB, microvascular thrombosis, and both vasogenic and cytotoxic cerebral edema [86,87].

Animal studies have suggested that, following antibiotic treatment, bacterial lysis induces inflammation in the subarachnoid space; when dexamethasone was used, the inflammatory changes were reduced, together with the sequelae seen [88]. Dexamethasone downregulates meningeal inflammation and reduces cerebral edema and therefore intracranial hypertension, thereby leading to a reduction in neurologic damage and the development of long-term sequelae. Adjunctive dexamethasone therapy has been shown to be beneficial for children with Hib meningitis who are at risk of deafness, and a meta-analysis has suggested a protective effect for those with pneumococcal meningitis if dexamethasone is administered at the same time as the initial antibiotic [89]. A study comparing early use of dexamethasone (administered before or with the first antibiotic dose) to placebo was undertaken with adults, with continued use for 4 days. Treatment with dexamethasone was associated with a reduction in both the risk of unfavorable outcome and mortality. There was an unfavorable outcome in 26% of the dexamethasone group compared with 52% of the placebo group [90]. A further adult study has reported a trend toward an improved outcome in the dexamethasone group, where 74% patients had no neurologic sequelae when compared with 52% of patients who did not receive corticosteroids [91]. This study was with adults with pneumococcal and meningococcal meningitis, and dexamethasone was administered up to 3 hr following antimicrobial therapy.

The potential pitfalls of the use of adjunctive corticosteroids include a reduction in BBB permeability, which may affect the penetration of antibiotics into the CSF, and the theoretical downregulation of potentially beneficial antiinflammatory cytokines such as IL-10. It was thought that, following corticosteroid administration, a dampened CSF inflammatory response would reduce vancomycin concentrations in the CSF and delay CSF sterilization; however, CSF vancomycin levels in children with bacterial meningitis were not reduced following adjunctive dexamethasone therapy [92]. To be able to offer any benefit, dexamethasone needs to be administered early in the course of the meningitis illness.

The use of corticosteroid therapy has been shown to be an effective adjunctive therapy for bacterial meningitis [93,94]. Although several other antiinflammatory agents, including polymyxin B, antibodies against TNF-α, IL-1β, recombinant bactericidal permeability/increasing protein (RBPI$_{21}$), have been used in studies of patients with sepsis, there has been no antiinflammatory agent assessed in patients with bacterial meningitis. These agents have been studied in various experimental models of bacterial meningitis and are discussed in further detail in the paragraphs below.

Experimental Therapies Targeting the Inflammatory Cascade

The effects of several nonsteroidal antiinflammatory compounds have been evaluated in experimental meningitis models, but data from clinical trials are scarce and to date none is currently recommended as routine adjunctive therapy. In rabbits with pneumococcal meningitis, no effect on CSF protein was seen with indomethacin, although adjunctive treatment with dexamethasone or oxindanac, another nonsteroidal antiinflammatory drug, was seen to produce the fastest reversion to normal CSF protein patterns [95]. Ketorolac, a nonsteroidal antiinflammatory drug, co-administered with ampicillin has been shown to reduce sensorineural hearing loss compared with placebo in an animal model [96]. However, ibuprofen, a widely used antipyretic agent, has itself been implicated in case reports as a cause of aseptic meningitis [97].

Interferon-γ activates macrophages, promotes cytotoxic T-cell differentiation, and stimulates B-cell production of complement fixing antibody to aid opsonization by macrophages and neutrophils. Production of IFN-γ is induced by IL-12 with TNF-α co-stimulation, and it is inhibited by IL-10. Levels of CSF IFN-γ have been measured in adults and children with bacterial, viral, and aseptic meningitis [98,99]. Higher levels of IFN-γ have been found in viral meningitis than in bacterial meningitis. However, greater rises in IFN-γ have been reported in children with pneumococcal meningitis than in those with Hib and meningococcal meningitis. Interferon-γ and its inducible chemokines have been shown to have antimicrobial effects in vitro [100]. Human glioblastoma cell lines inhibit the growth of group B streptococci when stimulated with IFN-γ [101]. Phase II clinical trials of recombinant IFN-γ as adjunctive therapy for meningitis are ongoing in the United States.

The proinflammatory cytokine TNF-α promotes the activation of macrophages and neutrophils and induces the production of IFNγ. Cerebrospinal fluid levels of TNF-α are significantly raised in bacterial meningitis when compared with clinical controls [102]. There is some evidence to suggest that the CSF level of TNF-α is related to the degree of BBB disruption and disease severity [103,104]. In a rat model, intracisternal administration of TNF-α resulted in dose- and time-dependent alterations in CSF penetration of radiolabeled albumin and in CSF white blood cells. The use of a monoclonal antibody (Mab) against TNF-α has been suggested as an adjuvant therapy in meningitis, modifying the acute inflammatory response and thereby reducing neuronal injury. In experimental E. coli meningitis in newborn piglets, Mab to TNF-α downmodulated CSF pleocytosis and reduced ICP but had no effect on CSF metabolism as measured by CSF lactate or lipid peroxidation products [105]. A Mab to TNF-α reduced only hippocampal neuronal apoptosis but not overall brain injury in a rat model of neonatal group B streptococcal meningitis [106]. Clinical trials of Mab to TNF-α in severe sepsis have had mixed results [107,108], and the experience in meningitis is limited at present to the animal models described earlier.

Pentoxifylline and thalidomide decrease the production of TNF-α. In experimental models they have had some beneficial effect in moderating CSF inflammation [109,110]. In a rabbit model of bacterial meningitis the antiinflammatory cytokine IL-10 has shown some benefit in reducing TNF-α production and CSF inflammation, with maximal effect shown when IL-10 was combined with dexamethasone [111].

Reactive oxygen intermediates, including superoxide anions and hydrogen peroxide, are generated by the inflammatory response in the CSF [112]. The antioxidants ascorbate and reduced glutathione are depleted in experimental meningitis models [113]. It has been suggested that clinically available antioxidants may reduce parenchymal brain injury caused by oxidative stress. In experimental pneumococcal meningitis in a rat model, the antioxidants N-acetylcysteine, desferroxamine, and tirilazad-mesylate have been shown to decrease cortical injury [114]. N-acetylcysteine also atten-uated the increase in brain water content, ICP, and CSF pleocytosis in advanced pneumococcal meningitis in rats [115].

The polysaccharide fucoidin is a selectin blocker that inhibits leukocyte rolling along endothelial cells, thereby preventing leukocyte recruitment into CSF. In an experimental model of rabbit meningitis induced by intracisternal injection of live pneumococci, fucoidin significantly reduced the accumulation of leukocytes and plasma proteins into CSF [116]. Animal studies have also shown a variable reduction in the CSF level of the proinflammatory cytokines IL-1β and TNF-α but required the early administration of fucoidin, 4 hr after the induction of meningitis by intracisternal injection of pneumococcal cell wall components in rabbits [117]. However, in rabbits treated with ampicillin 16 hr after induction of meningitis by intracisternal injection of live pneumococci, fucoidin had little effect on CSF levels of IL-1β and TNF-α [118].

Junctional adhesion molecule (JAM) is a member of the immunoglobulin superfamily found selectively concentrated at the tight junctions of endothelial cells. Varied reports exist on the efficacy of inhibition of plasma leukocyte migration through endothelial cells into the meninges in experimental meningitis models [119,120]. In a cytokine-induced mouse meningitis model, a Mab against JAM significantly inhibited CSF leukocyte accumulation and reduced BBB permeability. However anti-JAM antibodies in L. monocytogenes meningitis in mice failed to prevent leukocyte migration into the CSF.

The intercellular adhesion molecule-1 (ICAM-1) is a cell surface receptor involved in immune cell interactions and in leukocyte migration to inflamed tissues. In rat brain endothelial cell cultures, ICAM-1 expression is upregulated in response to bacterial cell wall products [121]. Patients with bacterial meningitis have been shown to have increased serum and CSF levels of soluble ICAM-1 [122]. In an experimental rat model of the early phase of bacterial meningitis induced by pneumococcal cell wall products, Mab to ICAM-1 significantly inhibited rises in ICP and brain water content [123].

Labradamil (receptor-mediated permeabilizer-7 [RMP-7]) is a nonapeptide that binds to B2 kinin receptors on endothelial cells of the BBB, therefore triggering nitric oxide and cyclic guanosine monophosphate pathways. This results in a brief relaxation of endothelial tight junctions, leading to a temporary increase in BBB permeability [124]. Receptor-mediated permeabilizer-7 has been developed to improve CNS penetration of existing chemotherapeutics and antiinfectives in brain tumours [125], ocular disease, and meningitis. Experimental tumor models have shown increased carboplatin delivery [126]. Phase I/II trials of amphotericin B in HIV-related cryptococcal meningitis [127] and pilot studies of CNS ganciclovir delivery showed that RMP-7 was reasonably, well tolerated with side effects of flushing, warmth, nausea, and vomiting consistent with kinin receptor activation [128]. A phase II clinical trial of RMP-7 as an adjunct to antibacterial therapy in meningitis is ongoing in the United States.

Hypothermia

Induced hypothermia in experimental models of meningitis has been shown to attenuate the inflammatory response and to be neuroprotective. In such models hypothermia reduces changes in CSF glucose, protein, lactate, excitatory neurotransmitters, TNF-α, and leukocytes [129,130]. A reduction in ICP and cerebral edema and an improvement in cerebral perfusion have been demonstrated in a rabbit model of severe group B streptococcal meningitis [131]. Similar neuroprotective benefits have been proposed for the adjunctive treatment of severe head injury with hypothermia. There are proposals for the use of moderate hypothermia (35°C) as an adjunctive treatment of bacterial meningitis in humans.

Prevention

The widespread introduction of Hib vaccine in the developed world has had a dramatic impact on the epidemiology of Hib meningitis, with virtual eradication of Hib as a cause of invasive disease in vaccinated groups [132]. The recent introduction of conjugated group C meningococcal vaccine in the United Kingdom has caused a reduction of around 80% in the incidence of group C meningococcal meningitis, with 90%–95% protection in immunized groups in the first year after vaccination [133]. It is likely that this vaccine will be introduced into other countries with a high incidence of group C meningococcal infection. Unfortunately, worldwide, groups A, B, W135, and Y meningococci are the major causes of severe infection. A quadrivalent group A/C/W135/Y-conjugated vaccine is under development and may become useful, particularly in view of the recent outbreaks of group A disease in Africa [134], W135 disease associated with the Hajj [135], and the recent increase in incidence of group Y disease in the United States [136].

Development of a vaccine for the prevention of meningococcal serogroup B disease remains a priority. The group B capsular polysaccharide is poorly immunogenic in humans, and it cross reacts with a human neural cell adhesion molecule (NCAM) that is highly expressed in infancy, thereby raising theoretical concerns that efforts to induce antibody to the polysaccharide would cause autoimmune disease. Several candidate vaccines have been produced or are in phase II/III evaluation. The most advanced are vaccines based on outer membrane proteins (OMP) of the meningococcus. Unfortunately, although two vaccines have shown efficacy in phase III studies in 10–16 year olds, they consist of a single Por A OMP serosubtype and therefore are highly specific for only one strain of organism [137,138]. In most countries, numerous B serosubtypes cause disease, and these vaccines are unlikely to offer any cross protection. In an attempt to produce an OMP vaccine that is cross-protective against multiple B serosubtypes, a genetically engineered vaccine that contains 6 Por A OMPs has been produced in the Netherlands and has undergone phase II studies. Good antibody responses were achieved to only two of the Por A proteins following immunization at 2, 3, and 4 months of age, although a fourth dose at 1 year produced responses to all six Por A OMPs, suggesting induction of immunologic memory [139].

To counteract theoretical problems raised by induction of antibody responses to the group B polysaccharide, one approach has been to chemically modify the polysaccharide and then conjugate it too an immunogenic protein carrier. Antibodies to the n-propionyl group B polysaccharide-tetanus toxoid conjugate vaccine showed little or no cross-reactivity to the polysialic acid carried by the NCAM in mice [140] and were immunogenic in primates. These vaccines are now in phase I trials in humans [141]. Thus the prospect for a successful group B meningococcal vaccine is improving.

Most pneumococcal meningitis occurs in children <5 years and in the elderly, apart from in those who are immunocompromised. A polysaccharide vaccine has been available for many years but is poorly immunogenic in children <2 years and in the immunocompromised. A 7-valent conjugated pneumococcal vaccine has recently been licensed in the United States and United Kingdom and is recommended to be given in three doses in the first year of life followed by a booster at 1 year [142]. From 65% to 80% of disease-causing serotypes in Europe and the United States would be covered by this vaccine. 9-Valent and 11-valent conjugated pneumococcal vaccines are also available and are under phase II evaluation. These would be likely to provide protection against a significantly higher proportion of invasive pneumococcal infections than the current 7-valent vaccine, and they would provide protection against the majority of penicillin and macrolide-resistant strains [143]. With all the newer vaccines, there is concern that vaccine introduction will have effects on the epidemiology of disease (such as the shifting of the likely age of infection into the adult age group in Hib disease) and on the ecology of the organism by replacement of vaccine serotypes with nonvaccine serotypes.

Viral Meningitis

Viral meningitis is an infection of the leptomeninges with viral particles. Many viruses may cause viral meningitis in children. Before the introduction of the combined MMR vaccine (measles, mumps, rubella), mumps was the most common cause of meningitis in children in England and Wales; although recent outbreaks of infection with mumps have been reported, there have been no reported cases of mumps meningitis. The common causes of viral meningitis include the enteroviruses, herpes viruses, lymphocytic choriomeningitis, cytomegalovirus (CMV), adenovirus, rubella, varicella, the arboviruses, influenza, and Epstein-Barr virus [144]. There is some overlap between meningitis and encephalitis; however, the majority of organisms generally lead to either meningitis or encephalitis. Death following viral meningitis is rare.

The enteroviruses are thought to be responsible for the majority of cases of viral meningitis. At least 70 different enteroviruses have been found, and those most likely to cause meningitis are polio, coxsackie (types A, B), and ECHO (enteric cytopathogenic human orphan) viruses [145]. These viruses are transmitted via the fecal, oral, and respiratory routes, and viral particles are shed in stools and may be detected for several weeks following infection. The enteroviruses generally lead to gastrointestinal upset; however, when present in the bloodstream, they show predominance for different organ systems, including the CNS. The enteroviral serotypes that have been found in the majority of CSF isolates are A9, E7, E9, E11, E19, and E30 [146]. Recent outbreaks of E13 have been associated with meningitis in the United States [147]. In Taiwan, an epidemic of enterovirus 71 has been associated with complications including meningitis and encephalitis [148].

Children with viral meningitis usually have fever, headache, neck stiffness, photophobia, vomiting, irritability, and lethargy. Neonates demonstrate nonspecific signs and symptoms. There may be associated signs such as a maculopapular rash, which is more common in ECHO virus infections, a parotitis in mumps or coxsackie infections, and a myalgia with coxsackie infections.

An LP usually confirms the diagnosis (Table 10.5); at the onset of disease, there is often a polymorphonuclear predominance (with up to 1,000 WBC/mm^3), which becomes lymphocytic within the next 12 hr; this is seen typically with enteroviral infections. Specimens should be obtained for viral culture from CSF, blood, and stool, if appropriate. Viral culture has a relatively low sensitivity for diagnosis of enteroviral meningitis and the poor growth of some enteroviral phenotypes [149]. Serology requires acute and convalescent samples and is therefore a relatively slow process. Techniques that use polymerase chain reaction–based assays of CSF are more sensitive and diagnostically accurate.

TABLE 10.5. Cerebrospinal fluid findings in different types of meningitis.

Condition	Leukocytes/mm³	Glucose mmol/L	Protein g/L	Specific tests
Bacterial meningitis	100–500 (sometimes thousands) Polymorphs	1.1–1.6 <0.5 <40%–60% of simultaneous blood glucose	0.4–1.5	Gram stain, rapid antigen screen positive
Tuberculous meningitis	25–100 Lymphocytes/monocytes predominate	<2.2 May be normal in early stages	Progressive increase to very high	Acid-fast organism on smear
Viral meningitis	25–500 Usually lymphocytes. Sometimes polymorphs in first 24 hr	Usually normal	Mild increase <1	Viral culture, polymerase chain reaction
Fungal meningitis	0–500 Lymphocytes	Mildly reduced/normal in early stages	Moderate increase	Fungal culture India ink, cryptococcal antigen
Partially treated bacterial meningitis	100–5,000 Polymorphonuclear/lymphocytes (50/50)	Low/mildly reduced	Mild to moderate increase	Cultures negative, rapid antigen and Gram-stain positive
Parameningeal infection	Up to 100 s Variable mononuclear and polymorphonuclear cells	Normal/mildly reduced	Mild to moderate increase	Cultures negative, cerebral imaging

Often bacterial and viral meningitis are indistinguishable, and, as bacterial disease is associated with high long-term morbidity and mortality, it is prudent to start treatment with an appropriate broad-spectrum antibiotic. The management of viral meningitis includes the support of systems that are affected with modalities such as neurointensive care, management of seizures, and airway protection. Some antivirals are available and may be considered for specific viruses or for immunocompromised hosts.

Tuberculous Meningitis

Tuberculous meningitis (TBM) is a severe complication of infection with *Mycobacterium tuberculosis*. Tuberculous meningitis has been reported worldwide and is an important public health problem in many developing countries and in poorer socioeconomic groups in developed countries. Where HIV is endemic, an ever-increasing number of patients are developing infection with tuberculosis (up to 18% of HIV-positive patients reported in endemic areas) [150]. It is associated with both high morbidity and mortality. The tubercle bacteria reach the CNS through hematogenous spread from a primary pulmonary focus; this hematogenous seeding can lead to other syndromes, including tuberculoma, tuberculosis brain abscess, and spinal cord tuberculous leptomeningitis [151]. Tuberculous meningitis arises following the rupture of a caseous focus into the ventricles or meninges.

Tuberculous meningitis usually has an insidious onset. The presentation is nonspecific with a variable fever, headache, and neck stiffness, often with an altered mental status, seizures, and focal changes [152]. Because of this nonspecific presentation, there is often a delay in evaluation and diagnosis. Diagnosis is confirmed by LP (see Table 10.5). A Mantoux test is positive in the majority of patients, and a chest radiograph may be abnormal in up to 50% of cases. Therapy should not be delayed while awaiting microbiologic confirmation of the diagnosis. Bacilli may be present in the CSF following the start of treatment; cultures will confirm the diagnosis, but these results can take several weeks to become positive. Cranial CT scan may be of value in making the diagnosis; characteristic appearances include basal enhancement, cortical thrombophlebitis, and tuberculomas, together with ventricular dilatation in up to 84% of cases [153,154].

The outcome of TBM depends on the stage at which appropriate treatment is commenced [155], and, of course, when this is delayed, neurologic sequelae will result. The most important factor appears to be delay in presentation before admission to the hospital. Although most studies show that appropriate therapy is started within 4 days of admission, there is no clear evidence that delay beyond this is associated with a poorer outcome. It may be that children, when there is this degree of delay, are already in a poor prognostic group, so any further delay does not significantly worsen outcome. The presence of hydrocephalus on scanning is particularly associated with advanced stage of disease and a poorer outcome [156]. The presence of HIV infection does not appear to be a significant factor as long as therapy for the TBM is not significantly delayed.

The optimal treatment has been under considerable discussion; since the advent of bactericidal drugs that penetrate the BBB well, this has avoided the need for intrathecal therapy. Isoniazid (INH), rifampin, and pyrazinamide penetrate the BBB well, whether or not there is meningeal inflammation [157], whereas ethambutol and streptomycin only achieve therapeutic levels when meningeal inflammation is present. Current regimens involve a combination of INH, rifampin, and pyrazinamide, together with ethambutol or streptomycin, as INH resistance is becoming increasingly common. Monitoring of liver function is essential during the early weeks. Treatment is recommended for 12 months [158] and, when tuberculomas are present, up to 24 months [159].

The use of dexamethasone is a subject of debate and a recent Cochrane Review looking at the adjunctive use in the management of TBM reviewed six studies assessing the effects of corticosteroids on death and disability in these patients [160]. Corticosteroids were associated with fewer deaths and a reduced incidence of severe residual disability. Although these studies were small, adjunctive corticosteroid treatment is now recommended in the first few weeks of treatment for TBM. Neurosurgical intervention may be required when obstructive hydrocephalus is revealed on cerebral imaging.

Fungal Meningitis

Fungal meningitis is more common in the immunocompromised population. Cryptococcal meningitis has been more commonly identified, and the population at highest risk includes those with HIV infection [161]. Cryptococcal infection is less common in children than in adults and is more commonly seen in adolescents.

Symptoms include headache, fever, neck stiffness, photophobia, focal findings (e.g., VI nerve palsy), and subtle neurologic signs. There may be other lesions in extraneural areas, including liver, lymph nodes, and the lungs. Diagnosis is by the identification of *Cryptococcus neoformans* in culture specimens of CSF or cryptococcal antigen test in serum or CSF. When the diagnosis has been confirmed, treatment with amphotericin B and/or flucytosine or fluconazole is recommended. The choice of therapy depends on the severity of disease and degree of immunocompromise. A communicating hydrocephalus may complicate cryptococcal meningitis, and serial LPs to relieve pressure or place a lumbar CSF drain may be required; these procedures have their own risks, including introduction of infection, and should be carried out weighing risks versus benefits for this population. The duration of therapy is lifelong in patients with HIV infection. Intrathecal treatment with amphotericin B is indicated for some patients.

Encephalitis

Encephalitis is inflammation of the brain parenchyma and presents as diffuse or focal neuropsychological dysfunction. It can occur following any infective process; the more common organisms include *Mycoplasma pneumoniae*, herpes simplex virus (HSV), the enteroviruses, adenoviruses, influenza viruses, and Japanese B virus [162,163]. The CNS may be affected, leading to a variety of *syndromes*, which vary from the more benign to catastrophic CNS illness and postinfectious encephalopathies.

Pathophysiology

Viruses spread to the CNS via hematogenous or neuronal routes [164,165]. Hematogenous spread is more common and leads to an alteration in the BBB, as seen in arthropod-borne viral infections. Following an insect bite, there is a local viral replication in the skin, followed by transient viremia and seeding of the reticuloendothelial system (and occasionally muscle tissue). Continued replication and secondary viremia leads to infection of other organs. In acute viral encephalitis, capillary and endothelial inflammation of cortical vessels is observed within the gray matter or at the gray–white junction. Perivascular lymphocytic infiltration occurs following passive transfer of a virus across the endothelium at pinocytic junctions of the choroid plexus or because of active viral replication in the capillary endothelial cells.

Viruses also move into the CNS via intraneuronal routes, for example, the herpes virus [166]. Other data suggest the olfactory tract is a route of access [167]. On reaching the brain, either the virus lies dormant or replication can take place intraneuronally or can lead to cell-to-cell or extracellular spread. Encephalitis caused by *M. pneumoniae* may occur following direct bacterial invasion of the brain parenchyma or an autoimmune or thromboembolic phenomenon [168]. The organism has been isolated following brain culture in a patient who died from disseminated infection. In other patients with encephalitis, *M. pneumoniae* has been cultured or identified by polymerase chain reaction.

Clinical Presentation

The classic features of acute encephalitis are fever, headache, and altered level of consciousness, which frequently follows a viral prodrome. Several other findings include disorientation, behavioral disturbances, focal neurologic signs, and seizures, including status epilepticus [169]. The clinical signs and symptoms represent disease progression and specific areas of brain involvement, which may be caused by the action of the specific microbe (e.g., HSV has a predilection for the temporal lobe).

When searching for an infecting pathogen, it is important to establish certain epidemiologic features, including time of year, travel, and contacts. For example, in temperate climates, enteroviral infections are predominant during late summer and early winter [170]. As long as there are no contraindications, an LP is essential. Typical findings include pleocytosis (mononuclear cells predominate) with an increase in CSF protein. Some patients (3%–5%) may have normal CSF, and, under these circumstances, the diagnosis is made using assays to detect viral antigens or nucleic acids, as viral culture is of limited use. Cerebral imaging is a valuable tool, and magnetic resonance imaging (MRI) changes may be present early in the disease. Characteristic changes may be present on an electroencephalogram (EEG); for example, the periodic high-voltage spike wave activity seen coming from the temporal lobes and slow-wave complexes at 2–3 sec internals are characteristic of HSV infection [171].

Management

It is not always possible to isolate the causative organism. In such circumstances, it is prudent to commence treatment with broad-spectrum antimicrobials and to cover the more common causative agents. When identification has been possible, therapy must be tailored for appropriate treatment. There are some specific therapies available for specific organisms as described later. Appropriate supportive intensive care may be required, including the use of neuroprotective strategies. Newer antivirals are continually being identified and may be more useful in the future. When organisms that cause encephalitis, such as Japanese B virus, are endemic, the availability of vaccination programs will lead to a reduction in prevalence and incidence of disease.

Common Causes of Encephalitis

Mycoplasma Pneumoniae Encephalitis

Mycoplasma pneumonia is thought to be responsible for up to 10% of acute childhood encephalitis cases in Europe and North America; one group reported *M. pneumoniae* associated with 70% of patients with a confirmed etiology. The association of CNS complications with *M. pneumoniae* infection were confirmed in the past 25 years, following isolation of the organism in the brain and CSF [172]. There are no specific CSF, EEG, or neuroimaging findings that typically follow *Mycoplasma* infection. Pneumonia may occur in only 10%–40% of cases.

The diagnosis of *M. pneumoniae* infection may be confirmed by several methods, including culture of the organism itself, polymerase chain reaction, and serology [173,174]. *Mycoplasma pneumoniae* replicates slowly and may take up to 4 weeks for isolation. The investigations are labor intensive, and overall the yield is better in respiratory secretions; CSF culture is rarely positive. Several polymerase chain reaction assays have been described, and these have a more rapid turnaround time and are more sensitive tests. The mainstay of diagnosis of infection with *Mycoplasma* is with the use of serology. This is a complement fixation test, and, for respiratory disease, the tests have good sensitivity and specificity; however, for nonrespiratory infections, the specificity is reduced. Immunoglobulin M (IgM) complement-fixing antibodies may be detected 1 week after the onset of the illness, while immunoglobulin G antibodies are present 5 days later [175]. The peak immunoglobulin M response is from day 10 to 30, usually falling to undetectable levels by 3 to 6 months [176].

For patients with *M. pneumoniae* encephalitis, a temporal clinical improvement has been reported in children treated with antibiotics [177]. On the other hand, some children recovered without antibiotics [178]. Macrolides are considered the antibiotic of choice for infection with *M. pneumoniae*. The disadvantages of macrolides lies in their poor penetrance of the BBB in order to achieve therapeutic levels within the CNS, although azithromycin has been found to achieve a high concentration in brain tissue [179,180]. Other agents that have been used for CNS disease include erythromycin, clarithromycin, tetracycline, doxycycline, chloramphenicol, ciprofloxacin, and streptogamins. The choice of antibiotic is based on several factors. When there is likely direct CNS invasion, based on clinical presentation, and detection of *M. pneumoniae* in CSF, then antibiotics that achieve therapeutic levels in the CNS should be used. Where there is no direct CNS invasion and the clinical syndrome is caused by an autoimmune or thromboembolic process, then the need to achieve high CNS levels is less urgent. However, if there is any doubt, appropriate antibiotics should be commenced while awaiting diagnostic reports.

Herpes Simplex Encephalitis

Herpes simplex virus is the most common cause of acute viral encephalitis [181]. It is characterized by an often focal necrotizing process, although in neonates there is more widespread tissue destruction. The estimated frequency is 1 case per 250,000–500,000 population per year, with 30% of cases affecting individuals under 20 years old [182]. Without effective treatment the mortality rate is greater than 70% [183]. In immunocompetent adults, over 90% of cases of herpes simplex encephalitis are caused by HSV-1 infection, and the remainder are caused by HSV-2 infection [184]. A large majority of these are caused by reactivation of latent HSV-1.

Herpes simplex virus infection in neonates is a particularly devastating disease. In the United Kingdom the incidence is 1.65 per100,000 live births [185], with a higher incidence in the United States of 20–50 per100,000 live births. Infection may result from either HSV-1 or HSV-2, and disease associated with HSV-2 has been shown to have a worse outcome [186]. Herpes simplex virus type 2 is the type found in 70% of neonatal cases of HSV infection worldwide. Neonatal HSV infection is largely acquired during vaginal delivery from virus that was shed in the maternal genital tract. Up to 5% of cases may be congenitally acquired infections, following either ascending infection or transplacental transmission. Infection may be acquired postnatally in up to 10% of cases, usually following contact with an environmental source of HSV. Herpes simplex virus infection in neonates classically leads to one of three different disease patterns: (1) disease localized to the skin, eye and mouth; (2) CNS disease (with or without skin, eye, and mouth involvement); and (3) disseminated disease with multiorgan failure [187].

Whenever HSV encephalitis is suspected, appropriate treatment must be commenced, as antiviral treatment is effective and reduces the morbidity and mortality. Polymerase chain reaction assay of the CSF is the gold standard investigation. In one study, CSF polymerase chain reaction was positive in 98% of patients, with biopsy-proven disease; this equates to a sensitivity of 98% and specificity of 94% [188]. After 10 days of treatment, HSV DNA may not be detectable in CSF, and polymerase chain reaction results will be negative. Cerebrospinal fluid antibody measurements may be then useful for retrospective analyses or when CSF was obtained late, and therefore the polymerase chain reaction was negative. In addition, viral cultures are of value only for patients older than 6 months. In HSV encephalitis, the following abnormalities are typically seen on examination of the CSF: elevated mononuclear cells, elevated protein, a lymphocytic pleocytosis of 10–500 cells/mm^3 (present in 85%), an increase in red blood cells (10–500/mm^3), and a reduction in glucose.

The majority of patients have abnormal neuroimaging, with MRI changes early in the course of the illness. The typical findings observed include edema and necrosis of the temporal lobes [189]. An EEG typically shows changes consistent with nonspecific slow-wave activity early in the illness, moving to paroxysmal sharp waves or triphasic complexes in the temporal lobes. In some cases periodic-lateralizing epileptiform discharges arise from the temporal lobe at 2–3 Hz.

Acyclovir is the treatment of choice. The current standard of care for adults and children over the age of 3 months is intravenous acyclovir at a dose of 10–20 mg/kg every 8 hr for 21 days. Neonates should be treated with 20 mg/kg every 8 hr or 500 mg/m^2 every 8 hr for 21 days. With this regimen, mortality from neonatal HSV encephalitis has fallen to 5%; 40% of survivors develop normally.

Outcome depends on age of patient, level of consciousness at presentation, duration of encephalitis, and viral load in patients treated with acyclovir. If the GCS is <7, outcome is universally poor. When treatment was instituted less than 4 days following the onset of symptoms, the survival at 18 months increased from 72% to 92% [190]. Relapse may occur despite appropriate therapy, with some studies quoting relapses in up to 26% of patients [191]. In neonates with HSV encephalitis treated with acyclovir 10 mg/kg every 6 hr for only 10 days, virologic relapse is not infrequent. Relapses tend to occur between 1 week and 3 months following an initial improvement after a course of treatment lasting between 10 and 14 days. When treatment regimens last for 21 days at higher doses, relapse has not been documented. It is recommended that CSF polymerase chain reaction be repeated following completion of therapy in order to monitor treatment response. This may be challenging to do with a clinically improved child! Currently there is a clinical trial looking at the use of oral valaciclovir as adjunctive therapy for 90 days following an intravenous course of aciclovir, which is being conducted by the Collaborative Antiviral Study Group (CASG 204). The study is being undertaken to determine if prolonged treatment will improve outcome from HSV encephalitis.

Enteroviral Encephalitis

The enteroviruses include poliovirus, coxsackie viruses, and echoviruses [192], and infection with these lead to a wide variety of clinical illnesses. Infection with some of these pathogens results in a neurologic syndrome (e.g., poliomyelitis). As discussed previously, enteroviral infection may result in aseptic meningitis and, less commonly in infancy, encephalitis.

In 1998, cases of enteroviral encephalitis caused by enterovirus 71 were reported in Taiwan [193]; the majority of patients were less than 5 years old, with a reported mortality rate of 19.3% in this group. The enterovirus 71 was isolated in 75% of patients and in 92% patients who did not survive. The clinical syndrome at presentation was rhombencephalitis with myoclonus, tremors, ataxia, and cranial nerve involvement. Some children had brain stem dysfunction, which was associated with a poor prognosis. Magnetic resonance imaging scans from these patients revealed high-intensity lesions localized to the midbrain, medulla, and pons. There was a high incidence of long-term neurologic sequelae among survivors.

Rabies

Rabies follows infection with a rhabdovirus and is virtually uniformly fatal. It can be prevented by appropriate immunization (active and passive) even when infection has occurred [194]. The primary vector for infection is an infected dog, but transmission can also occur from bats and wild terrestrial mammals [195]. The incubation period is typically between 20 and 60 days but may vary from 5 days to several months [196]. The prodrome with fever, malaise, anxiety, and itching at the site of inoculation is followed by an encephalitis or paralytic illness. This is then followed by coma, cardiorespiratory failure, and death. The diagnosis is made by detection of the rabies virus RNA in saliva using reverse transcriptase polymerase chain reaction or by biopsy of brain showing viral antigen [197]. Management of infected patients is supportive. A case of rabies in a 15 year old girl reported a clinical improvement following neuroprotection with induction of a medical coma and no rabies vaccine [198].

Arthropod-Borne Viral Encephalitis

Bites from arthropods are major causes of encephalitis worldwide. The viruses transmitted by arboviruses are from the following families: Togaviridae—alphavirus (eastern equine, western equine, Venezuelan equine); Flaviviridae—West Nile complex (St. Louis, Japanese, Murray Valley, West Nile, Ilheus, Rocio); tick-borne complex—Far Eastern, Central European, Kyasanur Forrest, Lopuing-III, Powassan, Negishi; Bunyaviridae—bunyavirus (California, La Crosse, Jamestown Canyon, Snowshoe Hare, Tahyna, Inkoo), phlebovirus (Rift Valley); and Reoviridae—orbivirus (Colorado tick fever). Japanese encephalitis, which is transmitted by the *Culex* species of mosquitoes, is responsible for the majority of cases of arthropod-borne viral encephalitis. Japanese encephalitis is concentrated largely in China and Southeast Asia, although it has been spreading to India, Pakistan, Russia, the Philippines, and Australia [199]. Children are predominantly affected. The typical disease presentation is a nonspecific illness followed by headache, vomiting, and altered mental status, with seizures reported in 85% of children. There is a coarse tremor, dystonia, rigidity, and a characteristic "mask-like" facies. Magnetic resonance imaging shows a pattern of mixed intensity or hypodense lesions in the thalamus, basal ganglia, and midbrain [200]. An LP confirms the diagnosis with the presence of immunoglobulin M in the CSF [201]. Therapy is supportive only. There is a mortality rate of 30%; 50% of survivors are left with severe neurologic sequelae. Management of the other arthropod-transmitted infection is support of organ systems.

Cerebral Malaria

Malaria is the most common parasitic disease worldwide, affecting about 5% of the world's population at a single time, leading to 0.5–2.5 million deaths each year [202]. *Plasmodium falciparum*

is responsible for the majority of deaths and long-term sequelae. Those at highest risk include the local populations in endemic areas and travellers to those regions. The incubation period of cerebral malaria is 2 weeks, and without treatment it is rapidly fatal, with up to 50% mortality [203].

Pathophysiology

At autopsy, the brain is usually edematous, and there may be features of cerebral herniation; brain slices are slate gray, and petechial haemorrhages are present [204]. The characteristic histopathologic features include the engorgement of cerebral capillaries and venules with parasitized red blood cells (PRBCs) and nonparasitized RBCs (NRBCs) [204]. On microscopy, no endothelial damage is visible; however, on immunohistochemical staining there is evidence of endothelial activation together with disruption of the BBB [205,206]. It is thought that red cells that contain the more mature forms of the parasite in the microvasculature lead to the complications of falciparum disease [207].

The sequestration of these PRBCs in venous beds encourages parasite growth, preventing these cells from splenic destruction. This sequestration is thought to occur via a process of cytoadherence in which an interaction takes place between PRBCs and the vascular endothelium [208]. This is mediated by *Plasmodium*-derived proteins expressed on the PRBC membranes and modified erythrocyte wall proteins and ligands on endothelial cells. With parasite growth, RBCs become more deformed [209], leading to stagnation of microvascular blood flow and subsequent end-organ dysfunction. These sequestered parasites are thought to compete for substrates such as glucose. In addition, levels of proinflammatory cytokines [210,211], such as TNF-α, are increased and are associated with coma, hypoglycemia, hyperparasitemia, and death.

Clinical Presentation

Cerebral malaria has been defined as a coma in the presence of a *P. falciparum* asexual parasitemia after the correction of hypoglycemia and exclusion of other encephalopathies [202]. Typically cerebral malaria presents with a 1–4 day history of fever and seizures; the seizures often proceed to coma [212]. The more commonly seen seizures are focal motor and generalized tonic–clonic seizures, although subclinical seizures may be seen on EEG. There may be other features of disease present, including headache, malaise, vomiting, and diarrhea, followed by the development of jaundice, anemia, thrombocytopenia, and splenomegaly, together with a marked metabolic acidosis. Neurologic signs seen in children are consistent with a diffuse encephalopathy, with symmetric upper motor neuron and brain stem signs. Some of the signs may be attributable to hypoglycemia, which must be urgently sought and corrected if present. Raised ICP is present because of an increase in cerebral blood volume and the sequestration of PRBCs in the vascular compartment. Neurologic sequelae can vary from devastating global injury to transient abnormalities. The sequelae are associated with prolonged seizures, coma, hypoglycemia, and in some studies severe anemia.

Management

Immediate treatment involves management of airway, breathing, and circulation together with management of intracranial hypertension as described previously. Any hypoglycemia must be corrected immediately, and acid–base and other electrolyte abnormalities should be corrected. Meticulous fluid management is warranted in view of the associated renal impairment. Fever should be managed with appropriate cooling techniques. Seizures must be managed, and recent studies have demonstrated a reduction in seizures when phenobarbital has been used.

Parenteral quinine is the first line of treatment for severe falciparum disease, but there are alternatives that should be considered for those exposed in areas of quinine resistance, including artemisinin derivatives. Quinine must be administered with an adequate loading dose (20 mg/kg of the dihydrochloride salt infused over 4 hr); this guarantees a parasiticidal concentration in the blood as soon as possible [213,214]. Following this initial loading dose, 30 mg/kg/day is administered for 7 days (typically in 2–4 hr infusions of 10 mg/kg every 8 hr). Drug therapy should be guided by up-to-date information based on known resistance patterns. Other adjunctive therapies include exchange transfusions and are used when patients are on maximal therapy with a high peripheral parasitemia, but no trials have been undertaken to evaluate these.

Brain Abscess/Subdural Empyema

Intracranial collections of pus, although eminently treatable, are serious and potentially life-threatening conditions for which the consequences of delay in diagnosis can be catastrophic. Optimal management requires close cooperation among the pediatric intensivist, neuroradiologist, neurosurgeon, and infectious disease specialist. Intracranial pus collection results from the invasion of infectious organisms as a consequence of spread of contiguous infection from non-neural tissue, of hematogenous spread from a remote site, or of direct mechanical introduction following penetrating trauma or surgical procedure. In children with normal immunity, brain abscess most commonly occurs in those with chronic suppurative upper respiratory tract infection—in particular of the sinuses, middle ear, and mastoid air cells. Other common etiologies include infection of the soft tissues of the face, orbit, or scalp; penetrating skull injury; comminuted fracture of the skull; cranial surgery, including the insertion of a ventriculoperitoneal (VP) shunt; congenital lesions of the head and neck, including dermal sinuses usually located over the posterior fossa; and cyanotic congenital heart disease. It is relatively uncommon for bacterial meningitis to be complicated by abscess formation in children, but bacterial meningitis is the most common cause of brain abscess in neonates and infants [215]. Children with defects in cellular immunity, such as occur in HIV infection and AIDS or in children following therapy for malignancy or bone marrow transplantation, are at increased risk of cerebral abscess caused by the protozoal pathogen *Toxoplasma gondii* or by fungi such as *Aspergillus* species. This is a group noted to be at increased risk of brain abscess in recent years. About 15% of brain abscesses seem to occur without any clear predisposing factor [215–217]. Subdural empyema, as in brain abscess, is also associated with chronic upper respiratory tract infection but, in contrast to brain abscess, has a strong association with bacterial meningitis, particularly that caused by *H. influenzae* and *Strep. pneumoniae*.

Both brain abscess and subdural empyema are rare. The incidence of brain abscess at all ages has been estimated at about 1 per 100,000, and subdural empyema appears to be even more rare [218]. The incidence of brain abscess varies considerably among popula-

tions, particularly in relation to the different predisposing conditions. It is relatively more common where chronic upper respiratory tract infection is widely found, and in childhood it occurs particularly in adolescents with chronic sinus or mastoid disease. When antibiotics are routinely prescribed for upper respiratory infection, the incidence of brain abscess has declined, and the majority of cases occur in children with congenital heart disease, although even in this condition it is rare below the age of 2 years [219]. In a prospective study of 483 infants with congenital heart disease, Piper et al. [220], found an overall annual incidence of 0.45% but a year-on-year increasing age-specific incidence of up to 1.75% at 12 years. In their first two decades, patients with tetralogy of Fallot—the most common association with brain abscess—have a risk of brain abscess of 12.1%. In congenital heart disease, the risk of brain abscess correlates with the degree of hypoxia [220].

Pathophysiology

At the histologic level, pyogenic brain abscess formation is typified by a number of sequential pathologic changes that have been elucidated using experimental animal models. In humans, staging has been based on findings obtained using CT and MRI scans. There are four histologic stages. The early stage is that of evolving cerebritis (usually days 1–3), typified by neutrophil accumulation, tissue necrosis, and edema. Microglial and astrocyte activation is also evident at this stage. The late cerebritis stage (days 4–9) is associated with a predominant macrophage and lymphocyte infiltration, leading to central liquefaction with early formation of a capsule of vascular connective tissue (days 10–13) and later maturation of this capsule (day 14 onward), effectively sequestering the lesion and protecting the surrounding brain parenchyma from additional damage. In addition to limiting the extent of infection, the immune response that is essential for abscess formation also destroys surrounding normal brain tissue [221,222].

In the context of chronic suppurative upper respiratory tract infection, the initiating event is probably thrombophlebitis spreading from an extracranial focus via penetrating emissary veins to a venous sinus, leading to congestion and inflammation of the underlying brain. Abscesses that occur in this scenario are usually single and predictably located—frontal or occasionally temporal when related to paranasal sinusitis and temporal or occasionally cerebellar when associated with ear infection. Children with CHD are at risk of developing microscopic areas of brain infarction because of severe hypoxemia, coupled with the increased viscosity of polycythemic blood, in particular when reduced blood flow in brain microcirculation becomes critical during episodes of dehydration or cardiac dysfunction. Episodes of low-grade bacteremia are common as right-to-left shunting of blood bypasses the pulmonary capillary bed filter, and seeding of these devitalized areas establishes foci of cerebritis. In these conditions, abscesses are often multiple and may be located anywhere, although they are most commonly found in the distribution of the middle cerebral artery. In addition, brain abscess has been reported as a complication of skin infection of the scalp, pulmonary infection, dental abscess, and bacterial endocarditis.

In contrast to the focal nature of infection in brain abscess, in subdural empyema infection can spread widely over the surface of the brain in the potential space defined by the dural and arachnoid membranes. Extradural suppurative collections occur when the dura is not breached by infection. Subdural empyema occurs where the dura is breached by the infection, most commonly following sinusitis. When associated with sinusitis, intracranial extension of inflammation again is thought to spread via penetrating emissary veins. In subdural empyema complicating bacterial meningitis, the pathogenesis is secondary infection of a subdural effusion, a common association of *H. influenzae* and *Strep. pneumoniae* meningitis.

Microbiology

Understanding of the microbiology of brain abscess is complex as patient populations and degrees of microbiologic investigation reported are variable. With careful and prolonged aerobic and anaerobic culture, organisms can nearly always be identified in aspirates of pus from brain abscesses [223]. Polymicrobial infections are not unusual, reflecting spread from upper airway focal infection. Gram-positive organisms, particularly streptococcal and staphylococcal species, account for up to 60% of isolates from brain abscesses in most series, in particular *Staph. aureus*, *Strep. millerii*, and other anaerobic/microphilic streptococci, often associated with sinusitis. In addition, the anaerobic *Bacteroides* spp. and fusobacteria, which are also common in congenital heart disease–associated brain abscess, reflect the origin of transient bacteremia from the mouth and upper respiratory tract. Aerobic Gram-negative bacterias, including *Proteus mirabilis*, *Klebsiella pneumoniae*, *E. coli*, and *Haemophilus* spp., are also relatively common (up to 30% of isolates) particularly in abscesses associated with ear foci [224–226]. Brain abscesses complicating head injury not surprisingly often contain *Staph. aureus* and other skin commensals. The unusual Gram-negative pathogen *Citrobacter diversus* has a particular propensity to cause abscess as a complication of neonatal meningitis [226]. Anaerobic streptococci, *Bacteroides*, and *Staph. aureus* in pure or mixed culture are often found in subdural empyema associated with sinusitis. In subdural empyema associated with meningitis, the organism is usually that causing the meningitis. A major concern in recent years has been the increasing incidence of multiresistant organisms being found in intracranial abscesses, particularly methicillin-resistant *Staph.* (MRSA) and extended spectrum β-lactamase–producing Gram-negative organisms [227].

Clinical Presentation

Clinical presentation of intracranial abscess depends on the site, size, number of lesions, and any associated secondary cerebral injury. Headache, fever, focal neurologic deficit, and altered sensorium are among the most common features. Headache is obviously difficult to elicit in infants, and, in a retrospective study, these classic features were found in only 28% of 101 children [228]. Fever and vomiting are common initial symptoms, later progressing to signs of raised ICP and focal neurologic signs (seen in 42% of cases in this series). Seizures are common (up to 50%) and are often generalized. Table 10.6 lists the most common signs and symptoms of children with brain abscess. A leukocytosis in peripheral blood and raised sedimentation rate may be found in up to 75% of cases, but acute phase markers are not sensitive indicators of intracranial pus collections [230]. The progression of disease may be insidious, and symptoms may precede diagnosis by many days; in the above series the mean time to diagnosis was 13 days (range 3–120).

Brain abscess should always be considered as part of the differential diagnosis of a febrile child with congenital heart disease or chronic upper respiratory tract infection, and delay in making the

TABLE 10.6. Signs and symptoms in children with brain abscess: a compilation from series of reports between 1945 and 1990.

Symptoms and signs	Percentage of children
Headache	65
Fever	55
Vomiting	53
Papilledema	48
Focal neurologic deficit	47
Change in mental status	43
Meningeal irritation	36
Seizure	34

Source: Data are from Woods [229].

diagnosis usually represents a failure to consider the diagnosis when the presentation is with a nonspecific illness, aggravated by a lack of ready access to CT imaging of the brain. Cases may occasionally present in a more fulminant fashion, with signs of rapidly progressive raised ICP, leading quickly to coma and impending herniation. As the presentation is essentially that of an intracranial mass lesion, tumor is important in the differential diagnosis. Viral encephalitis (particularly those with a predilection for a focal encephalitis, such as herpes simplex) can present with a similar constellation of symptoms and signs. Bacterial meningitis generally presents more acutely, but there are important examples with an insidious onset, such as tuberculous and cryptococcal meningitis. Similarly, acute vascular events, such as infarction and hemorrhage, may present with similar features, as may acute hydrocephalus.

Subdural empyema usually presents in a more acute fashion than abscess. Typically a child with sinusitis, not necessarily clinically obvious, develops signs of meningitis, rapidly progressing to focal neurologic signs and often seizures. The child may have clear signs of raised ICP [231]. Where subdural empyema occurs as a complication of bacterial meningitis, the presentation is typically of secondary fever and neurologic deterioration, which may be dramatic.

In the face of focal neurological signs and signs of raised ICP, LP is *absolutely* contraindicated. If CSF is obtained during neurosurgical intervention, or LP when it is deemed safe, the laboratory findings are nonspecific, with a moderate pleocytosis (usually <100 cells/mL), minimally elevated protein, and possibly reduced glucose. C-reactive protein levels may be elevated but again are nonspecific. Definitive diagnosis is accomplished by urgent imaging of the brain, with either CT or MRI. Brain abscesses are characteristically seen on CT as mass lesions with surrounding edema. These lesions *ring enhance* following injection of intravenous contrast medium, the highlighted vascular capsule suggesting that the mass lesion is an abscess rather than neoplastic. Magnetic resonance imaging is more sensitive than CT in detecting cerebritis and the extent of accompanying edema [232]. The same considerations apply to the investigation of subdural empyema.

Management

The aims of treatment are to eliminate the infectious process; to reduce the mass effect within the confined bony cavity of the skull and thus avoid or minimize a secondary cerebral injury; and to treat the infection with appropriate antimicrobial therapy. For adequate treatment of brain abscess, neurosurgical intervention is virtually always required in addition to prolonged antibiotic therapy. It is unlikely that antibiotics alone can ever be sufficient once cavitation occurs, although there have been convincing successes when diagnosis has been made early, in the cerebritis stage.

There is continuing controversy over the relative merits of stereotactic/CT-guided repeated aspiration of abscess cavities versus their complete excision, although the former approach is the most widely used and the latter considered by many to carry unacceptable risk for the postoperative morbidities of brain scarring and epilepsy [233]. In addition, excision is inappropriate in the cerebritis stage and for those abscesses without a well-developed capsule, and it is not advised for deep-seated or multiple abscesses or for those in critical areas of the brain. Excision should be considered for children with traumatic brain abscesses, because these may contain foreign bodies, and for those who are thought to have fungal brain abscess. More recently there has been excellent experience with neuroendoscopic management, which appears to offer more complete drainage and lavage of abscess cavities [234].

Nonsurgical management of intracranial abscesses is controversial. Selected cases may be suitable if the lesion(s) are small or multiple and/or the surgical risk is high.

Cranial CT is useful not only in helping to make the diagnosis but also in monitoring response to therapy. If therapy with aspiration and antimicrobial therapy is successful, repeated CT scanning should show decreases in degree of ring enhancement, edema, mass effect, and size of lesion. The majority of abscesses that will resolve with antibiotics alone will do so within 4 weeks.

Antibiotic choice is directed initially by the likely microorganisms involved, later modified by results of microbiologic evaluation. The usual empiric recommended regimen consists of a third-generation cephalosporin (such as cefotaxime or ceftriaxone), metronidazole, and an antistaphylococcal penicillin (such as flucloxacillin). However, this may be modified depending on the child's underlying immune status, the presumed etiology of the abscess, and the local resistance patterns. Once aspiration and culture have been performed, antimicrobials should be adjusted accordingly.

The place of intracavitary antibiotic therapy is not clearly defined and carries the risk of direct cerebral toxicity of high concentrations of antibiotics on surrounding brain tissue. In the acute phase of the illness, when surrounding cerebral edema may contribute to dangerously raised ICP, measures such as intravenous mannitol, or placement of an intraventricular drain, and the use of high-dose steroid therapy may be life saving. There are no data regarding the use of corticosteroid therapy in the routine management of cerebral abscesses.

The mainstay of management of subdural empyema has long been prompt neurosurgical intervention combined with appropriate antibiotics, selected on the same basis as above. Surgical drainage of any associated extracranial pus should also be considered.

Outcome and Complications

When the diagnosis has been made promptly by appropriate imaging, the mortality rate is around 10%–15%, with about 50% of survivors having significant long-term neurologic deficits. Rupture of an abscess into the ventricular system is a particularly dangerous complication, with high mortality. The rare, more aggressive subdural empyema has a mortality rate of around 30% and substantial morbidity in terms of hydrocephalus, focal brain damage, and epilepsy. Extensive cerebral thrombophlebitis and cerebral infarction are the serious complications in what remains a disease with a very gloomy prognosis.

The mortality rate has declined in the past few decades, probably in part due to the introduction of cranial CT, improvements in neurosurgical technique, and advances in antimicrobial therapy. Intracranial abscesses often cause significant morbidity, including epilepsy, motor or sensory dysfunction, visual field defects, and personality change.

Shunt Infection

The treatment of many CNS diseases involves gaining access to the CSF. Indications for such access can be classified as diversion, drainage, or monitoring. All of these involve prosthetic implants, which may be temporary or permanent. The usual reason is for continuous CSF diversion or *shunting* for the treatment of hydrocephalus. The risk of infection continues to be a major cause of morbidity and mortality for patients with CSF shunts.

As patients who require CSF shunting usually require their shunt for life, and those with benign diseases will probably require several shunt revisions for noninfectious reasons, a distinction must be made between *case infection rate* and *operative infection rate*. The former refers to the infection rate per patient, and the latter refers to the infection rate per procedure. Even if the operative infection rate remained constant, the case infection rate increases as the patient gets older and requires more revisions. In recent years the case infection rate has ranged from 10% to 40% and the operative infection rate from 5% to 14% [235–238]. Two studies have reported a greater operative infection rate for shunt revision [236,237]. In the United States about 33,000 CSF shunts are placed each year, with about half of these being shunt revisions [239]. While the proportion of revisions has remained fairly constant, the proportion involving shunt removal has decreased in recent years from about 23% in 1988 to 17% in 1991, which may reflect a decline in the operative infection rate [240]. Factors that are implicated in this include changes in materials used in shunt manufacture; changes in packaging and sterilization procedures; fewer pre-shunting invasive procedures (LP, pneumoencephalography, ventricular tap); improvements in operating room facilities; improvements in surgical technique and preoperative patient preparation; and reduced duration of surgery. There is an increased risk of infection for patients undergoing shunt revision following treatment for shunt infection, with an operative incidence of 10% to 20%. In these, the same organism is cultured in up to 50% of cases [235,241].

Shunt infection occurs in a bimodal distribution from the time of shunt placement; 70%–80% of infections occur within 6 months of the placement, with a second peak after 12 months [238]. The most important of the host factors that determine the incidence of shunt infection is age: children <6 months old at the time of first surgery, and particularly neonates, are at increased risk [237].

Table 10.7 lists the most common organisms isolated from infected shunts. Most infections are caused by skin or bowel flora. There is no difference in the distribution of organisms associated with acute or delayed infection. There is also no obvious contribution from the position of the distal end of the shunt. The only identifiable association is when the distal end of a ventriculoperitoneal shunt has perforated a hollow viscus, resulting in infection by mixed Gram-negative species. Infection by organisms usually associated with bacterial meningitis (*H. influenzae, N.*

TABLE 10.7. Most common etiologies of shunt infections.

Organism	Infection rate (%)
Gram positive	
Coagulase-negative staphylococci	45–70
Staphylococcus aureus	10–30
Streptococci	8–10
Diphtheroids	1–15
Gram negative	
Escherichia coli	8–10
Klebsiella species	3–8
Pseudomonas/Proteus	2–8
Anaerobes	6
Mixed cultures	10–15

Source: Adapted from Kaufman and McLone [243].

meningitides, and *Strep. pneumoniae*) only cause about 5% of shunt infections, although there is some suggestion that patients with shunts are more susceptible to these organisms [241].

Pathophysiology

Four mechanisms have been postulated by which shunt becomes infected. Probably the most frequent cause of shunt infection is colonization at the time of surgery. This is suggested by the fact that most shunt infections occur within a few weeks of surgery, usually with skin-colonizing organisms [238]. The initial step in shunt infection must be attachment of bacteria to the shunt material. Once bacteria have adhered to a catheter, they are not easily removed. Breakdown of surgical wounds or of skin overlying the shunt allows direct access of microbes to the shunt. Extensions of tissue infections adjacent to the shunt are also included in this category. Hematogenous seeding of shunts is probably uncommon. Shunts with their distal end in the venous system (e.g., ventriculoatrial shunts) are at continuous risk of infection due to bacteremia. Transient or asymptomatic bacteremia has not been definitively associated with shunt infection. It seems that sustained bacteremia, recent shunt surgery, and the presence of devitalized tissue and hematoma are necessary. Even then, shunt infection in these circumstances is rare [243].

There are several reports of *H. influenzae* shunt infections that occur relatively late after surgery, have an extra-CNS source of infection, and usually have positive blood cultures. These probably do not represent true shunt infection, but direct hematogenous CNS infection, with secondary shunt infection [238,244]. Retrograde infection is usually associated with infection of externalized devices where organisms invade directly from the exit site.

Clinical Presentation

Clinical presentation varies depending on the causative organism and the type of shunt. Symptoms are usually caused by shunt malfunction secondary to infection and include headache, nausea, lethargy, and deteriorating mental status. Fever and pain are not uniformly present. Signs are related to the site where the infection originated. Proximal infection may cause shunt malfunction or obstruction. As the shunt lies within the CSF space, infection results in meningitis or ventriculitis. With ventricular shunts, meningitis is rare, as there is usually no communication between the ventricles and the meninges. Distal infections usually have

symptoms specific to the location of the end. Infected vascular shunts have associated bacteremia. A complication of this may be shunt nephritis, which develops in about 4% of infected vascular shunts [238]. It is an immune complex–mediated disease, similar to that seen in bacterial endocarditis. Infected shunts that terminate in the pleural or peritoneal space will usually present with failure of CSF absorption. In the peritoneum, encystment of the catheter and loculation of pockets of CSF (CSF-oma) can occur. These may become large and palpable, particularly in infants. If more severe, peritonitis may develop [245]. Some shunt infections are insidious in onset, causing few symptoms. There may be only low-grade, intermittent malaise or fever. This is often the case when patients have received repeated courses of antibiotics for intercurrent infections.

The main principle in the diagnosis of shunt infection is to have a high index of suspicion. Infection should be considered for any patient with a CSF shunt who develops fever, although only rarely will fever be caused by shunt infection. The diagnostic procedure of choice is direct culture of CSF from within or around the shunt. All other investigations, apart from blood cultures in the presence of an intravascular shunt, are indirect pointers of shunt infection [246]. Most implanted devices have an access reservoir that can be sampled. The only risk of accessing these reservoirs is the introduction of infection. Any positive culture should be carefully evaluated. If the CSF is infected, a pleocytosis and variable biochemical changes may be found. In most shunt infections, culture of the tapped fluid is positive, even sometimes without a positive Gram stain, with a normal cell count and normal chemistry [238,247]. The culture may take several days or even weeks to become positive, particularly in those with infection caused by fastidious organisms, and the result may be confounded by prior antibiotic therapy. In distal shunt infection without shunt malfunction, the CSF may be completely normal. There may only be localized signs in the peritoneum, ranging from mild discomfort to frank peritonitis. In all cases, correlation of the clinical features, laboratory findings, and culture must be made. Because of the often insidious presentation of shunt infection, any positive culture result should be taken extremely seriously.

Management

There are no published well-conducted studies of any method of therapy for shunt infection. However, removal of the infected shunt is absolutely necessary for successful treatment [237,238]. Antibiotic therapy usually begins without positive bacteriologic diagnosis. Coverage is selected for the most likely organisms. Most infections are caused by staphylococci; therefore, appropriate antistaphylococcal therapy is necessary. Gram-negative aerobes are also relatively common and may be suggested by a more severe clinical course. Bacteriologic evaluation, with culture and sensitivities, will allow therapy to be modified appropriately.

Vancomycin has been shown to be effective in therapy of staphylococcal shunt infection. Its efficacy is increased by the addition of rifampicin, which penetrates CSF well. Rifampicin should not be used alone as resistance to it develops rapidly. For coverage for Gram-negative organisms, a third-generation cephalosporin, such as ceftriaxone or ceftazidime, penetrate inflamed meninges reasonably well. Aminoglycosides do not penetrate even inflamed meninges well, and their use should be restricted to *Pseudomonas* infection for which they should be used in combination with an antipseudomonal penicillin or ceftazidime [248]. Direct instillation of antibiotics into CSF is achieved through a ventriculostomy or via a reservoir. The most commonly used intraventricular antibiotics are vancomycin and gentamicin, but detailed studies of efficacy and pharmacokinetics are not available, so dosage and frequency are empirical.

Treatment of an infected shunt should include parenteral antibiotic therapy, complete removal of the infected shunt at the beginning of treatment, and placement of an external ventriculostomy, which can also be used for antibiotic instillation. This may have a cure rate of >90%. Duration of therapy is guided by the infecting organism, response to therapy, and duration of positive cultures. Usually 7–10 days of therapy following the last positive culture and removal of the infected device is sufficient. Shunt revision is usually carried out following 72 hr of observation off antibiotic therapy [242].

Prevention/Prophylaxis

There are reports of a reduction in shunt infection from 7.8% to <0.2% with a number of procedures aimed at risk reduction, such as restricting operating room personnel, operating early in the day, soaking the shunt in antibiotic fluid, using prophylactic antibiotics [249].

References

1. Overturf GD. Defining bacterial meningitis and other infections of the central nervous system. Pediatr Care Med 2005;6(Suppl):S14–S18.
2. Kaplan SL. Clinical presentations, diagnosis, and prognostic factors of bacterial meningitis. Infect Dis Clin North Am 1999;13:579–594.
3. Segretti J, Harris AA. Acute bacterial meningitis. Infect Dis Clin North Am 1996;10:707–809.
4. Wenger JD, Hightower AW, Facklam RR, et al. Bacterial meningitis in the United States, 1986: report of a multistate surveillance study. The Bacterial Meningitis Study Group. J Infect Dis 1990;162:316–323.
5. Schuchat A, Robinson K, Wenger JD, et al. Bacterial meningitis in the United States in 1995. N Engl J Med 1997;337:970–976.
6. Tikhomirov E, Santamaria M, Esteves K. Meningococcal disease: public health burden and control. World Health Stat Q 1997;50(3–4):170–177.
7. Pong A, Bradley JS. Bacterial meningitis and the newborn infant. Infect Dis Clin North Am 1999;13:711–713.
8. Gold R. Epidemiology of bacterial meningitis. Infect Dis Clin North Am 1999;13:515–525.
9. Williams AJ, Nadel S. Bacterial meningitis. Current controversies in approaches to treatment. CNS Drugs 2001;15:909–919.
10. Lieb SL, Tauber MG. Pathogenesis of bacterial meningitis. Infect Dis Clin North Am 1999;13:527–548.
11. Quagliarello V, Scheld WM. Bacterial meningitis: pathogenesis, pathophysiology and progress. N Engl J Med 1992;327:864–872.
12. Waage A, Halstensen A, Shalaby S, et al. Local production of tumour necrosis factor alpha, interleukin 1 and interleukin 6 in meningococcal meningitis. J Exp Med 1989;170:1859–1867.
13. Tauber MG, Moser B. Cytokines and chemokines in meningeal inflammation: biology and clinical implications. Clin Infect Dis 1999;28:1–12.
14. Ramilio O, Saez-Llorens X, Mertosola J, et al. Tumor necrosis factor alpha/cachectin and interleukin 1 beta initiate meningeal inflammation. J Exp Med 1990;172:4367–4375.
15. Fassenbender K, Schminke HF, Reiss S, et al. Endothelial-derived adhesion molecules in bacterial meningitis: association to cytokine release and intrathecal leucocyte recruitment. J Neuroimmunol 1997;74:130–134.
16. Kim KS, Wass CA, Cross AS, Opal SM. Modulation of blood–brain barrier permeability by tumour necrosis factor and antibody to tumour necrosis in the rat. Lymphokine Cytokine Res 1992;11:293–298.
17. Sharief MK, Ciardi M, Thompson EJ. Blood–brain barrier damage in patients with bacterial meningitis: association with tumour necrosis factor-α but not interleukin-1β. J Infect Dis 1992;166:350–358.
18. Tauber MG. Brain oedema, intracranial pressure and cerebral blood flow in bacterial meningitis. Pediatr Infect Dis J 1989;8:915–917.
19. Foster C, Nadel S. New therapies and vaccines for bacterial meningitis. Expert Opin Invest Drugs 2002;11:1051–1060.
20. Geiseler PJ, Nelson KE, Levin S, et al. Community-acquired purulent meningitis: a review of 1316 cases during the antibiotic era, 1954–1976. Rev Infect Dis 1980;2:725–745.
21. Saez-llorens X, McCracken GH Jr. Bacterial meningitis in neonates and children. Infect Dis Clin North Am 1990;44:623–644.
22. Radetsky M. Duration of symptoms and outcome in bacterial meningitis: an analysis of causation and the implications of a delay in diagnosis. Pediatr Infect Dis J 1992;11:694–698.
23. Oliver WJ, Shope TC, Kuhns LR. Fatal Lumbar Puncture: Fact versus fiction—an approach to a clinical dilemma. Pediatrics 2003;112:e174–e176.
24. Rennick G, Shann F, de Campo J. Cerebral herniation during bacterial meningitis in children. BMJ 306;953–955.
25. Behrman RE, Kleigman RM, Arvin RM. Nelson Textbook of Pediatrics, 15th ed. Philadelphia: WB Saunders; 1996.
26. El Bashir H, Laundy M, Booy R. Diagnosis and treatment of bacterial meningitis. Arch Dis Child 2003;88:615–620.
27. Kanegaye JT, Soliemanzadeh P, Bradley JS. Lumbar puncture in pediatric bacterial meningitis: defining the time interval for recovery of cerebrospinal fluid pathogens after parenteral antibiotic pretreatment. Pediatrics 2001;108:1169–1174.
28. Nadel S, Joarder R, Gibson M, et al. Emergency cranial computed tomography in the management of acute febrile encephalopathy in children. J Accid Emerg Med 1999;16:403–406.
29. Friedland IR, Paris MM, Rinderknecht S, et al. Cranial computed tomographic scans have little impact on management of bacterial meningitis. Am J Dis Child 1992;146:1484–1487.
30. Archer BD. Computed tomography before lumbar puncture in acute meningitis: a review of the risks and benefits. CMAJ 1993;148:961–965.
31. Stovring J, Snyder RD. Computed tomography in childhood bacterial meningitis. J Pediatr 1980;96:820–823.
32. Cabral DA, Flodmark O, Farrell K, et al. Prospective study of computed tomography in acute bacterial meningitis. J Pediatr 1987;111:201–205.
33. Packer RJ, Bilaniuk LT, Zimmerman RA. CT parenchymal abnormalities in bacterial meningitis: clinical significance. J Comput Assist Tomogr 1982;6:1064–1068.
34. Feldman WE. Concentrations of bacteria in cerebrospinal fluid of patients with bacterial meningitis. J Pediatr 1976;88:549–552.
35. Zwahlen A, Nydegger UE, Vaudaux P, et al. Complement mediated opsonic activity in normal and infected human cerebrospinal fluid: early response during bacterial meningitis. J Infect Dis 1982;145:635–646.
36. Madagame ET, Havens PL, Bresnahan BS, et al. Survival and functional outcome of children requiring mechanical ventilation during therapy for acute bacterial meningitis. Crit Care Med 1995;23:1279–1283.
37. Odio CM, Faingezicht I, Paris M, et al. The beneficial effects of early dexamethasone administration in infants and children with bacterial meningitis. N Engl J Med 1991;324:1525–1531.
38. Guidelines for the acute medical management of severe traumatic brain injury in infants, children and adolescents. Resuscitation of blood pressure and oxygenation and prehospital brain-specific therapies for the severe pediatric traumatic brain injury patient. Crit Care Med 2003;31:S428–S434.

39. Guidelines for the acute medical management of severe traumatic brain injury in infants, children and adolescents. Use of hyperventilation in the acute management of severe pediatric traumatic brain injury. Crit Care Med 2003;31:S461–S464.

40. Huynh T, et al. Positive end-expiratory pressure alters intracranial and cerebral perfusion pressure in traumatic brain injury. J Trauma 2002;53:488–493.

41. Tasker RC, et al. Monitoring in non-traumatic coma. Part 1: invasive intracranial measurements. Arch Dis Child 1988;63:888–894.

42. Johnston AJ, et al. Effect of cerebral perfusion pressure augmentation with dopamine and norepinephrine on global and focal brain oxygenation after traumatic brain injury. Intensive Care Med 2004;30: 791–797.

43. Steiner LA, et al. Direct comparison of cerebrovascular effects of norepinephrine and dopamine in head-injured patients. Crit Care Med 2004;32:1049–1054.

44. Guidelines for the acute medical management of severe traumatic brain injury in infants, children and adolescents. The role of temperature control following severe pediatric traumatic brain injury. Crit Care Med 2003;31:S469–S470.

45. Holzer M, et al. Mild therapeutic hypothermia to improve the neurologic outcome after cardiac arrest. N Engl J Med 2002;346:549–556.

46. Barnard S, et al. Treatment of comatose survivors of out-of-hospital arrest with induced hypothermia. N Engl J Med 2002;346:557–563.

47. Duke T. Fluid management of bacterial meningitis in developing countries. Arch Dis Child 1998;79:181–185.

48. Singhi SC, Singhi PD, Srinivas B, et al. Fluid restriction does not improve the outcome of acute meningitis. Pediatr Infect Dis J 1995;14:495–503.

49. Guidelines for the acute medical management of severe traumatic brain injury in infants, children and adolescents. Use of hyperosmolar therapy in the management of severe pediatric traumatic brain injury. Crit Care Med 2003;31:S456–S446.

50. Guidelines for the acute medical management of severe traumatic brain injury in infants, children and adolescents. Use of hyperventilation in the acute management of severe pediatric traumatic brain injury. Crit Care Med 2003;31:S461–S464.

51. Feldman WE. Concentrations of bacteria in cerebrospinal fluid of patients with bacterial meningitis. J Pediatr 1976;88:549–552.

52. Peltola H, Anttila M, Renkonen OV. Randomised comparison of chloramphenicol, ampicillin, cefotaxime and ceftriaxone fro childhood bacterial meningitis. Finnish Study Group. Lancet 1989;1(8650): 1281–1287.

53. Sande MA. Factors influencing the penetration and activity of antibiotics in experimental meningitis. J Infect 1981;3(1 Suppl):33–38.

54. Chavez-Bueno S, McCracken GH Jr. Bacterial meningitis. Pediatr Clin North Am 2005;52:795–810.

55. Huang CR, Lu CH, Chang WN. Adult *Enterobacter* meningitis: a high incidence of coinfection with other pathogens and frequent association with neurosurgical procedures. Infection 2001;29(2):75–79.

56. Vandecasteele SJ, Verhaegen J, Colaert J, Van Caster A, Devlieger H. Failure of cefotaxime and meropenem to eradicate meningitis caused by an intermediately susceptible *Streptococcus pneumoniae* strain. Eur J Clin Microbiol Infect Dis 2001;20:751–752.

57. Esen S, Leblebicioglu H, Sunbul M, Eroglu C. Repeated relapses in a meropenem-treated *Pseudomonas aeruginosa* meningitis. J Chemother 2002;14:535–536.

58. Cottagnoud P, Tauber MG. Fluoroquinolones in the treatment of meningitis. Curr Infect Dis Rep 2003;5:329–336.

59. Krueger WA, Kottler B, Will BE, Heininger A, Guggenberger H, Unertl KE. Treatment of meningitis due to methicillin-resistant *Staphylococcus epidermidis* with linezolid. J Clin Microbiol 2004;42:929–932.

60. Steinmetz MP, Vogelbaum MA, De Georgia MA, Andrefsky JC, Isada C. Successful treatment of vancomycin-resistant *Enterococcus* meningitis with linezolid: case report and review of the literature. Crit Care Med 2001;29:2383–2385.

61. Hansman D, Bullen MM. A resistant *Pneumococcus*. Lancet 1967;2: 264–265.

62. National Committee for Clinical Laboratory Standards. Performance standards for antimicrobial testing. Fifth International Supplement M10-S5. Villanova, PA: National Committee for Clinical Laboratory Standards, 1994.

63. Marton A, Gulyas M, Mumoz R, et al. Extremely high incidence of antibiotic resistance of *Streptococcus pneumoniae* in Hungary. J Infect Dis 1991;163:524–548.

64. Fenoll AI, Jado D, Vicioso A, et al. Evolution of *Streptococcus pneumoniae* serotypes and antibiotic resistance in Spain: update (1990–1996). J Clin Microbiol 1998;36:3447–3454.

65. Hoffman J, Cetron MS, Farley MM, et al. The prevalence of drug resistant *Streptococcus pneumoniae* in Atlanta. N Engl J Med 1995; 333:481–486.

66. Reacher MH, Shah A, Livermore DM, et al. Bacteraemia and antibiotic resistance of pathogens reported in England and Wales between 1990 and 1998: trend analysis. BMJ 2000;320:213–216.

67. Enright MC, Fenoll A, Griffiths D, et al. The three major Spanish clones of penicillin-resistant *Streptococcus pneumoniae* are the most common clones recovered in recent cases of meningitis in Spain. J Clin Microbiol 1999;37:3210–3216.

68. John CC. Treatment failure with the use of third generation cephalosporin for penicillin-resistant pneumococcal meningitis: case report and review. Clin Infect Dis 1994;18:188–193.

69. Pallares R, Linares J, Vadillo M, et al. Resistance to penicillin and cephalosporin and mortality from severe pneumococcal pneumonia in Barcelona, Spain. N Engl J Med 1995;333:474–480.

70. Tan TQ, Mason EO, Barson WJ, et al. Clinical characteristics and outcome in children with pneumonia attributable to penicillin-susceptible and penicillin-nonsusceptible *Streptococcus pneumoniae*. Pediatrics 1998;102:1369–1375.

71. Tan TQ, Schutze GE, Mason OE, et al. Antibiotic therapy and acute outcome in meningitis due to *Streptococcus pneumoniae* considered immediately susceptible to broad-spectrum cephalosporins. Antimicrob Agents Chemother 1994;38:918–923.

72. American Academy of Pediatrics. Committee on Infectious Diseases. Therapy for children with invasive pneumococcal infection. Pediatrics 1997;99:289–299.

73. Viladrich PF, Guidole F, Linares J, et al. Evaluation of vancomycin for therapy of adult pneumococcal meningitis. Antimicrob Agents Chemother 1991;35:2467–2472.

74. Paris MM, Hickey SM, Uscher MI, et al. Effect of dexamethasone of therapy of experimental penicillin-resistant and cephalosporin-resistant pneumococcal meningitis. Antimicrob Agents Chemother 1994;38:1320–1324.

75. Klugman KP, Friedland IR, Bradley JS, et al. Bactericidal activity against cephalosporin-resistant *Streptococcus pneumoniae* in cerebrospinal fluid of children with acute bacterial meningitis. Antimicrob Agents Chemother 1995;39:1988–1992.

76. Saez-Nieto JA, Lujan R, Berron S, et al. Epidemiology and molecular basis of penicillin-resistant *Neisseria meningitidis* in Spain: a 5 year history (1985–1990). Clin Infect Dis 1992;14:394–402.

77. Kaplam SL, Mason EO Jr. Management of infections due to antibiotic-resistant *Streptococcus pneumoniae*. Clin Mic Rev 1998;11:628–644.

78. Saez-Nieto, Klugman KP, Madhi SA. Emergence of drug resistance: impact on bacterial meningitis. Infect Dis Clin North Am 1999;13: 637–646.

79. Mandelman PM, Caugent DA, Kaltzoglou G, et al. Genetic diversity of penicillin G resistant *Neisseria meningitidis*. Clin infect Dis 1997;57: 1025–1029.

80. Oppenheimer BA. Antibiotic resistance in *Neisseria meningitidis*. Clin Infect Dis 1997;24:S98–S101.

81. Lucas Cubells C, Garcia Garcia JJ, Roca Martinez J, et al. Clinical data in children with meningococcal meningitis in a Spanish hospital. Acta Paediatr 1997;86:26–29.

82. Almog R, Block C, Gdalevitch M, et al. First recorded outbreaks of meningococcal disease in the Israeli defence force: three clusters due to serogroup C and the emergence of resistance to rifampicin. Infection 1994;22:67–71.

83. Gruneberg RN, Flemingham D. Results of the Alexander project: a continuing, multicentre study of antimicrobial susceptibility of community acquired lower respiratory tract bacterial pathogens. Diagn Microbiol Infect Dis 1996;25:169–184.

84. Johnson AW, Mokuolu OA, Onile BA. Chloramphenicol resistant *Haemophilus influenzae* meningitis in young urban Nigerian children. Acta Paediatr 1992;81:941–943.

85. Campos J, Hernando M, Roman F, Perez-Vazquez M, Aracil B, Oteo J, Lazaro E, de Abajo F. Group of invasive *Haemophilus* infections of the autonomous community of Madrid, Spain: analysis of invasive *Haemophilus influenzae* infections after extensive vaccination against *H. influenzae* type b. J Clin Microbiol 2004 Feb;42(2):524–529.

86. Arditi M, Manogue KR, Caplan M, et al. Cerebrospinal fluid cachectin/tumour necrosis factor-alpha, and platelet activating factor concentrations and severity of bacterial meningitis in children. J Infect Dis 1990;162:139–147.

87. Waage A, Halstensen A, Shalaby R, et al. Local production of tumour necrosis factor alpha, interleukin 1 and interleukin 6 in meningococcal meningitis: relation to the inflammatory response. J Exp Med 1989;170:1859–1867.

88. Scheld WM, Dacey RG, Winn R, Welsh JE. Cerebrospinal fluid outflow resistance in rabbits with experimental meningitis. J Clin Invest 1980;66:243–253.

89. McIntyre PB, Berkey CS, King SM, et al. Dexamethasone as adjunctive therapy in bacterial meningitis: a meta-analysis or randomised clinical trials since 1988. JAMA 1997;278:925–931.

90. De Gans J, Van de Beek for the European Dexamethasone in Adulthood Bacterial Meningitis Study Investigators. Dexamethasone in adults with bacterial meningitis. N Engl J Med 2002;347:1549–1556.

91. Thomas R, Le Tulzo Y, Bonget C, et al. Trial of dexamethasone for severe bacterial meningitis in adults. Adult Meningitis Steroid Group. Intensive Care Med 1999;25:475–480.

92. Tunkel AR, Scheld WM. Corticosteroids for everyone with meningitis? N Engl J Med 2002;347:1613–1615.

93. McIntyre PB, Berkey CS, King SM, et al. Dexamethasone as adjunctive therapy in bacterial meningitis: a meta-analysis or randomised clinical trials since 1988. JAMA 1997;278:925–931.

94. De Gans J, Van de Beek for the European Dexamethasone in Adulthood Bacterial Meningitis Study Investigators. Dexamethasone in adults with bacterial meningitis. N Engl J Med 2002;347:1549–1556.

95. Cerebrospinal fluid protein profile in experimental pneumococcal meningitis and its alteration by ampicillin and anti-inflammatory agents. J Infect Dis 1995;159:26–34.

96. Rappaport JM, Bhatt SM, Burkard RF, et al. Prevention of hearing loss in experimental pneumococcal meningitis by the administration of dexamethasone and ketorolac. J Infect Dis 1999;179:264–268.

97. Chez M, Sila CA, Ransohoff RM, Longworth DL, Weida C. Ibuprofen-induced meningitis: detection of intrathecal IGG synthesis and immune complexes. Neurology 1990;40:866–867.

98. Chez M, Kornelisse RF, Ohga S, Aoki T, Okada K, et al. Cerebrospinal fluid concentrations of interleukin-1 beta, tumour necrosis factor-alpha and interferon gamma in bacterial meningitis. Arch Dis Child 1994;70:123–125.

99. Glimaker M, Olcen P, Andersson B. Interferon gamma in cerebrospinal fluid from patients with viral and bacterial meningitis. Scand J Infect Dis 1994;26:141–147.

100. Cole AM, Ganz T, Liese AM, et al. Cutting edge: IFN-inducible ELR-CXC chemokines display defensin-like antimicrobial activity. J Immunol 2001;167:623–627.

101. Mackenzie CR, Willberg CB, Daubener W. Inhibition of group B streptococcal growth by IFNgamma-activated human glioblastoma cells. J Neuroimmunol 1998;89:191–197.

102. Van Furth AM, Seijmonsberg EM, Langermans JA, et al. High levels of interleukin-10 and tumour necrosis factor-alpha in cerebrospinal fluid during onset of bacterial meningitis. Clin Infect Dis 1995;21:220–222.

103. Kim KS, Wass CA, Cross AS, Opal SM. Modulation of blood–brain barrier permeability by tumor necrosis factor and antibody to tumor necrosis factor in the rat. Lymphokine Cytokine Res 1992;11:293–298.

104. Sharief MK, Ciardi M, Thompson EJ. Blood–brain barrier damage in patients: association with tumor necrosis factor-α but not interleukin-1 B. J Infect Dis 1992;166:350–358.

105. Park WS, Chang YS, Ko SY, et al. Efficacy of anti-tumor necrosis factor-alpha antibody as an adjunctive therapy in experimental *Escherichia coli* meningitis in the newborn piglet. Biol Neonate 1999;75:377–387.

106. Bogden I, Leib SL, Bergeron M, Chow L, Tauber MG. Tumor necrosis factor-alpha contributes to apoptosis in hippocampal neurons during experimental group B streptococcal meningitis. J Infect Dis 1997;176:693–697.

107. Abraham E, Wunderlink R, Silverman H, et al. Efficacy and safety of monoclonal antibody to human tumor necrosis factor alpha in patients with sepsis syndrome. A randomised, controlled, double-blinded, multicentre clinical trial. TNF-alpha Mab Sepsis Study Group. JAMA 1995;273:934–941.

108. Cohen J, Carlet J, et al. INTERSEPT: an international, multicentre, placebo-controlled trial of monoclonal antibody to human tumor necrosis factor alpha in patients with sepsis. International Sepsis Trial Study Group. Crit Care Med 1996;24:1413–1440.

109. Saez-llorens X, Ramilo O, Mustafa MM, et al. Pentoxyphylline modulates meningeal inflammation in experimental bacterial meningitis. Antimicrob Agents Chemother 1990;34:837–843.

110. Burroughs M, Tsenova-Berkova L, Sokol K, et al. Effect of thalidomide on the inflammatory response in cerebrospinal fluid in experimental bacterial meningitis. Microb Pathol 1995;19:245–255.

111. Paris MM, Hickey SM, Trujillo M, et al. The effect of interleukin-10 on meningeal inflammation in experimental bacterial meningitis. J Infect Dis 1997;176:1239–1246.

112. Ray G, Aneja S, Jain M, Batra S. Evaluation of the free radical status in CSF in childhood meningitis. Ann Trop Paediatr 2000;20:115–120.

113. Christen S, Schaper M, Lykkesfeldt J. Oxidative stress in bacterial meningitis: Differential effects of (alpha)-phenyl-tert-butyl nitrone and N-acetylcysteine treatment. Free Rad Biol Med 2001;31:754–762.

114. Auer M, Pfeister L-A, Leppert D, Tauber MG, Leib SL. Effects of clinically used antioxidants in experimental pneumococcal meningitis. J Infect Dis 2000;182:347–350.

115. Koedel U, Pfeister H-W. Protective effects of the antioxidant N-acetyl L-cysteine in pneumococcal meningitis in rats. Neurosci Lett 1997;225:33–36.

116. Garnet C, Raud J, Xie X, Lindquist L, Lindbom L. Inhibition of leucocyte rolling with polysaccharide fucoidin prevents pleocytosis in experimental meningitis in the rabbit. J Clin Invest 1994;93:929–936.

117. Garnet C, Raud J, Lindquist L. The polysaccharide fucoidin inhibits the antibiotic-induced inflammatory cascade in experimental pneumococcal meningitis. Clin Diagn Lab Immunol 1998;54:322–324.

118. Garnet C, Raud J, Waage A, Lindquist L. Effects of the polysaccharide fucoidin on cerebrospinal fluid interleukin-1 and tumor necrosis factor alpha in pneumococcal meningitis in the rabbit. Infect Immunol 1999;67:2071–2074.

119. Del Maschio A, De Luigi A, Martin-Padura I, et al. Leukocyte recruitment in the cerebrospinal fluid of mice with experimental meningitis is inhibited by an antibody to junctional adhesion molecule (JAM). J Exp Med 1999;190:1351–1356.

120. Lechner F, Sahrbacher U, Suter T, et al. Antibodies to the junctional adhesion molecule cause disruption of endothelial cells and do not prevent leukocyte influx into the meninges after viral or bacterial infection. J Infect Dis 2000;182:978–982.

121. Freyer D, Manz R, Zeigenhorn A, et al. Cerebral endothelial cells release TNF-alpha after stimulation with cell wall so *Streptococcus pneumoniae* and regulate inducible nitric oxide synthase and ICAM-1 expression via autocrine loops. J Immunol 1999;163:4308–4314.

122. Lewczuk P, Reiber H, Tumani H. Intracellular adhesion molecule-1 in cerebrospinal fluid—the evaluation of blood-derived and brain-derived fractions in neurological diseases. J Neuroimmunol 1998; 87:156–161.

123. Weber JR, Angstwurm K, Burger W, Einhaupl KM, Dirnagl U. Anti ICAM-1 (CD 54) monoclonal antibody reduces inflammatory changes in experimental bacterial meningitis. J Neuroimmunol 1995;63: 63–68.

124. Alavi A, Shoa L, Lattanand C, et al. Brain tumor permeability enhanced by RMP-7, a novel bradykinin agonist. Can J Infect Dis 1995;6SC:abstr 4153.

125. Elliot PJ, Hayward NJ, Huff MR, et al. Unlocking the blood–brain barrier: a role for RMP-7 in brain tumor therapy. Exp Neurol 1996;141: 214–224.

126. Bartus R, Elliot P, Hayward N, et al. RMP-7 selectively increase the uptake of carboplatin into rat brain tumors. Can J Infect Dis 1995;6SC: abstr 4152.

127. Washburn RG, Bartlett JA, Forthal DN, Graney WF. Phase I/II study of RMP-7 and amphotericin B for cryptococcal meningitis in AIDS. 35th Interscience conference on Antimicrobial Agents and Chemotherapy. San Francisco, 1995. Abstract A51.

128. Snodgrass PA, Emerich DF, Lafreniere DL, Bartus RT. Obligatory tachyphylaxis of bradykinin B2 receptors following increased permeability of blood brain barrier by intravenous report. Soc Neurosci Abstr (New Orleans) 2000;26: abstr 127.4.

129. Park WS, Chang YS, Lee M. Effect of hypothermia on brain cell membrane function and energy metabolism in experimental *Escherichia coli* meningitis in the newborn piglet. Neurochem Res 2001;26: 369–374.

130. Irazuzta JE, Olson J, Kiefaber MP, Wong H. Hypothermia decreases excitatory neurotransmitter release in bacterial meningitis in rabbits. Brain Res 2000;847:143–148.

131. Irazuzta JE, Pretzlaff R, Rowin M, et al. Hypothermia as an adjunctive treatment for severe bacterial meningitis. Brain Res 2000;881:88–97.

132. Peltola H. Prophylaxis of bacterial meningitis. Infect Dis Clin North Am 1999;13:685–710.

133. Ramsey ME, Andrews N, Kaczmarski EB, Miller E. Efficacy of meningococcal serotype C conjugate vaccine in teenagers and toddlers in England. Lancet 2001;195–196.

134. Mohammed I, Nasidi A, Alkali AS, et al. A severe epidemic of meningococcal meningitis in Nigeria, 1996. Trans R Soc Trop Med Hyg 2000; 94:265–270.

135. Popovic T, Sacchi CT, Reeves MW, et al. *Neisseria meningitidis* serogroup W135 isolates associated with the Et-37 complex. Emerg Infect Dis 2000;6:428–429.

136. Anonymous. Serotype Y meningococcal—Illinois, Connecticut, and selected areas, United States, 1989–1996. MMWR 1996;45:1010–1013.

137. Bjune G, Hoiby EA, Gronnesby JK, et al. Effect of an outer membrane vesicle vaccine against group B meningococcal disease in Norway. Lancet 1991;338:1093–1096.

138. Sierra GVG, Campa HC, Varcacel NM, et al. Vaccine against group B *Neisseria meningitidis*: protection trial and mass vaccination results in Cuba. NIPH Ann 1991;14:195–207.

139. Cartwright K, Morris R, Rumke H, et al. Immunogenicity and reactogenicity of a novel meningococcal vesicle vaccine containing multiple class 1 (Por A) outer membrane proteins. Vaccine 1999;17:2612–2619.

140. Coquillat D, Bruge J, Danve B, et al. Activity and cross-reactivity of antibodies induced in mice by immunization with a group B meningococcal conjugate. Infect Immun 2001;69:7131–7139.

141. Fusco PC, Michon F, Tai JY, Blake MS. Preclinical evaluation of a novel group B meningococcal conjugate vaccine that elicits bactericidal activity in both mice and nonhuman primates. J Infect Dis 1997;175: 364–372.

142. Black S, Shinefiled H, Fireman B, et al. Safety, immunogenicity and efficacy of a heptavalent pneumococcal conjugate vaccine in infancy. Pediatr Infect Dis J 2000;19:187–195.

143. George R, Mellagaro A. Invasive pneumococcal infection: England and Wales 1999. CDC Wkly Rep 2001;11:21.

141. Whitley RJ, Gnann JW. Viral encephalitis: familiar infections and emerging pathogens. Lancet 2002;359:507–514.

145. Davison KL, Ramsay ME. The epidemiology of acute meningitis in England and Wales. Arch Dis Child 2003;88:662–664.

146. Atkinson PJ, Sharland M, Maguire H. Predominant enteroviral serotypes causing meningitis. Arch Dis Child 1998;78:373–374.

147. Centers for Disease Control and Prevention. Echovirus type 13—United State, 2001. JAMA 2001;286:1831–1832.

148. Monto H, et al. An epidemic of enterovirus 71 infection in Taiwan. N Engl J Med 1999;341:929–935.

149. Sawyer MH. Enterovirus infections: diagnosis and treatment. Semin Pediatr Infect Dis 2002;13:40–47.

150. Berenguer J, Moreno S, Laguna F, et al. Tuberculous meningitis in patients infected with the human immunodeficiency virus. N Engl J Med 1992;326:668.

151. Udani PM, Parekh UC, Dastur DK. Neurological and related syndromes in CNS tuberculosis: clinical features and pathogenesis. J Neurol Sci 1971;14:341–357.

152. Levin M, Walters S. Infections of the nervous system. In: Brett EW, ed. Pediatric Neurology, 3rd ed. New York: Churchill Livingstone; 1997.

153. Stevens Dl, Everett ED. Sequential computerized axial tomography in tuberculous meningitis. JAMA 1978;239:642–643.

154. Witrak BJ, Ellis GT. Intracranial tuberculosis: manifestations on computerized tomography. South Med J 1985;78:386–392.

155. Fallon RJ, Kennedy DH. Treatment and prognosis in tuberculous meningitis. J Infect 1981;3:39–44.

156. Eng-King Tan, Michael W.L. Chee, Ling-Ling Chan, Yah-Leng Lee. Culture positive tuberculous meningitis: clinical indicators of poor prognosis. Clin Neurol Neurosurg 1999;101:157–160.

157. Ellard GA, Humphries MJ, Allen BW. Cerebrospinal fluid concentrations and the treatment of tuberculous meningitis. Am Rev Respir Dis 1993;148:650–655.

158. American Academy of Pediatrics. Report of the Committee of Infectious Diseases, Elk Grove Village, Illinois, 23rd ed. Tuberculosis 480–500.

159. Humphries M. The management of tuberculous meningitis. Thorax 1992;47:577–581.

160. Prasad K, Volmink J, Menon GR. Steroids for treating tuberculous meningitis. Cochrane Database System Rev 2000;3:CD002244.

161. Bicanic T, Harrison TS. Cryptococcal meningitis. Br Med Bull 2004;72:99–118.

162. Lin W-C, et al. *Mycoplasma pneumoniae* encephalitis in childhood. J Microbiol Immunol Infect 2002;35:173–178.

163. Candler PM, Dale RC. Three cases of central nervous system complications associated with *Mycoplasma pneumoniae*. Pediatr Neurol 2004;31:133–138.

164. Johnson RT. The pathogenesis of acute viral encephalitis and postinfectious encephalitis. J Infect Dis 1987;155:359–364.

165. Johnson RT, Mims CA. Pathogenesis of viral infections of the nervous system. N Engl J Med 1968;278:23–30, 84–92.

166. Jamieson GA, Maitland NJ, Wilcock GK, Craske J, Itzhaki RF. Latent herpes simplex virus type I in normal and Alzheimer's disease brains. J Med Virol 1991;33:224–227.

167. Barnett EM, Jacobsen G, Evans G, Cassell M, Perlman S. Herpes simplex encephalitis in the temporal cortex and limbic system after trigeminal nerve inoculation. J Infect Dis 1994;169:782–786.

168. Bitnun A, et al. *Mycoplasma pneumoniae* encephalitis. Semin Pediatr Infect Dis 2003;14:96–107.

169. Holtkamp M, Othman J, Buchheim K, Meierkord H. Predictors and prognosis of refractory status epilepticus treated in a neurological intensive care unit. J Neurol Neurosurg Psychiatry 2005;76:534–539.

170. Sawyer MH. Enterovirus infections: diagnosis and treatment. Semin Pediatr Infect Dis 2002;13:40–47.

171. Ch'ien LT, Boehm RM, Robinson H, Liu C, Frenkel LD. Characteristic early electroencephalographic changes in herpes simplex encephalitis. Arch Neurol 1977;34:361–364.

172. Koletsky RJ, Weinstein AJ. Fulminant *Mycoplasma pneumoniae* infection. Report of a fatal case, and a review of the literature. Am Rev Respir Dis 1980;122:491–496.

173. Kenny GE, Kaiser GG, Cooney MK, et al. Diagnosis of *Mycoplasma pneumoniae* pneumonia: sensitivities and specificities of serology with lipid antigen and isolation of the organism on soy peptone medium for the identification of infections. J Clin Microbiol 1990;28:2087–2093.

174. Tjhie JH, van Kupperveld FJ, Roosendaal R, et al. Direct PCR enables detection of *Mycoplasma pneumoniae* in patients with respiratory tract infections. J Clin Microbiol 1994;32:11–16.

175. Vikerfors T, Brodin G, Grandien M, et al. Detection of specific IgM antibodies for the diagnosis of *Mycoplasma pneumoniae* infections. A clinical evaluation. Scand J Infect Dis 1988;20:601–610.

176. Moule JH, Caul EO, Wreghitt TG. The specific IgM response to *Mycoplasma pneumoniae* infection: interpretation and application to early diagnosis. Epidemiol Infect 1987;99:685–692.

177. Lin W-C, Lee P-I, Lu C-Y, et al. *Mycoplasma pneumoniae* encephalitis in childhood. J Microbiol Immunol Infect 2002;35:173–178.

178. Thomas NH, Collins JE, Robb SA, et al. *Mycoplasma pneumoniae* infection and neurological disease. Arch Dis Child 1993;69:573–576.

179. Steigbigel NH. Macrolides and clindamycin. In: Mandell Gl, Bennett JE, Dolin R, eds. Principles and Practice of Infectious Diseases. New York: Churchill Livingstone; 2000:366–382.

180. Jaruratanasirikul S, Hortiwakul R, Tantisarasart T, et al. Distribution of azithromycin into brain tissue, cerebrospinal fluid and aqueous humor of the eye. Antimicrob Agents Chemother 1996;40:825–826.

181. Whitley RJ. Herpes simplex virus. In: Scheld WM, Whitley RJ, Durack DT, eds. Infections of the Central Nervous System, 2nd ed. Philadelphia: Lippincott-Raven; 1998:73–89.

182. Whitley RJ, Roizman B. Herpes simplex virus infections. Lancet 2001;357:1513–1518.

183. Tyler KL. Herpes simplex virus infections of the central nervous system: encephalitis and meningitis, including Mollaret's. Herpes 2004;S2:57A–64A.

184. Aurelius E, Johansson B, Skolden berg B, Forsgren M. Encephalitis in immunocompetent patients due to herpes simplex virus type 1 or 2 as determined by type specific polymerase chain reaction and antibody assays of cerebrospinal fluid. J Med Virol 1993;39:179–186.

185. Tookey P, Peckham CS. Neonatal herpes simplex virus infection in the British Isles. Paediatr Perinat Epidemiol 1996;10:432–442.

186. Kimberlin DW, Lin CY, Jacobs RF, Powell DA, Frenkell LM, Gruber WC, et al. Natural history of neonatal herpes simplex viral infections in the aciclovir era. Pediatrics 2001;108:223–229.

187. Kimberlin D. Herpes simplex virus, meningitis and encephalitis in neonates. Herpes 2004;11S2:65A–76A.

188. Lakeman FD, Whitley RJ. Diagnosis of herpes simplex encephalitis: application of polymerase chain reaction to cerebrospinal fluid from brain-biopsied patients and correlation with disease. National Institute of Allergy and Infectious Diseases Collaborative Antiviral study Group. J Infect Dis 1995;171:857–863.

189. Dominigues RB, Fink MCD, Tsanaclis AMC, et al. Diagnosis of herpes simplex encephalitis by magnetic resonance imaging and polymerase chain reaction assay of cerebrospinal fluid. J Neurol Sci 1998;157:148–153.

190. Whitley RJ, Alford Ca, Hirsch MS, et al. Vidarabine versus acyclovir therapy in herpes simplex encephalitis. N Engl J Med 1986;314:144–149.

191. De Tiege X, Rozenberg F, Des Portes V, et al. Herpes simplex encephalitis relapses in children. Neurology 2003;61:241–243.

192. Atkinson PJ, Sharland M, Maguire H. Predominant enteroviral serotypes causing meningitis. Arch Dis Child 1998;78:373–374.

193. Ho M, Chen E-R, Hsu K-H, et al. An epidemic of enterovirus 71 infection in Taiwan. N Engl J Med 1999;341:929–935.

194. Moran GJ, Talan DA, Mower W, et al. Appropriateness of rabies post-exposure prophylaxis treatment for animal exposures. Emergency ID Net Study Group. JAMA 2000;284:1000–1007.

195. Anonymous. World survey of rabies. Wkly Epidemiol Rec 1997;74:381–384.

196. Plotkin SA. Rabies. Clin Infect Dis 2000;30:4–12.

197. Noah DL, Drenzek CL, Smith JS, et al. Epidemiology of human rabies in the United States, 1980–1996. Ann Intern Med 1998;128:922–930.

198. Willoughby RE, et al. Survival after treatment of rabies with induction of coma. N Engl J Med 2005;352:2508–2514.

199. Solomon T, Dung NM, Kneen R, Gainsborough M, Vaughn DW, Khanh VT. Japanese encephalitis. J Neurol Neurosurg Psychiatry 2000;68:405–415.

200. Kalita J, Mista UK. Comparison of CT scan and MRI findings in the diagnosis of Japanese encephalitis. J Neurol Sci 2000;174:3–8.

201. Solomon T, thao LT, Dung NM, et al. Rapid diagnosis of Japanese encephalitis by using an immunoglobulin M dot enzyme immunoassay. J Clin Microbiol 1998;36:2030–2034.

202. Newton CRJC, Hein TT, White N. Cerebral malaria. J Neurol Neurosurg Psychiatry 2000;69:433–441.

203. Maitland K, Nadel S, Pollard A, et al. The management of severe malaria in children: proposed guidelines for the UK. BMJ 2005;331:337–343.

204. MacPherson GG, Warrell MJ, White NJ, et al. Human cerebral malaria. A quantitative ultrastructural analysis of parasitised erythrocyte sequestration. Am J Pathol 1985;119:385–401.

205. Turner GDH, Morrison H, Jones M, et al. An immunohistochemical study of the pathology of fatal malaria. Am J Pathol 1994;145:1057–1069.

206. Brown H, Hien TT, Day N, et al. Evidence of blood–brain barrier dysfunction in human cerebral malaria. Neuropathol Appl Neurobiol 1999;25:331–340.

207. White NJ, Ho M. The pathophysiology of malaria. Adv Parasitol 1992;31:83–173.

208. Kaul DK, Liu XD, Nagel RL, et al. Microvascular haemodynamics and in vivo evidence for the role of intracellular adhesion molecule-1 in the sequestration of infected red blood cells in a mouse model of lethal malaria. Am Trop Med Hyg 1998;58:240–247.

209. Cranston HA, Boylan CW, Carroll GL, et al. *Plasmodium falciparum* maturation abolishes physiologic red cell deformability. Science 1984;223:400–403.

210. Grau GE, Taylor TE, Molyneux ME, et al. Tumour necrosis factor and disease severity in children with falciparum malaria. N Engl J Med 1989;320:1586–1591.

211. Kwiatkowski D, Hill AV, Sambou I, et al. TNF concentrate in fatal cerebral, nonfatal cerebral and uncomplicated *Plasmodium falciparum* malaria. Lancet 1990;336:1201–1204.

212. Marsh K, Forster D, Waruiru C, et al. Indicators of life threatening malaria in African children. N Engl J Med 1995;332:1399–1404.

213. White NJ. The treatment of malaria. N Engl J Med 1996;335:800–806.

214. Phillips RE, Solomon. Cerebral malaria in children. Lancet 1990;336:1355–1360.

215. Goodkin HP, Pomeroy SL. Parameningeal infections. In: Feigin RD, Cherry JD, Demmler GJ, Kaplan SL, eds. Textbook of Pediatric Infectious Diseases, 5th ed. Philadelphia: WB Saunders; 2003:475–483.

216. Wong TT, Lee LS, Wang HS, Shen EY, Jaw WC, Chiang CH, Chi CS, Hung KL, Liou WY, Shen YZ. Brain abscesses in children—a cooperative study of 83 cases. Child's Nerv Syst 1989;5:19–24.

217. Brook I. Brain abscess in children: microbiology and management. J Child Neurol 1995;10:283–288.

218. Nicolisi A, Hauser WA, Beghi E, Kurland LT. Epidemiology of central nervous system infections in Olmstead County, Minnesota 1950–1981. J Infect Dis 1986;154:399–408.

219. Osenbach RK, Loftus CM. Diagnosis and management of brain abscess. Neurosurg Clin North Am 1992;3:403–420.

220. Piper C, Horstkotte D, Arendt G, Strauer BE. Brain abscess in children with cyanotic heart defects. Z Kardiol 1994;83:188–193.

221. Britt RH, Enzmann DR, Yeager AS. Neuropathological and computerised tomographic findings in experimental brain abscess. J Neurosurg 1981;55:590–603.

222. Kielian T. Immunopathology of brain abscess. J Neuroinflammation 2004;1:1–16–26.

223. Brook I. Aerobic and anaerobic bacteriology of intracranial abscesses. Pediatr Neurol 1992;8:210–214.

224. de Louvois J, Gortvai P, Hurley R. Bacteriology of abscesses of the central nervous system: a multicentre prospective study. BMJ 1977; 2:981–984.

225. Ciurea AV, Stoica F, Vasilescu G, Nuteanu L. Neurosurgical management of brain abscesses in children. Child's Nerv Syst 1999;15: 309–317.

226. Goodkin HP, Harper MB, Pomeroy SL. Intracerebral abscess in children: historical trends at Children's Hospital, Boston. Pediatrics 2004;113:1765–1770.

227. Roche M, Humphreys H, Smyth E, Phillips J, Cunney R, McNamara E, O'Brien D, McArdle O. A twelve-year review of central nervous system bacterial abscesses; presentation and aetiology. Clin Microbiol Infect 2003;9:803–809.

228. Saez-Llorens XJ, Umana MA, Odio CM, McCracken GH Jr, Nelson JD. Brain abscess in infants and children. Pediatr Infect Dis J 1989;8: 449–458.

229. Woods CR. Brain abscess and other intracranial suppurative complications. Adv Pediatr Infect Dis 1995;10:41–80.

230. Loeser E Jr, Scheinberg L. Brain abscesses: a review of 99 cases. Neurology 1957;7:601–606.

231. Skelton R, Maixner W, Isaacs D. Sinusitis-induced subdural empyema. Arch Dis Child 1992;67:1478–1480.

232. Smith RR. Neuroradiology of intracranial infection. Pediatr Neurosurg 1992;18:92–104.

233. Shahzadi S, Tasker RR, Guha A, Bernstein M, Lozano AM. Stereotactic management of bacterial brain abscesses. Can J Neurol Sci 1996; 23:34–39.

234. Fritsch M, Manwaring KH. Endoscopic treatment of brain abscess in children. Minim Invasive Neurosurg 1997;40:103–106.

235. Ersahin Y, McLone DG, Storrs BB, Yogev R. Review of 3017 procedures for the management of hydrocephalus in children. Concepts Pediatr Neurosurg 1989;9:21–28.

236. George R, Leibrock L, Epstein M. Long-term analysis of cerebrospinal fluid shunt infections: a 25 year experience. J Neurosurg 1979;51: 804–811.

237. Odio C, McCracken GH, Nelson JD. CSF shunt infections in pediatrics. Am J Dis Child 1984;138:1103–1108.

238. Schoenbaum SC, Gardner P, Shillito J. Infections of cerebrospinal fluid shunts: epidemiology, clinical manifestations and therapy. J Infect Dis 1975;131:543–552.

239. Bondurant CP, Jiminez DF. Epidemiology of cerebrospinal fluid shunting. Pediatr Neurosurg 1995;23:254–259.

240. Sainte-Rose C, Hoffman HJ, Hirsch JF. Shunt failure. In: Marlin AE, ed. Concepts in Pediatric Neurosurgery, vol 9. Basel: Karger; 2000:7–20.

241. Meirovitch J, Kitae-Cohen Y, Keren G, Fiendler G, Rubenstein G. Cerebrospinal fluid shunt infections in children. Pediatr Infect Dis J 1987;6:921–924.

242. Kaufman BA, McLone DG. Infections of cerebrospinal fluid shunts. In: Scheld WM, Whitley RJ, Durack DT, eds. Infections of the Central Nervous System. New York: Raven Press; 1991:561–585.

243. Shurtleff DB, Christie D, Foltz EL. Ventriculoauriculostomy-associated infection: a 12 year study. J Neurosurg 1971;35:686–694.

244. Lerman SJ. *Haemophilus influenzae*: infections of cerebrospinal fluid shunts. J Neurosurg 1981;54:261–263.

245. James HE. Infections associated with cerebrospinal fluid prosthetic devices. In: Sugarman B, Young EJ, eds. Infections Associated with Prosthetic Devices. Chicago: CRC Press; 1984:23–42.

246. Noetzel MJ, Baker RP. Shunt fluid examination: risks and benefits in the evaluation of shunt malfunction and infection. J Neurosurg 1984; 61:328–332.

247. Myers MG, Schoenbaum SC. Shunt fluid aspiration. Am J Dis Child 1975;129:220–222.

248. Everett ED, Strausbaugh LJ. Antimicrobial agents and the central nervous system. Neurosurgery 1980;6:691–714.

249. Choux M, Genitori L, Lang D, Lena G. Shunt implantation: reducing the incidence of shunt infection. J Neurosurg 1992;77:875–880.

11
Status Epilepticus

Richard F.M. Chin and Rod C. Scott

Introduction

Status epilepticus is the most common neurologic emergency in childhood [1,2] and may be convulsive (i.e., tonic, clonic, or tonic-clonic) or nonconvulsive in nature. As the majority of children admitted to a pediatric intensive care unit (PICU) for status epilepticus have convulsive status epilepticus (CSE), this is the focus of the current chapter.

There continues to be significant morbidity and mortality associated with CSE. The possible adverse outcomes from childhood CSE include subsequent epilepsy; permanent neurologic, developmental, and cognitive deficits; and death [3]. Among children admitted to the PICU for CSE, 5%–6% will die during their hospital admission, and neurologic sequelae ranging from minor impairment to persistent vegetative states are identified in about one third of children at discharge [4,5]. Mortality and morbidity associated with CSE is largely dependent on etiology [6–8] and on seizure length, with increasing seizure length being associated with a worse outcome [9–11]. Given that etiology is an important determinant of outcome, it can be hypothesized that early identification and prompt, effective treatment of the underlying etiology may improve the outcome of CSE. However, interventions that decrease seizure length may also reduce morbidity. Such interventions may occur in the prehospital setting, the emergency room, or the intensive care unit. It is either failure of initial therapy or respiratory depression that is responsible for admission to the intensive care unit in the majority of cases, and therefore it is important for intensive care physicians to be aware of treatment issues outside of the intensive care unit in order to plan effective therapy.

Definitions

The conventional definition of CSE is a seizure, or a series of seizures without recovery of consciousness between seizures, that lasts at least 30 min [12]. However, it is unacceptable to wait until a seizure has continued for at least 30 min before initiating treatment, as it is unethical to delay therapy, given that increasing seizure length is associated with increasing difficulty in seizure termination [13] and outcome worsens with increasing seizure length [9,11]. The majority of tonic-clonic epileptic seizures are self-limiting, lasting less than 2–3 min, and hence frequently do not require rescue therapy. However, approximately 95% of seizures that last at least 5 min will last at least 30 min unless there has been an appropriate intervention [14–16]. Therefore, a seizure that lasts 5 min is pathophysiologically similar to one that lasts 30 min and should be considered to be status epilepticus requiring emergency therapy. For these reasons it is frequently recommended that children whose seizures have not self-terminated within 5 min should receive rescue therapy [17], accepting that a few children would have had a seizure that would have stopped spontaneously.

As data from animal models of CSE suggest that brain injury can occur with seizures that have lasted at least 30 min [18,19], most studies that address the outcomes from CSE have used a 30-min definition. Thus, it can be considered that treatment initiated as soon as possible after onset of status epilepticus (with a 5-min definition) is necessary in order to reduce potential adverse outcomes associated with seizures that last at least 30 min.

Incidence

All epidemiologic studies reported to date that aim to estimate the incidence of CSE have used the 30-min definition described above. There are seven epidemiologic cohorts that have been reported, and all except one primarily or exclusively included adults [20–26]. These studies have recently been systematically reviewed [27]. Among children, the incidence of status epilepticus ranges from 4 to 38 episodes per 100,000 children per year. This wide range can be partly explained by differences in methodology and differences in ascertainment, but the incidence of status epilepticus in childhood ranges from 24 to 38 per 100,000 children per year even if the studies are of similar high quality [27]. This variation may be partly explained by the ethnic makeup of the populations, given that the

D.S. Wheeler et al. (eds.), *The Central Nervous System in Pediatric Critical Illness and Injury*,
DOI 10.1007/978-1-84800-993-6_11, © Springer-Verlag London Limited 2009

incidence is higher in nonwhite than in white populations, as well as socioeconomic factors. The North London Status Epilepticus in Childhood Surveillance Study (NLSTEPSS) is the only purely pediatric epidemiologic study on status epilepticus in Europe, and preliminary results from this study suggest that the incidence of status epilepticus in childhood is 18 per 100,000 children per year [27]. Among children with incident episodes of CSE, 47% will require admission to a PICU [26]. Thus, each year within the United Kingdom, of the estimated 4,000 children with a lifetime first episode of status epilepticus, approximately 2,000 will require admission to a PICU. This estimate does not include the population of children who would have had at least one previous episode of CSE and would have been admitted to a PICU for a subsequent episode, and hence the final estimate of admissions to the PICU for status epilepticus would be greater. Children admitted to a PICU for CSE account for 1.6%–4% of all admissions to pediatric intensive care [4,5]. It is hence likely that physicians working in the PICU will need to treat an episode of CSE several times per year.

Etiology

As the outcome of CSE is heavily dependent on etiology, it is important to address causation of CSE when planning therapy or when giving long-term prognoses. The etiology of CSE can be classified as prolonged febrile seizures, acute symptomatic, remote symptomatic, acute or remote symptomatic, or idiopathic epilepsy related (see Table 11.1 for definitions). Prolonged febrile seizures are the most common type of CSE in childhood, but because this diagnosis is conditional upon an absence of CNS infection, the diagnosis is one of exclusion. Because children with CSE (seizures lasting at least 30 min) associated with fever are much more likely to have acute bacterial meningitis than children with short seizures (less than 15 min) associated with fever (15%–18% vs. 1.2%) [28], there should be a low threshold for empirical treatment with antibiotics for such patients. Among acute symptomatic CSE in childhood, CNS infections, acute metabolic disturbances (including hyponatremia and hypocalcemia), drug usage, head injury,

hypoxia/anoxia, and cerebrovascular accidents are the most common causes [2]. Within the subgroup of children with idiopathic epilepsy–related CSE, the possibility of pyridoxine/pyridoxal phosphate-dependent epilepsy or an underlying metabolic cause should be considered.

Pathophysiology

Seizure Initiation, Prolongation, and Termination

For CSE to develop, a seizure must be initiated, and the putative mechanisms that terminate seizures must fail. Convulsive status epilepticus can be induced in animal models by creating an imbalance between inhibitory and excitatory neurotransmitter systems such that the ratio between the systems favors excitation [29]. The major inhibitory neurotransmitter is gamma-aminobutyric acid (GABA), and the major excitatory neurotransmitter in the brain is glutamate [30]. The effects of these systems may be modulated by the cholinergic and/or adenosinergic neurotransmitter systems [31–33]. Seizure onset in humans could also be a result of an endogenously created imbalance between excitatory and inhibitory neurotransmitter systems [29]. Human studies assessing mechanisms of seizure onset have only been performed in patients with lesional epilepsy undergoing presurgical evaluation. The excitatory neurotransmitters glutamate and aspartate increase at the seizure focus in adults with temporal lobe epilepsy as measured by in vivo intracerebral microdialysis [34,35]. Elevations of glycine and D-serine, which are both cotransmitters at the excitatory postsynaptic N-methyl-D-aspartate (NMDA) receptor, can also be identified [36]. Preictal decreases in GABA concentrations occur at the site of seizure onset [34]. There is, therefore, animal model and human evidence to support the view that excitatory/inhibitory imbalances initiate seizures.

It is possible that continuing imbalances between excitatory and inhibitory neurotransmitters would result in prolongation of seizures. However, animal models of CSE universally show a decrease in extracellular or whole brain glutamate concentrations during CSE [37–39], and, additionally, GABA concentrations may continue to rise throughout the period of epileptic activity [37,38], an effect that is more easily maintained in the developing than the developed brain [40]. These effects are more likely to be compensatory rather than seizure prolonging. These data therefore suggest that the mechanisms of seizure prolongation are different from the mechanisms of seizure initiation. Failures of the mechanisms that terminate seizures are likely to be responsible for seizure prolongation, and manipulation of these systems may be required for successful seizure termination.

Extracellular adenosine may also have seizure-modifying or terminating effects [41]. Injection of adenosine agonists or adenosine breakdown enzyme antagonists into rat prepiriform cortex protects against bicuculline (a $GABA_A$ antagonist)–induced seizures [42]. Adenosine receptor antagonism with aminophylline may account for the seizure-prolonging effects of this drug [43]. Adenosine agonists also block the CSE-inducing effects of pilocarpine in rats [44]. There are no current treatments that manipulate the adenosinergic system in order to terminate CSE.

Seizures are more likely to start and more likely to be prolonged in the developing brain than in the developed brain. This is well documented in animal models in which seizures are induced with global ischemia, pilocarpine, kainate, or electrical stimulation

TABLE 11.1. Classification of etiology of convulsive status epilepticus (CSE) in childhood.

Etiology	Definition
Prolonged febrile seizure	CSE in a previously neurologically normal child aged between 6 months and 5 years during a febrile (temperature above 38°C) illness and in the absence of defined central nervous system (CNS) infection
Acute symptomatic	CSE in a previously neurologically normal child, within 1 week of an identified acute neurologic insult, including head trauma, CNS infection, encephalopathy, cerebrovascular disease, and metabolic or toxic derangements
Remote symptomatic	CSE in the absence of an identified acute insult but with a history of a CNS insult more than 1 week before
Acute on remote symptomatic	CSE that occurred within 1 week of an acute neurologic insult or febrile illness and occurred in a child with a history of previous neurologic abnormality
Idiopathic epilepsy related	CSE that is not symptomatic (see above) and occurred in subjects with a prior diagnosis of epilepsy or when the episode of CSE is the second unprovoked seizure that has led to a diagnosis of idiopathic epilepsy
Unclassified	CSE that could not be classified into any other group

[45–47] and has been shown epidemiologically in humans. There are several potential reasons for this age-determined effect [48], and further understanding of these mechanisms may lead to appropriate age-related therapies. This may be most obvious for the treatment of neonatal CSE given that it is known that the GABA receptor is depolarizing in the developing brain and that many of the drugs used in the treatment of neonatal seizures (e.g., barbiturates and benzodiazepines) act at the GABA receptor.

On pathophysiologic grounds is not surprising that the incidence of CSE in the pediatric population is higher than in the young adult population. Despite this, most of the basic science research attempting to clarify mechanisms of seizure genesis and termination is performed in adult models. There are, however, increasing numbers of animal models assessing epileptogenesis in the immature brain. These may help to clarify some of the mechanisms responsible for the vulnerability of the developing brain to CSE [17] and may provide a framework for the development of new therapies for CSE.

Systemic Effects of Convulsive Status Epilepticus

The systemic effects of CSE need to be considered in the treatment of CSE, as inappropriate treatment may impair compensatory mechanisms or fail to adequately correct systemic effects that are potentially harmful. Once compensatory mechanisms have failed, it may be most appropriate for the child to be treated in the PICU. The early systemic effects of CSE are initially dominated by appar-

ent compensatory effects that may be neuroprotective. Blood pressure and central venous pressure rise, blood glucose increases, and the patient becomes tachycardic. Cerebral blood flow, blood glucose, and oxygen utilization increase in experimental models and in humans during this compensatory phase of CSE. These events attempt to ensure that metabolic demand is met by supply and that toxic metabolites are removed from the brain [49,50]. After approximately 30 min of continuous epileptic activity, the protective mechanisms described above begin to fail and subsequent events are potentially harmful to the brain. Cerebral blood flow declines during the course of CSE as there is failure of cerebral vascular autoregulation (i.e., the cerebral vasculature loses the ability to alter its diameter to ensure appropriate cerebral blood flow). Cerebral blood flow becomes dependent on systemic blood pressure, which also declines. Provision of oxygen and glucose for the brain becomes impaired. Respiratory and metabolic acidosis, electrolyte imbalance, hyperthermia, and rhabdomyolysis may also occur and are potentially harmful. This is the phase of decompensation [49,50] (see Figure 11.1 for further details on the pathophysiologic changes during the different phases of CSE).

Brain Injury Associated with Status Epilepticus

In addition to morbidity that may be associated with systemic decompensation, there is also evidence that CSE, in and of itself, can cause brain injury, particularly to the hippocampus. Although

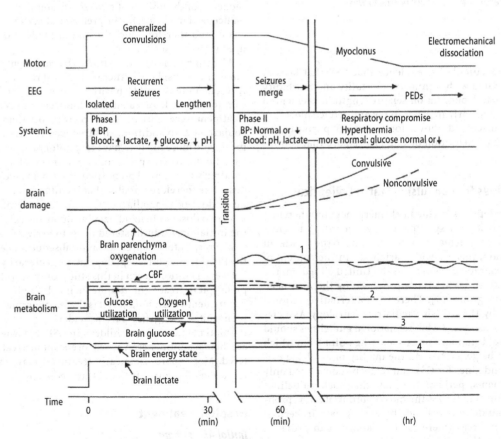

FIGURE 11.1. Pathophysiologic characteristics during the phases of compensation (within 30 min of onset) and decompensation (after 30 min of onset) of status epilepticus. BP, blood pressure; PEDs, periodic epileptiform discharges. (Adapted from Lothman E. The biochemical basis and pathophysiology of status epilepticus. Neurology 40[5 Suppl 2]:15. © 1990 with permission from Lippincott Williams & Wilkins.)

the most common site of pathologic brain injury is the hippocampus, many other brain regions, including the amygdala, cerebellum, thalamus, and cortex, may be injured by CSE [51]. The majority of work attempting to define brain damage associated with CSE has been carried out in animal models. The seminal studies that identified that CSE can result in widespread neuronal damage and neuronal death were carried out by Meldrum et al., using the $GABA_A$ antagonist bicuculline to induce CSE in adolescent baboons [52]. Subsequent models of CSE in which areas of neuronal damage occur manipulate other neurotransmitter systems. Glutamatergic drugs such as kainic acid, NMDA, quisqualate and domoic acid given to rats result in prolonged limbic seizures [53–57]. Cholinergic drugs such as pilocarpine also cause limbic CSE. Subsequently spontaneous recurrent seizures analogous to the situation in humans occur [19,58–61]. It could be argued that it is the drug used to induce CSE that is causing neuronal damage and not the CSE itself. However, in addition to the chemical models there are electrical stimulation models that also result in unilateral or bilateral hippocampal damage similar to that identified in the other models [62]. Thus, many different experimental paradigms result in damage to similar areas of the brain, which might suggest that CSE itself is responsible for the damage.

In humans there is increasing evidence from magnetic resonance imaging studies that CSE, particularly prolonged febrile seizure, can cause hippocampal injury in humans [63–66]. Studies addressing whether the children with evidence of acute hippocampal injury go on to develop temporal lobe epilepsy associated with mesial temporal sclerosis are currently underway.

Management

Given that there is accumulating evidence that CSE that lasts at least 30 min is associated with significant mortality and morbidity that is, at least in part, dependent on seizure length, it is essential that seizures are treated early in order to try and reduce mortality and morbidity. As discussed above, for treatment purposes, an appropriate operational definition of CSE is a seizure that continues for at least 5 min.

Treatment Guidelines for Convulsive Status Epilepticus

Convulsive status epilepticus is a medical emergency, and therefore it is important to treat in a systematic way, according to clear guidelines. However, as systematic studies relating to the treatment of CSE are uncommon, there is wide variability in the content of guidelines across geographic regions. In the United Kingdom, the most widely used guidelines are those produced by the Advanced Pediatric Life Support group [67]. There is an alternative national guideline produced by the British Paediatric Neurology Association [68]. This raises the issue of whether national guidelines should be considered as a gold standard or as a starting point from which local guidelines can be generated. As the quality of available evidence is such that guidelines for CSE can really be considered only as consensus statements, perhaps the view that such guidelines constitute a minimum standard is the most appropriate. It is probable that national guidelines will not be appropriate in certain environments (e.g., in areas where there is no access to pediatric intensive care services, the use of lidocaine may be more appropriate than the use of recurrent benzodiazepines or barbiturates as second line therapy, as it does not cause respiratory depression).

Some children may not respond to the usual treatments, and these children should have a personalized treatment protocol.

Prehospital Treatment

Most episodes of CSE begin in the community, and, as early treatment is likely to reduce morbidity, treatment should be initiated in the prehospital setting if possible. The most commonly used prehospital treatment is rectal diazepam, which has been used in Europe for many years. Although rectal diazepam is an effective agent, its use in the prehospital setting is falling out of favor, largely because it may be considered that giving rectal medication is socially unacceptable, particularly in public places, and teachers and caregivers are reluctant to administer rectal diazepam for fear of sexual abuse allegations [69]. It also may be difficult to administer to wheelchair users or during tonic seizures [70]. These factors have led to the development of agents that can be administered via a more socially acceptable route. Buccal midazolam is rapidly absorbed into the bloodstream and the brain [71] and is comparable to rectal diazepam in terms of efficacy [72]. Subsequent observational studies have also supported the view that buccal midazolam is an effective agent for treating CSE [73,74]. Another alternative to rectal diazepam is the nasal administration of midazolam, which has been shown to reduce epileptiform discharges in the electroencephalogram (EEG) [75], and it is similarly effective in terminating seizures compared with intravenous diazepam [76]. Potential problems with the use of nasal midazolam include pain as a consequence of the low pH of midazolam solution. There are, however, no licensed medications for prehospital use other than rectal diazepam, and therefore buccal or nasal medications still need to be used with caution.

Although prehospital treatment has apparent advantages, not all guidelines consider whether prehospital treatment has been given. A recent audit of children with status epilepticus requiring admission to the PICU revealed that children who received prehospital treatment were more likely to receive more than two doses of benzodiazepine. In addition, children who received prehospital treatment were more likely to have respiratory depression than children who did not receive prehospital treatment [5]. In this study, 55% of children who received prehospital treatment received an inadequate dose. It is therefore possible that if children were to receive an adequate dose of benzodiazepine in the community, as well as more than two doses of benzodiazepine upon arrival to the hospital (i.e., the initial dose administered prior to arrival is ignored), then the risk of respiratory depression and subsequent need for admission to the PICU will be unacceptably and unnecessarily increased.

Of even more concern in this study, only 51% of children received prehospital treatment despite being brought to the emergency department via ambulance. It is therefore germane to ask why some prehospital emergency care providers are not administering prehospital medications to children in CSE and why inadequate doses are being administered when prehospital treatment is administered. More appropriate early treatment may result in earlier termination of seizures [13] and thus reduce PICU admissions.

Hospital Treatment

Initial Assessment

The initial statement in many guidelines relates to the important assessment of airway, breathing, and circulation when a child arrives in the emergency department with an episode of CSE. Most children do not have underlying respiratory or cardiac abnormalities, and thus cardiorespiratory abnormalities identified during CSE are likely to be a result, rather than a cause, of the seizure itself [17]. This suggests that treatment is equally as important as assessing physiologic changes, because treating the seizure is likely to correct the cardiorespiratory insufficiencies. All children with CSE should have blood glucose estimation and correction if required. It is also important to determine whether there is an acute symptomatic etiology that requires treatment in its own right (e.g., meningitis or cerebrovascular accident).

First-Line Therapy

It is almost universally accepted that the most appropriate first-line agents are benzodiazepines. Many children will receive rectal diazepam upon arrival in the emergency department in the United Kingdom. However, in the United States, intravenous benzodiazepines are recommended unless intravenous access cannot be obtained. It remains uncertain which of these approaches is most appropriate, and further studies are required. The two most commonly used intravenous agents are diazepam and lorazepam [77]. In adults lorazepam is more effective than phenytoin alone as a first-line agent. It is similarly effective to diazepam plus phenytoin or phenobarbital [77]. However, lorazepam has a longer therapeutic half-life than diazepam and tends to be the agent of choice in developed countries. Although diazepam has a short therapeutic half-life, it has a long elimination half-life. This means that diazepam unbinds from the GABA$_A$ receptor in the brain soon after administration but is stored in body fat for many hours without offering a therapeutic effect. Administration of recurrent doses of diazepam may overload the stores with subsequent respiratory depression.

Second-Line Therapy

Although there is a reasonable amount of data to support the use of benzodiazepines as first-line agents for CSE, there are very sparse data providing guidance on appropriate subsequent agents. The most commonly used second-line agent for the treatment of CSE worldwide is phenytoin. In the United Kingdom, paraldehyde is frequently recommended. Although there is a justification for the administration of rectal paraldehyde to children in whom intravenous access has not been established, this justification is less obvious for children when intravenous access is secured. The disadvantages of rectal administration of drugs (intrafecal administration, expulsion, uncertainties about bioavailability) could be considered as outweighing the advantages when one is certain about administration of intravenous agents. This also needs to be considered in the development of local guidelines.

Phenytoin needs to be administered intravenously under continuous electrocardiographic monitoring over approximately 20 min, although it is often effective prior to completion of the infusion. An alternative is fos-phenytoin, which can be administered over 7–8 min. The active agent in fos-phenytoin is phenytoin. As fos-phenytoin has to be metabolized in order to obtain phenytoin the time it takes for phenytoin to enter the brain may be similar with fos-phenytoin and with phenytoin.

Subsequent Therapy

Once second-line treatments have failed, further medications will potentially depress respiration, and therefore respiratory monitoring is mandatory. This may be best achieved in the PICU, where there is a high level of nursing input and sophisticated technology for continual monitoring of physiologic parameters. It is important for all acute care units to have access to PICU facilities, as a small proportion of children will have (1) CSE associated with a severe systemic or neurologic disorder, (2) CSE refractory to first-line anticonvulsant agents, or (3) respiratory depression as a consequence of treatment.

Treatment of Status Epilepticus in the Pediatric Intensive Care Unit

A number of agents have been used to treat status epilepticus in the intensive care setting, but there is no clear evidence that any one treatment is superior to another. Comparative studies, ideally large multicenter, randomized, controlled trials, are urgently needed to clarify the optimal management of patients with status epilepticus. Until then, treatment will remain empirical and subject to personal experience and choice. In the next sections, we list commonly used anesthetic and nonanesthetic agents for the treatment of CSE in the PICU, including their pros and cons, as well as other agents that may be potentially beneficial in the future.

When seizure activity continues despite standard second-line anticonvulsants, it is usual practice to induce a state of general anesthesia in an attempt to terminate seizure activity. As the principles of therapy are similar for all anesthetic agents, it is possible that a wide range of barbiturate and nonbarbiturate anesthetic agents could be used in the treatment of CSE, but within the published literature there are few reported. There are also reports of the use of benzodiazepine infusions, conventional antiepileptic drugs, and other miscellaneous agents.

Barbiturates

Historically, the initial drugs used in intensive care are frequently barbiturates (e.g., phenobarbital, thiopentone, pentobarbital). These drugs have been widely used in clinical practice for many decades and have strong antiseizure actions but are potentially highly toxic, tend to have long half-lives, tend to accumulate, and have saturatable kinetics, and patients can become tolerant to the antiseizure effect [51]. The usual length of barbiturate coma is a few days, but there is a report of an 18-year-old male being maintained in a barbiturate coma for 53 days who had a good neurologic outcome [78]. The initial choice of barbiturate varies across geographic regions.

Phenobarbital

Phenobarbital has been widely used in clinical practice since 1912. Many intensive care units in Britain continue to use phenobarbital as the barbiturate of choice for children [79]. Its main advantages are its powerful antiepileptic action, long duration of action, and possible neuroprotective properties [80]. However, it is a powerful sedative, has a long elimination half-life, and may cause respiratory depression and hypotension.

Phenobarbital has a greater intrinsic anticonvulsant action than other barbiturates (including thiopentone and pentobarbital), which may be related to its cerebral distribution, high concentration in the motor cortex, or a specific physicochemical membrane-stabilizing action [81]. It is usually administered by the intravenous route, but it can also be administered by the rectal and intramuscular routes. A loading dose of 20 mg kg^{-1} followed by 10 mg^{-1}kg boluses every 30 min until the seizure cessation has been suggested [82]. Such a regimen will almost certainly lead to respiratory depression. After intravenous administration, phenobarbital is first concentrated in vascular organs and is then more evenly distributed throughout the body, with a low concentration in fat. It has a slow entry into the brain (maximal brain: blood level ratios reached in 12–60 min) compared with more lipid-soluble compounds such as diazepam (1 min) or thiopentone (30 sec) [51], but during seizure activity its rate of cerebral uptake is much faster and it may be preferentially concentrated in seizure foci [83]. High cerebral concentrations are maintained for a long period of time (60 min) despite falling blood levels [84]. The elimination half-life ranges from 50 to 150 hr [85], and one can expect the patient to have side effects for several days after a single intravenous dose. Excretion is reduced by liver or renal disease. Hypotension is possible, particularly at high or rapidly rising blood levels, but is easily controlled [82]. Some children may not develop respiratory depression even with high levels of phenobarbital, but respiratory depression is a common side effect. Children frequently develop acute tolerance to the respiratory depressing and sedative effects of phenobarbital but not without its antiseizure effect [82]. This is a significant advantage over benzodiazepines. Phenobarbital continues to be the mainstay treatment for seizures in the neonatal period [86], although the evidence suggests that no current anticonvulsant medication reliably works in this age group.

Thiopentone

Thiopentone is the favored barbiturate in the treatment of refractory CSE in Europe and Australia and has been used in the treatment of CSE for over 40 years. It is alkaline in solution, highly soluble in lipid, and also freely soluble in water. It is only administered by the intravenous route. Intramuscular injection causes severe local injury, skin sloughing may result from extravasation into subcutaneous tissue, and permanent palsy may result from injection adjacent to a nerve. Thiopentone can react with polyvinyl infusion bags and plastic giving sets. The continuous infusion should be made up in normal saline. Its alkalinity makes it incompatible with a large number of acidic or oxidizing substances, and therefore no additional drugs should be added to the infusions. Thiopentone is usually administered at an initial dose of 4–8 mg^{-1}kg followed by a maintenance infusion at the minimum dose (usually 3–5 mg^{-1}kg^{-1}hr) required to stop electrical (Figure 11.2) and clinical epileptic activity for 12–24 hr followed by an attempt to wean the drug. After an initial single dose of thiopentone, unconsciousness occurs in 10–20 sec, depth of anesthesia increases for approximately 40 sec, and then the depth decreases progressively until recovery of consciousness after 7–10 min, reflecting a rapid fall in blood levels as it is redistributed in the body (distribution half-life 2.5 min) [51]. The drug has a tendency to accumulate in lipid stores, and, when lipid stores are saturated, such as after long continuous infusions, the duration of action of thiopentone is dramatically increased (elimination half-life 18–36 hr) [87] and recovery times may be protracted. Thiopentone is metabolized in the liver, and, although the majority of its metabolites are inactive, one metabolite, pentobarbitone, has potent antiseizure activity. Thiopentone and pentobarbitone levels should be monitored in prolonged therapy (e.g., more than 3 days) [88]. Hypotension can be an adverse effect, and concomitant inotropic support is commonly required. An acute hypersensitivity reaction may

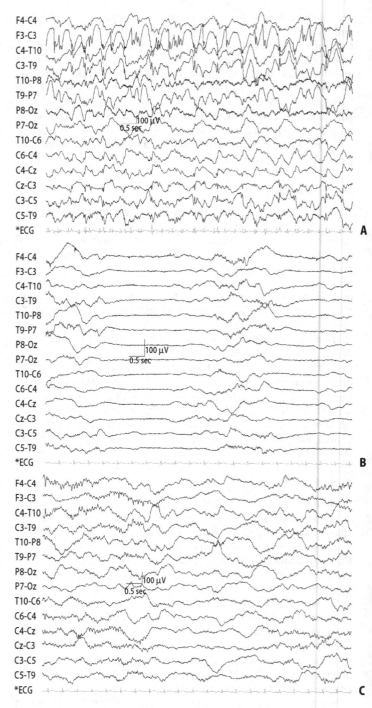

FIGURE 11.2. Electroencephalogram (EEG) features of a 20-month-old boy admitted to the PICU for status epilepticus and treated with thiopentone infusion. **(A)** He is already receiving thiopentone, but there remains irregular diffuse continuous epileptiform activity consistent with status epilepticus. **(B)** There is burst suppression with an increased dose of thiopentone, with absence of any spikes (i.e., cessation of electrical seizure activity). **(C)** He has reverted to a normal physiologic state after thiopentone was withdrawn, with bilateral sleep spindles and absence of any spikes on the EEG. (Courtesy of Dr. Stewart Boyd, Consultant Neurophysiologist, Great Ormond Street Hospital for Children NHS Trust, London, United Kingdom.)

occur (1 in 30,000 administrations, 50% mortality) with thiopentone, and prolonged therapy may result in pancreatitis and hepatic dysfunction. It should be used with caution in patients with hepatic, cardiac, or renal disease or with myotonic dystrophy and myasthenia gravis.

Pentobarbital

Pentobarbital has been the preferred barbiturate in the United States for the treatment of refractory status epilepticus, although there is little published experience with children. It is chemically similar to thiopentone, from which it is produced by desulfuration. Like thiopentone, it is administered only by the intravenous route, but it does not interact with plastic, and infusions may be prepared in normal saline or 5% dextrose. An intravenous loading dose of 5–20 mg^{-1} kg is administered at a rate no greater than 25 mg^{-1} min followed by a continuous infusion of 0.5–3 mg^{-1} kg^{-1} hr titrated to the minimum rate to stop all clinical and electrical seizures, followed by gradual weaning after 12 hr without any electrical seizure activity. Although it is similar to thiopentone, pentobarbital has theoretical advantages over thiopentone, including a shorter elimination half-life, nonsaturable kinetics, and GABAergic activity that may enhance neuroprotection, and it is less cardiotoxic in high doses. However, in practice, the use of pentobarbital has been associated with poor outcome [89]. In a meta-analysis of 37 patients treated with high-dose pentobarbitone, 32% died, and pentobarbitone was thought to contribute to the deaths of one third of the patients [89]. Among 12 patients, Osorio and Reed reported initial seizure control in all but this required hours or days [90]. Two patients in this series died (17%), and there was a marked tendency for breakthrough seizures when the drug was tapered too quickly [90]. Hypotension is as common as in thiopentone anesthesia, but, in addition, pentobarbitone has a negative inotropic effect and may cause a rapid fall in blood pressure. Thus, the overall outcome of patients with CSE treated with pentobarbital is a cause for concern, and further research on this agent is required.

Nonbarbiturate Anesthetic Agents

Apart from propofol, the nonbarbiturate anesthetics are rarely used in practice. The evidence to support their use is largely anecdotal.

Propofol

Propofol is a relatively new anesthetic agent with probable GABAergic effects that is becoming widely used in the intensive care treatment of CSE [91,92]. In status epilepticus, initial 2 mg^{-1} kg bolus doses are administered until seizures stop, followed by an infusion of 5–10 mg^{-1} kg^{-1} hr titrated against EEG or cerebral function analyzing monitor (CFAM) measurement. Its advantages include a rapid onset of action, a short half-life, and rapid elimination [93]. There are concerns about prolonged infusions during childhood, as it has been associated with severe metabolic acidosis, lipemia, and hypoxia of uncertain origin [94]. Rhabdomyolysis has also been reported during maintenance infusion [95]. The seizure-like behaviors myoclonus and opisthotonus have also been observed during propofol infusions. The debate on whether propofol can be convulsant as well as anticonvulsant continues [96]. Although propofol is a drug with potential, it should be used with caution in childhood.

Etomidate

Etomidate was the first nonbarbiturate intravenous anesthetic used to treat status epilepticus. It is an imidazole derivative and is widely used as an anesthetic throughout Europe and to a lesser extent in the United States. As etomidate interferes with adrenocortical function, corticosteroids must be co-administered and continued for 72 hr after etomidate infusions. Following intravenous boluses of 0.3 mg^{-1} kg until cessation of seizure activity, etomidate is usually administered as a continuous infusion made up in 5% dextrose at a rate of 20 μg^{-1} kg^{-1} min adjusted to a mean cortical activity of 5 μV on CFAM [97]. After 24 hr without seizure activity, the drug is tapered slowly. It has a low risk of cardiovascular toxicity and therefore is an excellent drug to be considered for patients with cardiovascular disease, although hypotension is common [98]. There remains uncertainty as to whether it has intrinsic anticonvulsant properties, but seizure-like movements and myoclonus have been reported with its usage, particularly in patients with preexisting epilepsy. Recurrence of seizures is common after the drug is weaned [99]. Preliminary studies on etomidate in the treatment of status epilepticus suggest that it has clinical potential, but further work with this agent is warranted.

Isoflurane

The first suggestion to use isoflurane in the treatment of CSE was made only two decades ago [100]. Since then, there have been few published reports, and experience with pediatric patients is slight. Isoflurane is administered at end tidal volume concentrations of 0.8%–2% to produce burst suppression on EEG (see Figure 11.2), with an interburst interval of 15–30 sec [101]. Termination of seizure activity is rapidly obtained with isoflurane administration, but this is not sustained, and seizure recurrence after withdrawal is common. Further disadvantages of isoflurane include the need for an inhalation anesthetic system in a PICU setting and its frequent association with hypotension requiring fluid and inotropic support. The role of inhalation anesthetics in the treatment of status epilepticus remains unclear. Further work in this area is needed to clarify its position.

Benzodiazepine Infusions

Both diazepam and midazolam infusions have been used in the intensive care management of CSE in childhood. Diazepam tends to be used in developing countries [102,103], probably because of the low cost, and midazolam tends to be used in the developed world.

Diazepam

For four decades, diazepam has been used in the treatment of status epilepticus, for which it has to be administered rectally or intravenously to be effective [51]. When diazepam is administered by a continuous infusion, infusions should be freshly prepared, as the drug is absorbed by polyvinyl plastics. Diazepam activity decreases on standing, so fresh solutions should be made up within 6 hr [104]. There are limited data on the optimum rate of infusion, but a rate of 10–30 μg^{-1} kg^{-1} min has been used [102]. It is metabolized by hepatic microsomal enzymes with an active antiepileptic metabolite that accumulates with continuous infusion therapy, and excretion is by the renal route. Diazepam is highly lipid soluble, resulting in a rapid uptake by cerebral tissue and consequent rapid onset of action, but its lipid solubility also causes rapid redistribution in lipid stores in the rest of the body, thereby creating a short duration of action after initial doses. With continuous infusions, this rapid redistribution does not occur and may result in high cerebral tissue concentrations with accompanying potential sudden cardiorespiratory collapse and CNS depression, adverse effects that have been reported in the literature [102,105]. For these reasons midazolam has become the favored benzodiazepine.

Midazolam

Midazolam is an injectable benzodiazepine used primarily as a premedicant, sedative, and anesthetic agent. The unique chemical structure of midazolam includes a fused imidazole ring, which accounts for its stability in an aqueous solution and rapid metabolism. Midazolam causes little, if any, local discomfort after administration and has been shown to have a wide safety margin with a broad therapeutic index. It also diffuses rapidly across the capillary wall into the central nervous system and can be mixed with saline or glucose solutions, thereby facilitating its administration as a continuous infusion [106]. At physiologic pH the compound becomes extremely lipophilic, which facilitates its rapid effect on brain tissue [107].

The antiepileptic properties of midazolam were identified during the late 1970s, and more recently the drug has emerged as an effective treatment for CSE. It remains uncertain why midazolam infusions can terminate seizure activity when diazepam and phenytoin/phenobarbital, as first- and second-line agents, have failed, but a more rapid rate of arrival at receptors governing seizure termination is hypothesized [108]. Effective doses of midazolam vary among patients, and EEG monitoring is beneficial to evaluate subclinical seizure activity [109]. Loading dosages from 0.02 to 0.38 mg^{-1} kg and infusion rates ranging from 60 to 1,080 mg^{-1} kg^{-1} hr have been reported as effective in seizure termination [110–112]. The mean time for seizure termination following administration is 65 min [111]. Hypotension can occur with midazolam [113,114] but is much less frequent and severe compared with high-dose barbiturates [109]. Hypoxia associated with respiratory depression [111,114] and increased pharyngeal secretions may occur with midazolam infusions [110].

Continuous midazolam and diazepam infusions are equally effective for control of refractory status epilepticus, but midazolam infusions are associated with greater seizure recurrence following initial termination of seizure activity in the PICU [114]. In a systematic review of treatment of refractory status epilepticus with pentobarbital, propofol, or midazolam, Claassen and colleagues found that, compared with treatment with midazolam and propofol, treatment with pentobarbital was associated with a lower frequency of short-term treatment failure and breakthrough seizures after seizure termination but a higher frequency of hypotension than the other agents [115]. These data would suggest that further study on the role of continuous midazolam infusion in the management of CSE in the PICU is required but that there are data that suggest that other traditional options may be superior. The nonbarbiturate agents (e.g., isoflurane, propofol, etomidate) are much less toxic than barbiturates without the cardiorespiratory-suppressing effects of barbiturates and much more convenient pharmacokinetics, but there is limited experience with them in the treatment of CSE. In addition, although the nonbarbiturate agents are strong anesthetic agents, they generally do not have antiseizure properties, and, at subanesthetic doses, isoflurane, propofol, and etomidate can precipitate seizures.

Conventional Antiepileptic Drugs

Conventionally antiepileptic agents are used to prevent the onset of seizures, and, given that the mechanisms of seizure onset and seizure termination are not necessarily the same, it may not be intuitive that antiepileptic drugs (AEDs) will be effective in the termination of CSE. However, there are some data to support the use of three AEDs.

Sodium Valproate

Sodium valproate is a branched chain fatty acid with a chemical structure similar to the inhibitory neurotransmitter GABA. The exact mechanism of action of this commonly used antiepileptic drug is unknown, but it is thought to have GABAergic actions and blocks sodium ion channels. It is normally administered orally or rectally, but intravenous sodium valproate became available in the 1980s initially for use in patients who were temporarily unable to tolerate oral therapy. However, since then there has been an emerging use of sodium valproate primarily in nonconvulsive status epilepticus [116,117] but also in the control of acute repetitive seizures and in the treatment of CSE [118]. In a retrospective study of 18 children with CSE, Yu and colleagues found that rapid intravenous loading with 25 mg^{-1} kg of valproate stopped seizures within 20 min of completion of the infusion [118]. All children remained seizure free up to 12 hr after treatment, and there were no adverse cardiovascular or respiratory effects. In particular, in their study, no child had hypotension [118]. Another study with adults and children also found no significant hypotensive effects with treatment with intravenous sodium valproate [119]. These findings are important as they contradict the findings of a case report of an 11-year-old girl who developed significant hypotension when treated with intravenous valproate [120]. Thus, valproate has potential, but further study would clarify its position in the emergency treatment of CSE.

Topiramate

Topiramate, first licensed in 1995, is a second-generation AED with multiple mechanisms of action, including GABAergic activity, inhibition of kainate-evoked currents, blockade of voltage-gated sensitive Na$^+$ and L-type Ca^{2+} channels, and inhibition of carbonic anhydrase isoenzymes [121]. Animal studies suggest that topiramate may have neuroprotective effects and thus makes it an interesting prospect in the treatment of CSE [122,123]. Two recent reports of adults, one a case report [124] and the other a series of three patients [125], demonstrated that enteral topiramate can be beneficial in the treatment of refractory CSE in adults. Topiramate was administered in daily doses of 300–1,600 mg, but termination occurred hours to 12 days after initiation of topiramate therapy. There is also a recent small retrospective case series showing its effectiveness in children with refractory CSE [126]. In three children, topiramate administered by the nasogastric route at an initial dose of 2–3 mg^{-1} kg^{-1} day and then titrated to a maintenance dose of 5–6 mg^{-1} kg^{-1} day, CSE was terminated within 24 hr of maintenance therapy. No adverse short-term effects were observed. However, topiramate at high doses or titrated rapidly is associated with psychomotor slowing and decline in attention and word fluency [127,128], and in one child such cognitive deficits were identified. Whether these deficits were due to topiramate or o the underlying pathology is unclear. Further studies on this drug in the treatment of status epilepticus are needed.

Lamotrigine

There is a single case report that lamotrigine may be effective is status epilepticus [129]. However, there is an animal study that reports that termination of CSE by lamotrigine requires therapeutic levels commonly in excess of the normal therapeutic levels in chronic epilepsy [130], and high levels of lamotrigine can precipitate myoclonic status epilepticus [131].

Miscellaneous Agents

Lidocaine

The local anesthetic agent lidocaine may also have a role in the management of CSE. Lidocaine is a common drug in the emergency department that is seldom considered in this context [132]. The major advantage is the absence of respiratory side effects, so that lidocaine can be administered safely to patients with limited respiratory reserve [51]. Lidocaine has also been used successfully in patients who have been resistant to benzodiazepines and phenytoin [133]. The initial dose needs to be followed up with an intravenous infusion, as its half life is very short [134,135]. If the infusion is given for only up to 12 hr, there is little risk of accumulation. Lidocaine has been used in neonates with some success, but there is a high recurrence rate after the infusion is stopped [136]. Lidocaine should be administered with ECG monitoring, as it may cause cardiac arrhythmias despite its acceptance as a drug for treating these cardiac problems. In high doses lidocaine may be convulsant, although this is not an expected side effect at the doses recommended.

Chlormethiazole

Chlormethiazole is a useful anticonvulsant used primarily in the United Kingdom, the rest of Europe, and Australia. It is almost never used in the United States. Although it has been primarily used is in the treatment of alcohol withdrawal and eclampsia [137], there are now alternative treatments for these conditions, and the use of chlormethiazole has fallen out of favor. The clinical effect is short, and therefore chlormethiazole needs to be administered as an intravenous infusion [138]. The dose can be titrated against seizure response in a minute-to-minute fashion during the initial stages. Accumulation in fat stores after approximately 12 hr negates this advantage [139]. Unfortunately, chlormethiazole needs to be administered in large volumes of fluid, and therefore it may be difficult to get adequate calories into a seriously ill child being treated with this drug. Nevertheless it can be useful in the neonatal intensive care unit [140]. It is also important to be certain that the patient's kidneys are functioning well before administering a large fluid load. Accepting these limitations, chlormethiazole has proved to be a very useful drug for CSE by avoiding the significant problems associated with barbiturates.

Ketamine

Ketamine is an NMDA blocker that may be neuroprotective [141]. In humans, its use has been largely restricted to treatment of non-convulsive status epilepticus [142], but animal models suggest that it may be effective in CSE in humans [143].

Levetiracetam

Levetiracetam is a novel AED that was licensed in 1999. It possesses a broad spectrum of anticonvulsant activity and a high therapeutic index in animal models of epilepsy [144,145]. Levetiracetam is also neuroprotective [146], an asset in the treatment of CSE, because it may not only stop seizures but also reduce seizure-induced brain damage. Furthermore, its potent and persistent antikindling activity [144,145] might be beneficial against the epileptogenic effects of status epilepticus [147] or against the "acute epileptogenesis" seen during status epilepticus. No human studies with levetiracetam in the treatment of CSE have been reported, but preliminary data from an animal study suggest that levetiracetam potentiates the anticonvulsant effect of diazepam [148] and may therefore have a potential role in the treatment of CSE.

Felbamate

Felbamate is an anticonvulsant active at NMDA receptors [149] and is also a potent neuroprotective agent [150,151]. It has been shown to be effective in treating animal models of status epilepticus [152], but, to the authors' knowledge, there are no published data on its use in status epilepticus in humans.

Role of Electrophysiology in the Pediatric Intensive Care Unit

There is a predictable sequence of EEG changes associated with ongoing CSE. These changes have been identified in at least six animal models and in adult humans. Secondarily generalized CSE begins with localized epileptic activity followed by isolated generalized bursts of seizure activity with normal EEG activity between events. If the patient does not regain consciousness between these episodes, then the patient will meet the clinical criteria for CSE. The isolated ictal discharges merge and become a continuous discharge after about 30 min. Discharges then fragment and become interspersed with flat periods. Ultimately, periodic epileptiform discharges, which may reflect underlying metabolic failure, will occur. The motor phenomena of CSE follow a similar pattern to the EEG changes. Recurrent seizures merge into continuous motor activity followed by fragmentation of the motor activity and myoclonus. If the seizure persists, then electromechanical dissociation, defined as continuing epileptiform abnormalities in the EEG with no associated motor phenomena, will occur. The prognosis for a good outcome declines as the patient moves through the continuum [49,153].

In the majority of children admitted to the PICU, clinical neurologic examination alone may be a reliable method of assessing cerebral function [154]. However, neurologic evaluation may be affected by administration of medications that affect CNS function and/or muscle function, such as hypnotics, sedatives, anxiolytics, or muscle relaxants, especially when the patient is in a comatose state. In such comatose children, the need for an objective measure of cerebral function is required [154]. Conventional EEG provides such a reliable such measure.

Confirmation of Seizure Termination

Termination of the motor manifestations of CSE does not necessarily imply that the abnormal brain electrical activity has also stopped. Such electromechanical dissociation is associated with a worsened prognosis, and it is therefore important not to miss it [158]. For the same reason, paralyzing drugs should be used cautiously in children with CSE. The only reliable means to identify this phenomenon of electromechanical dissociation is to obtain an EEG recording after termination of the motor manifestations. If this were to be done in all children who have required rescue therapy, EEG departments would be overloaded, and the rate at which significant abnormalities relating to electromechanical dissociation would be low. Children who recover quickly are extremely unlikely to have a continuing EEG abnormality. Therefore, children who do not regain consciousness as rapidly as expected and those who require intensive care should have at least a single EEG recording. A potential pitfall is overtreating children with long-standing frequent EEG abnormalities who have an episode of CSE in order to try and remove all epileptic discharges from the EEG.

Confirmation of a Burst-Suppression Pattern

It has long been suggested that children who require intensive care treatment for CSE should have doses of the chosen medication that result in a burst-suppression pattern in the EEG. This pattern should be maintained for approximately 24 hr before weaning of medication. In practice, many children are ventilated for only a few hours [5], and, as there is morbidity associated with ventilation, it would not be advantageous for an individual child to be ventilated for longer than necessary. Thus, children who are not tracheally extubated early should have EEG monitoring. Multichannel and single-channel EEG monitoring have been shown to be useful during thiopentone therapy [159,160] for status epilepticus. Multichannel EEGs have the advantage that global findings and changes are well represented, but, when there is continuous multichannel EEG monitoring over many days, they have considerable disadvantages, especially with large volumes of data and continuous bedside interpretations. A continuous single- or two-channel processed EEG such as a CFAM compresses processing and data on brain electrical activity and presents it in an easily interpretable form [161]. Consequently, the findings from CFAM may not reflect global cerebral function and not detect areas of single or multiple focal abnormalities. A combination of serial multichannel EEGs and continuous CFAM may be best, with a multichannel EEG for initial assessment and to determine the optimum montage for continuous CFAM and intermittent EEGs between to detect any global changes [160].

Conclusion

Convulsive status epilepticus is a common acute neurologic event and remains associated with significant morbidity and mortality. Early appropriate therapy in the prehospital, emergency department, and intensive care settings may improve its outcome. Currently, the precise mechanisms for seizure termination are not yet known, and there are limited comparative data on the optimum treatment of CSE, particularly that which requires PICU management. Therefore, research in these areas is urgently required to improve the management of children with CSE.

References

1. Leppik IE. Status epilepticus. Clin Ther 1985;7(2):272–278.
2. DeLorenzo RJ, Hauser WA, Towne AR, et al. A prospective, population-based epidemiologic study of status epilepticus in Richmond, Virginia. Neurology 1996;46(4):1029–1035.
3. Towne AR, Pellock JM, Ko D, DeLorenzo RJ. Determinants of mortality in status epilepticus. Epilepsia 1994;35(1):27–34.
4. Lacroix J, Deal C, Gauthier M, Rousseau E, Farrell CA. Admissions to a pediatric intensive care unit for status epilepticus: a 10-year experience. Crit Care Med 1994;22(5):827–832.
5. Chin RFM, Verhulst L, Neville BGR, Peters MJ, Scott RC. Inappropriate emergency management of status epilepticus in children contributes to need for intensive care. J Neurol Neurosurg Psychiatry 2004;75(11):1584–1588.
6. Aicardi J, Chevrie JJ. Convulsive status epilepticus in infants and children. A study of 239 cases. Epilepsia 1970;11(2):187–197.
7. Yager JY, Cheang M, Seshia SS. Status epilepticus in children. Can J Neurol Sci 1988;15(4):402–405.
8. Maytal J, Shinnar S, Moshe SL, Alvarez LA. Low morbidity and mortality of status epilepticus in children. Pediatrics 1989;83(3):323–331.
9. Logroscino G, Hesdorffer DC, Cascino G, Annegers JF, Hauser WA. Short-term mortality after a first episode of status epilepticus. Epilepsia 1997;38(12):1344–1349.
10. Sagduyu A, Tarlaci S, Sirin H. Generalized tonic-clonic status epilepticus: causes, treatment, complications and predictors of case fatality. J Neurol 1998;245(10):640–646.
11. Logroscino G, Hesdorffer D, Cascino G, Annegers JF, Bagiella E, Hauser AW. Long-term mortality after a first episode of status epilepticus. Neurology 2002;58:537–541.
12. Celesia GG. Modern concepts of status epilepticus. JAMA 1976;235(15):1571–1574.
13. Knudsen FU. Rectal administration of diazepam in solution in the acute treatment of convulsions in infants and children. Arch Dis Child 1979;54(11):855–857.
14. Lowenstein DH, Bleck T, Macdonald RL. It's time to revise the definition of status epilepticus. Epilepsia 1999;40(1):120–122.
15. Shinnar S, Berg AT, Moshe SL, Shinnar R. How long do new-onset seizures in children last? Ann Neurol 2001;49(5):659–664.
16. DeLorenzo RJ, Garnett LK, Towne AR, et al. Comparison of status epilepticus with prolonged seizure episodes lasting from 10 to 29 minutes. Epilepsia 1999;40(2):164–169.
17. Scott RC, Surtees RA, Neville BG. Status epilepticus: pathophysiology, epidemiology, and outcomes. Arch Dis Child 1998;79(1):73–77.
18. Meldrum B, Brierley JB. Prolonged epileptic seizure in primates: ischaemic cell changes and its relation to ictal physiological events. Arch Neurol 1973;28:10–17.
19. Cavalheiro EA. The pilocarpine model of epilepsy. Ital J Neurol Sci 1995;16(1–2):33–37.
20. DeLorenzo RJ, Pellock JM, Towne AR, Boggs JG. Epidemiology of status epilepticus. J Clin Neurophysiol 1995;12(4):316–325.
21. Hesdorffer DC, Logroscino G, Cascino G, Annegers JF, Hauser WA. Incidence of status epilepticus in Rochester, Minnesota, 1965–1984. Neurology 1998;50(3):735–741.
22. Coeytaux A, Jallon P, Galobardes B, Morabia A. Incidence of status epilepticus in French-speaking Switzerland: EPISTAR. Neurology 2000;55(5):693–697.
23. Knake S, Rosenow F, Vescovi M et al. Incidence of status epilepticus in adults in Germany: a prospective, population-based study. Epilepsia 2001;42(6):714–718.
24. Wu YW, Shek DW, Garcia PA, Zhao S, Johnston SC. Incidence and mortality of generalized convulsive status epilepticus in California. Neurology 2002;58(7):1070–1076.
25. Trevathan E, Fitzgerald R, Wang D. The impact of convulsive status epilepticus on the risk of death varies by age. Epilepsia 2002;43(Suppl 7):75.
26. Chin RF, Neville BG, Bedford H et al. NLSTEPSS—A population-based study on convulsive status epilepticus in childhood. Epilepsia 2003;44(Suppl 9):163.
27. Chin RF, Neville BG, Scott RC. A systematic review of the epidemiology of status epilepticus. Eur J Neurol 2004;11(12):800–810.

28. Chin RFM, Neville BGR, Scott RC. Meningitis is a common cause of convulsive status epilepticus with fever. Arch Dis Child 2005;90(1): 66–69.

29. Wasterlain CG, Baxter CF, Baldwin RA. GABA metabolism in the substantia nigra, cortex, and hippocampus during status epilepticus. Neurochem Res 1993;18(4):527–532.

30. Feldman RS, Meyer JS, Quenzer LF. Principles of Neuropsychopharmacology. Sunderland, MA: Sinauer Associates; 1997.

31. Stringer JL, Lothman EW. A1 adenosinergic modulation alters the duration of maximal dentate activation. Neurosci Lett 1990;118(2): 231–234.

32. Herberg LJ, Rose IC, Mintz M. Effect of an adenosine A1 agonist injected into substantia nigra on kindling of epileptic seizures and convulsion duration. Pharmacol Biochem Behav 1993;44(1):113–117.

33. Malhotra J, Gupta YK. Effect of adenosine receptor modulation on pentylenetetrazole-induced seizures in rats. Br J Pharmacol 1997; 120(2):282–288.

34. During MJ, Spencer DD. Extracellular hippocampal glutamate and spontaneous seizure in the conscious human brain. Lancet 1993; 341(8861):1607–1610.

35. Ronneengstrom E, Hillered L, Flink R, Spannare B, Ungerstedt U, Carlson H. Intracerebral microdialysis of extracellular amino-acids in the human epileptic focus. J Cereb Blood Flow Metab 1992;12(5): 873–876.

36. Carlson H, Ronneengstrom E, Ungerstedt U, Hillered L. Seizure related elevations of extracellular amino-acids in human focal epilepsy. Neurosci Lett 1992;140(1):30–32.

37. Chapman AG. Regional changes in transmitter amino-acids during focal and generalized seizures in rats. J Neural Transm 1985;63(2): 95–107.

38. Walton NY, Gunawan S, Treiman DM. Brain amino acid concentration changes during status epilepticus induced by lithium and pilocarpine. Exp Neurol 1990;108(1):61–70.

39. Cavalheiro EA, Fernandes MJ, Turski L, Naffah-Mazzacoratti MG. Spontaneous recurrent seizures in rats: amino acid and monoamine determination in the hippocampus. Epilepsia 1994;35(1):1–11.

40. Sankar R, Shin DH, Wasterlain CG. GABA metabolism during status epilepticus in the developing rat brain. Brain Res Dev Brain Res 1997; 98(1):60–64.

41. During MJ, Spencer DD. Adenosine—a potential mediator of seizure arrest and postictal refractoriness. Ann Neurol 1992;32(5):618–624.

42. Murray TF, Franklin PH, Zhang G, Tripp E. A1 adenosine receptors express seizure-suppressant activity in the rat prepiriform cortex. Epilepsy Res Suppl 1992;8:255–261.

43. Dragunow M. Adenosine receptor antagonism accounts for the seizure-prolonging effects of aminophylline. Pharmacol Biochem Behav 1990;36(4):751–755.

44. George B, Kulkarni SK. Modulation of lithium-pilocarpine-induced status epilepticus by adenosinergic agents. Methods Find Exp Clin Pharmacol 1997;19(5):329–333.

45. Cavalheiro EA, Silva DF, Turski WA, Calderazzo-Filho LS, Bortolotto ZA, Turski L. The susceptibility of rats to pilocarpine-induced seizures is age-dependent. Brain Res 1987;465(1–2):43–58.

46. Stafstrom CE, Thompson JL, Holmes GL. Kainic acid seizures in the developing brain: status epilepticus and spontaneous recurrent seizures. Brain Res Dev Brain Res 1992;65(2):227–236.

47. McCown TJ, Breese GR. The developmental profile of seizure genesis in the inferior collicular cortex of the rat: relevance to human neonatal seizures. Epilepsia 1992;33(1):2–10.

48. Holmes GL. Epilepsy in the developing brain: lessons from the laboratory and clinic. Epilepsia 1997;38(1):12–30.

49. Fountain NB, Lothman EW. Pathophysiology of status epilepticus. J Clin Neurophysiol 1995;12(4):326–342.

50. Shorvon S. The outcome of tonic-clonic status epilepticus. Curr Opin Neurol 1994;7(2):93–95.

51. Shorvon S. Status Epilepticus: Its Clinical Features and Treatment in Adults and Children. Cambridge: Cambridge University Press; 1994.

52. Meldrum BS, Horton RW. Physiology of status epilepticus in primates. Arch Neurol 1973;28(1):1–9.

53. Ben-Ari Y. Limbic seizure and brain damage produced by kainic acid: mechanisms and relevance to human temporal lobe epilepsy. Neuroscience 1985;14(2):375–403.

54. Golden GT, Smith GG, Ferraro TN, Reyes PF. Rat strain and age differences in kainic acid induced seizures. Epilepsy Res 1995;20(2): 151–159.

55. Cendes F, Andermann F, Carpenter S, Zatorre RJ, Cashman NR. Temporal lobe epilepsy caused by domoic acid intoxication: evidence for glutamate receptor–mediated excitotoxicity in humans. Ann Neurol 1995;37(1):123–126.

56. Sperk G, Lassmann H, Baran H, Kish SJ, Seitelberger F, Hornykiewicz O. Kainic acid induced seizures: neurochemical and histopathological changes. Neuroscience 1983;10(4):1301–1315.

57. Haglid KG, Wang S, Qiner Y, Hamberger A. Excitotoxicity. Experimental correlates to human epilepsy. Mol Neurobiol 1994;9(1–3): 259–263.

58. Nagao T, Avoli M, Gloor P. Interictal discharges in the hippocampus of rats with long-term pilocarpine seizures. Neurosci Lett 1994;174(2): 160–164.

59. Liu Z, Nagao T, Desjardins GC, Gloor P, Avoli M. Quantitative evaluation of neuronal loss in the dorsal hippocampus in rats with long-term pilocarpine seizures. Epilepsy Res 1994;17(3):237–247.

60. Priel MR, dos SN, Cavalheiro EA. Developmental aspects of the pilocarpine model of epilepsy. Epilepsy Res 1996;26(1):115–121.

61. Fujikawa DG. The temporal evolution of neuronal damage from pilocarpine-induced status epilepticus. Brain Res 1996;725(1):11–22.

62. Lothman EW, Bertram EH, Kapur J, Stringer JL. Recurrent spontaneous hippocampal seizures in the rat as a chronic sequela to limbic status epilepticus. Epilepsy Res 1990;6(2):110–118.

63. VanLandingham KE, Heinz ER, Cavazos JE, Lewis DV. Magnetic resonance imaging evidence of hippocampal injury after prolonged focal febrile convulsions. Ann Neurol 1998;43(4):413–426.

64. Scott RC, Gadian DG, King MD et al. Magnetic resonance imaging findings within 5 days of status epilepticus in childhood. Brain 2002; 125(Pt 9):1951–1959.

65. Scott RC, King MD, Gadian DG, Neville BG, Connelly A. Hippocampal abnormalities after prolonged febrile convulsion: a longitudinal MRI study. Brain 2003;126(Pt 11):2551–2557.

66. Tien RD, Felsberg GJ. The hippocampus in status epilepticus: demonstration of signal intensity and morphologic changes with sequential fast spin-echo MR imaging. Radiology 1995;194(1):249–256.

67. The Advanced Life Support Group. Advanced Paediatric Life Support: The Practical Approach, 4th ed. London: Blackwell; 2005.

68. Appleton R, Choonara I, Martland T, Phillips B, Scott R, Whitehouse W. The treatment of convulsive status epilepticus in children. Arch Dis Child 2000;83(5):415–419.

69. Scott RC, Neville BG. Pharmacological management of convulsive status epilepticus in children. Dev Med Child Neurol 1999;41(3): 207–210.

70. Wilson MT, Macleod S, O'Regan ME. Nasal/buccal midazolam use in the community. Arch Dis Child 2004;89(1):50–51.

71. Scott RC, Besag FM, Boyd SG, Berry D, Neville BG. Buccal absorption of midazolam: pharmacokinetics and EEG pharmacodynamics. Epilepsia 1998;39(3):290–294.

72. Scott RC, Besag FM, Neville BG. Buccal midazolam and rectal diazepam for treatment of prolonged seizures in childhood and adolescence: a randomised trial. Lancet 1999;353(9153):623–626.

73. Wassner E, Morris B, Fernando L, Rao M, Whitehouse WP. Intranasal midazolam for treating febrile seizures in children. Buccal midazolam for childhood seizures at home preferred to rectal diazepam. BMJ 2001;322(7278):108

74. Kutlu NO, Dogrul M, Yakinci C, Soylu H. Buccal midazolam for treatment of prolonged seizures in children. Brain Dev 2003;25(4): 275–278.

75. O'Regan ME, Brown JK, Clarke M. Nasal rather than rectal benzodiazepines in the management of acute childhood seizures? Dev Med Child Neurol 1996;38(11):1037–1045.

76. Lahat E, Goldman M, Barr J, Bistritzer T, Berkovitch M. Comparison of intranasal midazolam with intravenous diazepam for treating febrile seizures in children: prospective randomised study. BMJ 2000;321(7253):83–86.

77. Treiman DM, Meyers PD, Walton NY, et al. A comparison of four treatments for generalized convulsive status epilepticus. Veterans Affairs Status Epilepticus Cooperative Study Group. N Engl J Med 1998;339(12):792–798.

78. Mirski MA, Williams MA, Hanley DF. Prolonged pentobarbital and phenobarbital coma for refractory generalized status epilepticus. Crit Care Med 1995;23(2):400–404.

79. Walker MC, Smith SJ, Shorvon SD. The intensive care treatment of convulsive status epilepticus in the UK. Results of a national survey and recommendations. Anaesthesia 1995;50(2):130–135.

80. Piatt JH, Jr., Schiff SJ. High dose barbiturate therapy in neurosurgery and intensive care. Neurosurgery 1984;15(3):427–444.

81. Raines A, Blake GJ, Richardson B, Gilbert MB. Differential selectivity of several barbiturates on experimental seizures and neurotoxicity in the mouse. Epilepsia 1979;20(2):105–113.

82. Crawford TO, Mitchell WG, Fishman LS, Snodgrass SR. Very-high-dose phenobarbital for refractory status epilepticus in children. Neurology 1988;38(7):1035–1040.

83. Walton NY, Treiman DM. Phenobarbital treatment of status epilepticus in a rodent model. Epilepsy Res 1989;4(3):216–221.

84. Ramsey RE, Hammond EJ, Perchalski RJ, Wilder BJ. Brain uptake of phenytoin, phenobarbital, and paraldehyde. Arch Neurol 1979;32:535–539.

85. Rust RS, Dodson WE. Phenobarbital: absorption, distribution and excretion. In: Levy RH, Dreifuss FE, Mattson RA, Meldrum BS, Penry JK, eds. Antiepileptic Drugs. New York: Raven Press; 1989:293–304.

86. Rennie JM, Boylan GB. Neonatal seizures and their treatment. Curr Opin Neurol 2003;16(2):177–181.

87. Turcant A, Delhumeau A, Premel-Cabic A, et al. Thiopental pharmacokinetics under conditions of long-term infusion. Anesthesiology 1985;63(1):50–54.

88. Watson WA, Godley PJ, Garriott JC, Bradberry JC, Puckett JD. Blood pentobarbital concentrations during thiopental therapy. Drug Intell Clin Pharm 1986;20(4):283–287.

89. Bleck TP. High-dose pentobarbital therapy of refractory status epilepticus: a meta-analysis of published studies. Epilepsia 1992;33(Suppl 3):4.

90. Osorio I, Reed RC. Treatment of refractory generalized tonic-clonic status epilepticus with pentobarbital anesthesia after high-dose phenytoin. Epilepsia 1989;30(4):464–471.

91. Hantson P, Van Brandt N, Verbeeck R, Guerit JM, Mahieu P. Propofol for refractory status epilepticus. Intensive Care Med 1994;20(8):611–612.

92. Stecker MM, Kramer TH, Raps EC, O'Meeghan R, Dulaney E, Skaar DJ. Treatment of refractory status epilepticus with propofol: clinical and pharmacokinetic findings. Epilepsia 1998;39(1):18–26.

93. Bansinath M, Shukla VK, Turndorf H. Propofol modulates the effects of chemoconvulsants acting at GABAergic, glycinergic, and glutamate receptor subtypes. Anesthesiology 1995;83(4):809–815.

94. Parke TJ, Stevens JE, Rice AS et al. Metabolic acidosis and fatal myocardial failure after propofol infusion in children: five case reports. BMJ 1992;305(6854):613–616.

95. Hanna JP, Ramundo ML. Rhabdomyolysis and hypoxia associated with prolonged propofol infusion in children. Neurology 1998;50(1):301–303.

96. Borgeat A, Wilder-Smith OH, Jallon P, Suter PM. Propofol in the management of refractory status epilepticus: a case report. Intensive Care Med 1994;20(2):148–149.

97. Yeoman P, Hutchinson A, Byrne A, Smith J, Durham S. Etomidate infusions for the control of refractory status epilepticus. Intensive Care Med 1989;15(4):255–259.

98. Guldner G, Schultz J, Sexton P, Fortner C, Richmond M. Etomidate for rapid-sequence intubation in young children: hemodynamic effects and adverse events. Acad Emerg Med 2003;10(2):134–139.

99. Wauquier A. Profile of etomidate. A hypnotic, anticonvulsant and brain protective compound. Anaesthesia 1983;38 (Suppl):26–33.

100. Ropper AH, Kofke WA, Bromfield EB, Kennedy SK. Comparison of isoflurane, halothane, and nitrous oxide in status epilepticus. Ann Neurol 1986;19(1):98–99.

101. Kofke WA, Young RS, Davis P et al. Isoflurane for refractory status epilepticus: a clinical series. Anesthesiology 1989;71(5):653–659.

102. Singhi S, Banerjee S, Singhi P. Refractory status epilepticus in children: role of continuous diazepam infusion. J Child Neurol 1998; 13(1):23–26.

103. Ogutu BR, Newton CR. Management of seizures in children with falciparum malaria. Trop Doct 2004;34(2):71–75.

104. MacKichan J, Duffner PK, Cohen ME. Adsorption of diazepam to plastic tubing. N Engl J Med 1979;301(6):332–333.

105. Leppik IE, Derivan AT, Homan RW, Walker J, Ramsay RE, Patrick B. Double-blind study of lorazepam and diazepam in status epilepticus. JAMA 1983;249(11):1452–1454.

106. Galvin GM, Jelinek GA. Midazolam: an effective intravenous agent for seizure control. Arch Emerg Med 1987;4(3):169–172.

107. Reves JG, Fragen RJ, Vinik HR, Greenblatt DJ. Midazolam: pharmacology and uses. Anesthesiology 1985;62(3):310–324.

108. Bleck TP. Advances in the management of refractory status epilepticus. Crit Care Med 1993;21(7):955–957.

109. Bebin M, Bleck TP. New anticonvulsant drugs. Focus on flunarizine, fosphenytoin, midazolam and stiripentol. Drugs 1994;48(2):153–171.

110. Rivera R, Segnini M, Baltodano A, Perez V. Midazolam in the treatment of status epilepticus in children. Crit Care Med 1993;21(7):991–994.

111. Koul RL, Raj AG, Chacko A, Joshi R, Seif EM. Continuous midazolam infusion as treatment of status epilepticus. Arch Dis Child 1997;76(5):445–448.

112. Ozdemir D, Gulez P, Uran N, Yendur G, Kavakli T, Aydin A. Efficacy of continuous midazolam infusion and mortality in childhood refractory generalised convulsive status epilepticus. Seizure 2005; 14(2):129–132.

113. Kumar A, Bleck TP. Intravenous midazolam for the treatment of refractory status epilepticus. Crit Care Med 1992;20(4):483–488

114. Singhi S, Murthy A, Singhi P, Jayashree M. Continuous midazolam versus diazepam infusion for refractory convulsive status epilepticus. J Child Neurol 2002;17(2):106–110.

115. Claassen J, Hirsch LJ, Emerson RG, Mayer SA. Treatment of refractory status epilepticus with pentobarbital, propofol, or midazolam: a systematic review. Epilepsia 2002;43(2):146–153.

116. Chez MG, Hammer MS, Loeffel M, Nowinski C, Bagan BT. Clinical experience of three pediatric and one adult case of spike-and-wave status epilepticus treated with injectable valproic acid. J Child Neurol 1999;14(4):239–242.

117. Jha S, Jose M, Patel R. Intravenous sodium valproate in status epilepticus. Neurol India 2003;51(3):421–422.

118. Yu KT, Mills S, Thompson N, Cunanan C. Safety and efficacy of intravenous valproate in pediatric status epilepticus and acute repetitive seizures. Epilepsia 2003;44(5):724–726.

119. Sinha S, Naritoku DK. Intravenous valproate is well tolerated in unstable patients with status epilepticus. Neurology 2000;55 (5):722–724.

120. White JR, Santos CS. Intravenous valproate associated with significant hypotension in the treatment of status epilepticus. J Child Neurol 1999;14(12):822–823.

121. Shank RP, Gardocki JF, Streeter AJ, Maryanoff BE. An overview of the preclinical aspects of topiramate: pharmacology, pharmacokinetics, and mechanism of action. Epilepsia 2000;41(Suppl 1):S3–S9.

122. Niebauer M, Gruenthal M. Topiramate reduces neuronal injury after experimental status epilepticus. Brain Res 1999;837(1–2):263–269.

123. Kudin AP, Debska-Vielhaber G, Vielhaber S, Elger CE, Kunz WS. The mechanism of neuroprotection by topiramate in an animal model of epilepsy. Epilepsia 2004;45(12):1478–1487.

124. Reuber M, Evans J, Bamford JM. Topiramate in drug-resistant complex partial status epilepticus. Eur J Neurol 2002;9(1):111–112.

125. Bensalem MK, Fakhoury TA. Topiramate and status epilepticus: report of three cases. Epilepsy Behav 2003;4(6):757–760.

126. Kahriman M, Minecan D, Kutluay E, Selwa L, Beydoun A. Efficacy of topiramate in children with refractory status epilepticus. Epilepsia 2003;44(10):1353–1356.

127. Martin R, Kuzniecky R, Ho S et al. Cognitive effects of topiramate, gabapentin, and lamotrigine in healthy young adults. Neurology 1999;52(2):321–327.

128. Tatum WO, French JA, Faught E et al. Postmarketing experience with topiramate and cognition. Epilepsia 2001;42(9):1134–1140.

129. Pisani F, Gallitto G, Di Perri R. Could lamotrigine be useful in status epilepticus? A case report. J Neurol Neurosurg Psychiatry 1991;54(9):845–846.

130. Walton NY, Jaing Q, Hyun B, Treiman DM. Lamotrigine vs. phenytoin for treatment of status epilepticus: comparison in an experimental model. Epilepsy Res 1996;24(1):19–28.

131. Guerrini R, Belmonte A, Parmeggiani L, Perucca E. Myoclonic status epilepticus following high-dosage lamotrigine therapy. Brain Dev 1999;21(6):420–424.

132. Teng E, Wilkins P. Lidocaine in status epilepticus. Ann Pharmacother 1994;28(11):1248–1249.

133. Brodtkorb E, Sand T, Strandjord RE. Neuroleptic and antiepileptic treatment in the mentally retarded. Seizure 1993;2(3):205–211.

134. Brown JK, Hussain IH. Status epilepticus. II: Treatment. Dev Med Child Neurol 1991;33(2):97–109.

135. Shepherd SM. Management of status epilepticus. Emerg Med Clin North Am 1994;12(4):941–961.

136. Sugiyama N, Hamano S, Mochizuki M, Tanaka M, Eto Y. [Efficacy of lidocaine on seizures by intravenous and intravenous-drip infusion.] No To Hattatsu 2004;36(6):451–454.

137. Braunwarth WD. [Indications for the use of chlormethiazole]. Fortschr Med 1990;108(26):504–506.

138. Browne TR. Paraldehyde, chlormethiazole, and lidocaine for treatment of status epilepticus. Adv Neurol 1983;34:509–517.

139. Robson DJ, Blow C, Gaines P, Flanagan RJ, Henry JA. Accumulation of chlormethiazole during intravenous infusion. Intensive Care Med 1984;10(6):315–316.

140. Miller P, Kovar I. Chlormethiazole in the treatment of neonatal status epilepticus. Postgrad Med J 1983;59(698):801–802.

141. Fujikawa DG. Neuroprotective effect of ketamine administered after status epilepticus onset. Epilepsia 1995;36(2):186–195.

142. Mewasingh LD, Sekhara T, Aeby A, Christiaens FJ, Dan B. Oral ketamine in paediatric non-convulsive status epilepticus. Seizure 2003;12(7):483–489.

143. Borris DJ, Bertram EH, Kapur J. Ketamine controls prolonged status epilepticus. Epilepsy Res 2000;42(2–3):117–122.

144. Loscher W, Honack D, Rundfeldt C. Antiepileptogenic effects of the novel anticonvulsant levetiracetam (ucb L059) in the kindling model of temporal lobe epilepsy. J Pharmacol Exp Ther 1998;284(2):474–479.

145. Klitgaard H. Levetiracetam: the preclinical profile of a new class of antiepileptic drugs? Epilepsia 2001;42(Suppl 4):13–18.

146. Hanon E, Klitgaard H. Neuroprotective properties of the novel antiepileptic drug levetiracetam in the rat middle cerebral artery occlusion model of focal cerebral ischemia. Seizure 2001;10(4):287–293.

147. Glien M, Brandt C, Potschka H, Loscher W. Effects of the novel antiepileptic drug levetiracetam on spontaneous recurrent seizures in the rat pilocarpine model of temporal lobe epilepsy. Epilepsia 2002;43(4):350–357.

148. Mazarati AM, Baldwin R, Klitgaard H, Matagne A, Wasterlain CG. Anticonvulsant effects of levetiracetam and levetiracetam-diazepam combinations in experimental status epilepticus. Epilepsy Res 2004;58(2–3):167–174.

149. McCabe RT, Wasterlain CG, Kucharczyk N, Sofia RD, Vogel JR. Evidence for anticonvulsant and neuroprotectant action of felbamate mediated by strychnine-insensitive glycine receptors. J Pharmacol Exp Ther 1993;264(3):1248–1252.

150. Wallis RA, Panizzon KL, Fairchild MD, Wasterlain CG. Protective effects of felbamate against hypoxia in the rat hippocampal slice. Stroke 1992;23(4):547–551.

151. Wasterlain CG, Adams LM, Wichmann JK, Sofia RD. Felbamate protects CA1 neurons from apoptosis in a gerbil model of global ischemia. Stroke 1996;27(7):1236–1240.

152. Mazarati AM, Sofia RD, Wasterlain CG. Anticonvulsant and antiepileptogenic effects of fluorofelbamate in experimental status epilepticus. Seizure 2002;11(7):423–430.

153. Treiman DM. Electroclinical features of status epilepticus. J Clin Neurophysiol 1995;12(4):343–362.

154. Price HL, Matthew DJ. Evaluation of pediatric intensive care scoring systems. Intensive Care Med 1989;15(2):79–83.

155. Janati A, Erba G. Electroencephalographic correlates of near-drowning encephalopathy in children. Electroencephalogr Clin Neurophysiol 1982;53(2):182–191.

156. Markand ON, Warren CH, Moorthy SS, Stoelting RK, King RD. Monitoring of multimodality evoked potentials during open heart surgery under hypothermia. Electroencephalogr Clin Neurophysiol 1984;59(6):432–440.

157. Tasker RC, Boyd S, Harden A, Matthew DJ. Monitoring in nontraumatic coma. Part II: Electroencephalography. Arch Dis Child 1988;63(8):895–899.

158. Treiman DM. Status epilepticus. Baillieres Clin Neurol 1996;5(4):821–839.

159. Amit R, Goitein KJ, Mathot I, Yatziv S. Prolonged electrocerebral silent barbiturate coma in intractable seizure disorders. Epilepsia 1988;29(1):63–66.

160. Tasker RC, Boyd SG, Harden A, Matthew DJ. EEG monitoring of prolonged thiopentone administration for intractable seizures and status epilepticus in infants and young children. Neuropediatrics 1989;20(3):147–153.

161. Maynard DE, Jenkinson JL. The cerebral function analysing monitor. Initial clinical experience, application and further development. Anaesthesia 1984;39(7):678–690.

12
Diseases of the Peripheral Nervous System

Cecil D. Hahn and Brenda L. Banwell

Introduction

The peripheral nervous system (PNS) is composed of anterior horn cells in the spinal cord, motor nerve processes, the neuromuscular junction, muscle, and peripheral sensory receptors and their corresponding sensory nerves. Neuromuscular weakness, particularly bulbar weakness or respiratory failure, may precipitate admission to the pediatric intensive care unit (PICU) as an acute acquired disease, an initial manifestation of a congenital disorder, or an acute deterioration in a child with a preexisting static or deteriorating PNS disease. These diseases are discussed in the first part of the chapter. Peripheral nervous system disease may also develop as a secondary consequence of systemic critical illness; these diseases are discussed in the second part of the chapter. In both parts of the chapter, disorders are grouped into sections based on the location of their primary pathology in the PNS: anterior horn cell disorders, peripheral neuropathies, disorders of the neuromuscular junction, and disorders of muscle. Each disease is then discussed in terms of epidemiology, clinical features, diagnostic evaluation, treatment, the role of the critical care physician, and outcome.

Peripheral Nervous System Diseases Presenting to the Pediatric Intensive Care Unit

Anterior Horn Cell Disorders

Spinal Muscular Atrophy

Epidemiology

Spinal muscular atrophy (SMA) is a relatively common genetic disease with a population incidence of 1 in 6,000–10,000 live births [1,2]. Spinal muscular atrophy is inherited as an autosomal recessive disease and represents a significant cause of infantile death and childhood disability. Spinal muscular atrophy is commonly classified into three subtypes based on clinical features (Table 12.1).

Type I SMA (Werdnig-Hoffman disease) is the most severe form, characterized by severe hypotonia and weakness either present at birth or developing by the age of 6 months. Death from respiratory failure usually occurs before age 2 years. Type II SMA becomes clinically apparent before age 18 months. Affected children are able to sit but are never able to stand or walk. Patients may survive into adulthood; in one series, survival rates were 98% at 5 years of age and 68% at 25 years of age [3]. Type III SMA (Kugelberg-Welander disease) is characterized by proximal muscle weakness, which becomes apparent after age 18 months and may manifest as late as early adulthood. By definition, patients with SMA type III achieve independent ambulation at some point in their lives, although progressive weakness may ultimately render them wheelchair dependent. The clinical features of some patients appear to overlap between type I and II or type II and III disease.

Genetics and Pathophysiology

Spinal muscular atrophy types I, II, and III are allelic disorders caused by mutations of the survival motor neuron (SMN) gene in an unstable and genetically complex region at chromosome 5q13. There are two copies of the SMN gene within this region: SMN1 or SMN_t, which is closer to the telomere, and SMN2 or SMN_c, which is closer to the centromere. Mutations in the SMN1 gene are responsible for the vast majority of SMA cases. The inheritance of SMA is autosomal recessive. Over 95% of SMA patients have homozygous deletions of all or part of the SMN1 gene, and most of the remaining patients are compound heterozygotes, having a deletion on one chromosome and a missense mutation on the other [4]. Based on this evidence, accurate pre- and postnatal genetic testing is available for diagnostic confirmation of SMA.

The clinical phenotypes of types I, II, and III SMA appear to be related to the overall amount SMN protein expression [4]. Patients with SMA I have little or no SMN production, whereas patients with type II or III have some SMN production, possible owing to increased copy numbers of the SMN_c gene. The SMN protein appears to be involved in RNA metabolism and is expressed in most tissue types. It is not known why motor neurons appear to be specifically dependent on SMN protein for their survival.

Diagnosis

Patients with SMA typically present with symmetric flaccid weakness most apparent in proximal muscles. Overall muscle bulk is

D.S. Wheeler et al. (eds.), *The Central Nervous System in Pediatric Critical Illness and Injury*,
DOI 10.1007/978-1-84800-993-6_12, © Springer-Verlag London Limited 2009

TABLE 12.1. Classification of cases of childhood spinal muscle atrophy (SMA).

SMA type I (Werdnig-Hoffmann)	Onset at birth to 6 months Never able to sit independently Death <2 years
SMA type II	Onset <18 months Able to sit, but never able to stand or walk independently Death >2 years
SMA type III (Kugelberg-Welander)	Onset >18 months Able to stand and walk independently Life expectancy is normal

Source: Adapted from Munsat [143].

reduced, and approximately 40% of patients will have tongue muscle fasciculations. Tendon reflexes are absent or markedly diminished. Electromyography reveals a chronic muscle denervation pattern, and nerve conduction studies demonstrate normal motor and sensory nerve conduction velocities. Diagnosis is confirmed by genetic analysis. Muscle biopsy (which is seldom necessary given the availability of genetic testing) shows muscle fiber atrophy, and the SMA type I patients also demonstrate group hypertrophy of type I fibers.

Treatment

There is no treatment available to delay or reverse the progressive muscular weakness associated with SMA. Management involves a multidisciplinary approach. Families require extensive counseling regarding expectations for survival and the role of mechanical ventilatory support. Infants with SMA type I develop poor sleep, nocturnal hypoventilation, and reduced energy to feed associated with tachycardia and diaphoresis. Gastrostomy tube feedings can significantly increase the quality of life. Nocturnal ventilatory support, either noninvasively in the form of bilevel positive airway pressure or via tracheostomy, is a complex decision, particularly for patients with SMA type I. Orthopedic support for kyphoscoliosis is typically required for patients with SMA type II and for more severely affected patients with SMA type III. It is important to remember that patients with SMA have normal cognitive and sensory functions.

The PICU medical team is often involved in the care of infants with SMA type I, who may have the diagnosis of SMA confirmed in the PICU setting, or children with SMA type II or III who experience acute decompensation in the context of intercurrent respiratory infection, aspiration, or postorthopedic procedures. The PICU team often plays an integral role in the planning of long-term respiratory care. Children with SMA II and III may recover from an acute illness and return to their previous level of functioning. Maximizing acute ventilatory support while minimizing the duration of mechanical ventilation is often critical to the success of tracheal extubation in these children. It is important that families are offered emotional and social supports by the hospital multidisciplinary care team. The Muscular Dystrophy Association is another invaluable resource.

Juvenile Amyotrophic Lateral Sclerosis

Epidemiology

Juvenile amyotrophic lateral sclerosis (ALS), defined by its onset prior to the age of 25 years, is exceedingly rare. Juvenile ALS is generally considered a familial disorder; both autosomal recessive [5] and autosomal dominant [6] kindreds have been described.

However, spontaneous cases do occur. In contrast to adult-onset ALS, juvenile ALS is a more chronic, slowly progressive disease. The mean age of symptom onset is 12 years (range 3–25 years) in the autosomal recessive form and 17 years (range 1–63 years) in the autosomal dominant form. Bulbar dysfunction occurs in a minority of patients with the autosomal recessive form only.

Genetics and Pathophysiology

The autosomal recessive form of juvenile ALS (termed ALS2) has been linked to chromosomes 2q33 and 15q15–22, whereas the autosomal dominant form (termed ALS4) has been linked to chromosome 9q34. Although mutations in the gene encoding superoxide dismutase 1 (SOD1) account for 20% of adult-onset familial ALS [7], they have not been implicated in juvenile ALS. The pathobiology of the disease involves progressive loss of anterior horn cells in the spinal cord, as well as degeneration of the corticospinal and corticobulbar pathways. The disease is thought to relate to excitotoxicity and subsequent cellular apoptosis, but the precise mechanisms underlying these processes have yet to be delineated.

Diagnosis

The hallmark of juvenile ALS is the slowly progressive development of combined upper and lower motor neuron symptoms and signs in the absence of significant sensory abnormalities or ataxia. Upper motor neuron dysfunction (which distinguishes ALS from SMA) is evident as spasticity, hyperreflexia, and extensor plantar responses. Lower motor neuron dysfunction is evident as progressive distally predominant muscular atrophy, weakness, and fasciculations, in addition to painful muscle cramps. Involvement of bulbar muscles does not occur in the dominant form (ALS4) but may occur in the recessive form (ALS2), resulting in dysarthria and dysphagia. Electromyography and nerve conduction studies reveal evidence of chronic muscle denervation with preservation of motor and sensory nerve conduction velocities.

Treatment

The management of ALS is primarily supportive. Riluzole, a glutamate antagonist, prolongs survival in adult ALS patients by 3–6 months [8] but has not been systematically studied in juvenile ALS. Vitamin E, coenzyme Q10 and creatine, and xaliproden are other unproven therapies. The question of whether and when to initiate mechanical ventilation is one of the central treatment decisions for ALS patients and their families. Progressive respiratory insufficiency first manifests as chronic nocturnal hypoventilation. Symptoms can be effectively managed by noninvasive intermittent positive pressure ventilation, which improves quality of life, and may even prolong life span [9]. Tracheostomy and continuous long-term mechanical ventilation are treatment options that many fully informed patients and families choose not to pursue. Timely discussion of these issues should occur while the patient is still able to communicate. The completion of advance directives is crucial in order to define the conditions for the emergency initiation of mechanical ventilatory support as well as the conditions for the withdrawal of mechanical ventilatory support.

West Nile Virus

Epidemiology

West Nile virus has been associated with North American epidemics between the months of July and December. Only 20% of infected individuals are symptomatic (fever, headache, anorexia, general malaise), and less than 1% of infections result in severe neurologic disease such as meningoencephalitis or acute flaccid paralysis [10]. Furthermore, neurologic disease is far less common in children than adults. Nervous system infection with West Nile virus, considered by some to represent the "polio of the 21st century," occurred in 3.6% of 4,146 cases reported in 2002 in the United States. West Nile virus is usually transmitted to humans by a mosquito vector from infected birds, but reports exist of transmission through organ transplantation, blood products, and transplacentally from mother to fetus. The incubation period is 2–14 days [11].

Diagnosis

The diagnosis of West Nile viral infection is through serologic assessment. For patients with meningoencephalitis, cerebrospinal fluid (CSF) analysis reveals IgM antibodies directed against the virus in CSF within 8 days of symptom onset [12]. Cerebrospinal fluid also shows elevated protein levels and pleocytosis (initially neutrophilic, then lymphocytic). Peripheral nervous system involvement, in the form of anterior horn cell infection leading to muscle weakness and areflexia, has been reported [13,14]. In one series, 54% of patients with West Nile infection demonstrated focal neuromuscular deficits [15].

Treatment

Treatment of West Nile virus CNS disease is largely supportive, focusing on respiratory support, management of cerebral edema in patients with meningoencephalitis, and prevention of secondary bacterial infection. Rehabilitation is critical for patients with anterior horn cell damage, although full recovery may be limited. There have been no controlled studies of ribavirin, interferon, intravenous immune globulin (IVIG), corticosteroids, or osmotic therapy for cerebral edema. Human vaccines are currently in development.

Poliomyelitis and Poliomyelitis-Like Syndromes

Epidemiology

Although poliovirus was eradicated from the Western hemisphere in 1994 and from all industrialized nations in 2002 [16], several other members of the enterovirus family can cause a poliomyelitis-like syndrome. As discussed earlier, in North America the most common of these is the West Nile virus. Outbreaks of Japanese encephalitis virus (JEV) and enterovirus 71 (E71) have most recently been reported in Asia. The last cases of paralytic poliomyelitis caused by endemic transmission of wild-type virus in the United States occurred in 1979. Vaccine-associated paralytic poliomyelitis was a rare adverse reaction to the live attenuated oral poliovirus vaccine but has not occurred in the United States since the exclusive use of the inactivated poliovirus vaccine in the year 2000.

Pathophysiology

Neurologic symptoms are caused by invasion of the enterovirus into the CNS. Infection of anterior horn cells in the ventral spinal cord causes acute flaccid paralysis and areflexia, with preservation of sensory function. Infection of the brain and brain stem causes encephalopathy and bulbar dysfunction and may disrupt respiratory control. Pathologic studies show inflammatory changes in the anterior horn cell region, which may extend into nerve roots [17].

Diagnosis

Because of the almost complete eradication of the poliovirus, poliomyelitis-like syndromes have become an uncommon cause of acute flaccid paralysis (AFP) compared with the more commonly encountered disorders Guillain-Barré syndrome (GBS) and transverse myelitis. It is important to distinguish these different causes of AFP for public health reasons and because they have different treatments and prognoses. Fortunately, it is usually possible to distinguish these conditions on the basis of clinical presentation, CSF examination, spinal magnetic resonance imaging (MRI), and electrodiagnostic testing (Table 12.2). The diagnosis of the poliomyeli-

TABLE 12.2. Differentiation of poliomyelitis-like syndromes from typical Guillain-Barré syndrome and transverse myelitis.

Characteristic	Poliomyelitis-like syndrome	Guillain-Barré syndrome	Transverse myelitis
Time of onset	During acute infection	Postinfection	Postinfection
Fever	Always present	Uncommon	Uncommon
Distribution of weakness	Asymmetric, proximal predominant; occasional monoplegia	Generally symmetric, proximal and distal; monoplegia rare	Symmetric; monoplegia rare
Sensory symptoms	Absence of numbness, paresthesias, sensory loss. May have back pain or myalgia	Painful distal paresthesias and sensory loss	Sensory level (cervical or thoracic)
Concurrent encephalopathy	Common	Absent	Present only in the context of ADEM
Respiratory insufficiency	Only if bulbar involvement	Common	Uncommon
Bowel and bladder involvement	Common for West Nile virus; rare for poliovirus	Rare	Common
Cerebrospinal fluid profile	Pleocytosis and elevated protein	Elevated protein without pleocytosis (albumino-cytologic dissociation)	Pleocytosis and elevated protein. May have oligoclonal bands
Spinal magnetic resonance imaging	Spinal cord and/or cauda equina (increased T2/FLAIR signal ± gadolinium enhancement	Cauda equina only (increased T2/FLAIR signal ± gadolinium enhancement)	Spinal cord only (increased T2/FLAIR signal ± gadolinium enhancement)
Electrodiagnostic features	Anterior horn cell/motor axon process: reduced/absent CMAPs, preserved SNAPs; asymmetric denervation	Demyelination: markedly slow conduction velocity; conduction block, temporal dispersion, reduced SNAPs	No abnormalities on nerve conduction or electromyography, but often shows delayed/absent somatosensory evoked responses

Note: ADEM, acute disseminated encephalomyelitis; CMAPs, compound muscle action potentials; SNAPs, sensory nerve action potentials.
Source: Data are from Sejvar et al. [18] and Al-Shekhlee and Katirji [19].

tis-like syndromes is confirmed by microbiologic and serologic investigations.

Enterovirus infection typically begins with a prodromal illness consisting of nonspecific upper respiratory tract or gastrointestinal tract symptoms, myalgia, and general malaise. In addition, E71 infection presents with herpangina or hand-foot-and-mouth disease. The AFP of poliovirus-like syndromes typically begins 1–10 days after the onset of prodromal symptoms. Paralysis usually worsens over 2–3 days, accompanied by loss of deep tendon reflexes. Weakness is usually asymmetric, typically proceeds proximally to distally in the affected limb(s), and involves the legs more often than the arms. Bulbar involvement (facial weakness and speech or swallowing impairment) may also occur, but rarely without accompanying limb weakness. Bowel and bladder impairment are rare in poliovirus, but common in WNV, JEV and E71 infection. Preservation of sensory function is the rule, and distinguishes poliomyelitis-like syndromes from GBS and transverse myelitis.

Both the poliovirus-like syndromes and transverse myelitis are associated with a primarily lymphocytic pleocytosis and elevated CSF protein levels. In contrast, the hallmark of GBS is elevated CSF protein in the absence of pleocytosis (termed albumino-cytologic dissociation).

Evidence of inflammation on MRI occurs in the form of increased signal on T2 and FLAIR sequences and gadolinium enhancement. In the poliomyelitis-like syndromes, these inflammatory changes are most prominent in the ventral spinal cord but may also extend into the ventral nerve roots [17]. In contrast, in children with GBS, these inflammatory changes are typically limited to the cauda equina, whereas in children with transverse myelitis inflammatory changes are limited to the spinal cord with a predilection for white matter, although inflammation may also extend into gray matter.

Nerve conduction and electromyographic studies are useful in distinguishing poliomyelitis-like syndromes from GBS, which is the most common cause of AFP. Poliomyelitis-like syndromes cause anterior horn cell injury, which results in reduced or absent compound muscle action potentials (CMAPs), whereas nerve conduction velocities are normal and sensory nerve action potentials are preserved [18,19]. Guillain-Barré syndrome causes peripheral nerve demyelination, resulting in slowing of conduction velocities and conduction block, usually affecting both motor and sensory nerve fibers. Transverse myelitis causes spinal cord demyelination, and therefore electrodiagnostic studies of the peripheral nerves are normal.

Viral isolation and detection of viral RNA by reverse-transcriptase polymerase chain reaction provide the most definitive diagnosis. Enteroviruses may be isolated from the stool, pharynx, and CSF. Because the viruses may be excreted intermittently, two stool samples should be collected at least 24 hr apart. Serologic diagnosis requires paired serum specimens collected during the acute illness and at least 2–3 weeks later. A fourfold or greater rise in antibody titers between acute and convalescent sera is generally considered diagnostic.

Treatment

Treatment of the poliomyelitis-like syndromes is primarily supportive. In cases affecting bulbar function or respiratory control, preemptive airway management and adequate respiratory support is critical. Immunomodulatory and antiviral therapies are currently experimental and unproven. The pediatric intensivist should anticipate the possible development of respiratory compromise in all patients presenting with limb weakness or cranial nerve palsies. Proactive airway protection and mechanical ventilatory support may prevent aspiration pneumonia. Because weakness following enterovirus infection is usually permanent, early consideration should be given to tracheostomy.

Outcome

Because the infected anterior horn cell neurons are postmitotic and cannot regenerate, the damage caused during the acute infection is permanent. The denervated muscles become atrophic over several weeks; no significant evidence of muscle reinnervation can be demonstrated on electromyography. Recovery from respiratory failure generally follows the *rule of thirds*, with one third of children experiencing complete recovery, one third suffering mild respiratory dysfunction, and one third developing chronic respiratory failure requiring chronic mechanical ventilatory support. Postpolio syndrome, which consists of muscle pain and the exacerbation of existing weakness, occurs in approximately one third of patients with poliomyelitis 30–40 years after their acute infection. The incidence of this syndrome following West Nile virus and other enteroviral poliomyelitis-like infections is still uncertain. The pathophysiology of postpolio syndrome is presumed to involve *overuse* failure of the residual anterior horn cells, which for many years have supplied larger than normal motor units as a compensatory mechanism following the original acute loss of anterior horn cells.

Peripheral Neuropathies

Guillain-Barré Syndrome

Guillain-Barré syndrome of AFP associated with areflexia and elevated cerebrospinal fluid protein was first described in 1916 by Guillain, Barré, and Strohl. The annual incidence is 1.3–1.9 per 100,000 (20). Guillain-Barré syndrome can occur at any age but is rare in infancy. It is the most common cause of AFP in children, the main differential diagnoses being transverse myelitis, cord compression, and the poliomyelitis-like syndromes (see Table 12.2) [21].

Classification

Although GBS was originally thought to be single entity, it is now considered to consist of several subtypes, each with a distinct pathophysiology (Table 12.3). The classic form of GBS most commonly encountered in Europe and North America is termed *acute inflammatory demyelinating polyneuropathy* (AIDP). Acute inflammatory demyelinating polyneuropathy is characterized by motor and sensory nerve demyelination, presents with both paralysis and sensory loss, may be acutely life threatening, but is associated with a relatively favorable prognosis. Two axonal variants of GBS have also been characterized. Acute motor-sensory axonal neuropathy (AMSAN) is characterized by motor and sensory axonal injury, which causes severe sensory loss and paralysis and slow, incomplete recovery. Acute motor axonal neuropathy (AMAN), first identified following outbreaks of *Campylobacter jejuni* in China, is characterized by motor axonal injury, causing severe paralysis in the absence of sensory findings, with variable recovery. The Miller-Fisher syndrome is a variant of GBS characterized by ataxia, areflexia, and ophthalmoplegia with preservation of strength, associated with a specific anti-GQ1b autoantibody directed at the oculomotor nerves, spinal nerve ganglia, and cerebellar neurons.

TABLE 12.3. Classification of Guillain-Barré syndrome subtypes.

Condition	Clinical features	Pathophysiology	Prognosis
Acute inflammatory demyelinating polyneuropathy	Weakness Areflexia Sensory loss	Demyelination of motor and sensory nerves Secondary axonal degeneration in severe cases Anti-GM2 antibodies	Often rapid and complete recovery
Acute motor axonal neuropathy	Weakness Areflexia Little or no sensory loss Muscle atrophy	Axonal degeneration in motor nerves Milder cases caused by functional conduction block by antibodies, without significant axonal injury Associated with *Campylobacter jejuni* infection Anti-GM1 antibodies directed at axon cell membrane	Variable
Acute motor-sensory axonal neuropathy	Weakness Areflexia Sensory loss Muscle atrophy	Axonal degeneration in motor and sensory nerves	Delayed and poor recovery
Miller-Fisher syndrome	Ataxia Areflexia Ophthalmoplegia ± nonreactive pupils	Associated with *Campylobacter jejuni* infection Anti-GQ1b antibodies directed at oculomotor nerves, sensory nerve ganglia, cerebellar neurons	Rapid and complete recovery

Pathophysiology

Guillain-Barré syndrome is the prototype of a postinfectious autoimmune neurologic illness. Two thirds of cases are preceded by a clinically apparent respiratory or gastrointestinal infection, which occurs 1–3 weeks before the onset of neurologic symptoms. There is convincing epidemiologic evidence for an association between GBS and preceding infection by the following organisms: cytomegalovirus, Epstein-Barr virus, varicella zoster virus, *C. jejuni*, and *Mycoplasma pneumoniae*. An association with preceding surgery and influenza vaccination has been reported but is less definitive [22].

The postulated mechanism of nerve injury in GBS is an autoimmune attack on peripheral nerves. This autoimmune process is believed to be triggered by molecular mimicry, a process in which shared epitopes between the organism responsible for the recent infection (i.e., *Campylobacter*), and the peripheral nerve fibers result in autoimmune cross-reactivity. The cross-reactive target epitopes frequently appear to be gangliosides, a component of the cell membranes of both axons and their surrounding myelin sheaths. Autoantibodies to various gangliosides have been detected in GBS patients, for example, anti-GM2 antibodies in AIDP patients, anti-GM1 in AMAN patients, and anti-GQ1b in patients with the Miller-Fisher syndrome. The autoimmune process likely involves both T-cell and antibody-mediated autoimmunity, in addition to complement-mediated destruction of the myelin sheath or axons. This process occurs both proximally and distally along the entire length of peripheral nerves.

In AIDP, the autoimmune attack is focused primarily on the myelin sheath; secondary axonal injury may occur but becomes significant only in severe cases of AIDP. Recovery from AIDP requires remyelination, which occurs relatively rapidly, usually within several weeks.

In the axonal forms of GBS (AMAN and AMSAN), the autoimmune attack is focused primarily on the axon. Injury occurs mainly at nodes of Ranvier and at the peripheral nerve terminal because these regions are unmyelinated, exposing cross-reactive epitopes on the axon surface to autoimmune attack. Axonal injury leads to Wallerian degeneration of disconnected distal nerve segments, resulting in denervation of associated muscles and profound muscle

atrophy. Recovery from axonal forms of GBS is much slower because it requires axonal regeneration, which occurs from the intact proximal nerve segment at a rate of approximately 1 mm/day. Furthermore, because of scar tissue in the degenerated distal nerve segment, nerve regeneration is frequently incomplete.

In the Miller-Fisher syndrome, the characteristic anti-GQ1b antibodies found in the majority of patients have been shown to bind specifically to the oculomotor nerves, to sensory neurons in the dorsal root ganglia, and to cerebellar neurons. This binding pattern corresponds to the characteristic symptoms of ophthalmoplegia, areflexia, and ataxia in this variant of GBS.

Diagnosis

The diagnosis of GBS is primarily clinical, based on the characteristic history and findings on physical examination. Guillain-Barré syndrome patients typically present with symmetric, both proximal and distal weakness and areflexia 1–3 weeks following a prodromal respiratory or gastrointestinal illness. Weakness can develop acutely within several days or subacutely over a period lasting up to 4 weeks. Respiratory compromise may develop rapidly or insidiously and results from a combination of intercostal and diaphragmatic muscle weakness. Cranial nerve involvement is not infrequent, presenting as unilateral or bilateral facial weakness, or bulbar dysfunction, which may impair speech, swallowing, and control of the airway. Ophthalmoplegia and pupillary dysfunction are most commonly seen in the Miller-Fisher variant of GBS. Sensory involvement is common in AIDP and AMSAN, presenting as distal-predominant paresthesias and sensory loss. Pain occurs in the majority of patients and may be the predominant early symptom. This may present a particular diagnostic challenge in young children if they are unable to communicate the nature of the pain: these patients may present with nonspecific irritability and may even appear encephalopathic [23]. The absence of deep tendon reflexes is an important diagnostic clue in such situations.

Lumbar puncture is a useful initial diagnostic test. The classic CSF profile is that of elevated protein in the context of a normal cell count, so-called albumino-cytologic dissociation. However, CSF protein levels may be normal in up to 20% of patients during the first week of the disease [23]. The presence of pleocytosis should suggest other diagnoses such as a poliomyelitis-like syndrome or demyelination triggered by acute human immunodeficiency virus (HIV) infection.

Electrodiagnostic testing is helpful to differentiate among the subtypes of GBS. Acute inflammatory demyelinating polyneuropathy, the primarily demyelinating form of GBS, is associated with increased latency of distal nerve conduction, delayed or absent F waves, and a slowing of nerve conduction velocities with temporal dispersion and nerve conduction block. The axonal forms of GBS, AMAN and AMSAN, are associated with markedly reduced or absent CMAPs in the setting of relatively normal conduction velocities. Patients with severe forms will demonstrate progressive loss of electrical excitability of muscle.

The differential diagnosis of GBS includes poliomyelitis-like syndromes, acute HIV infection, botulism, tick paralysis, acute toxic neuropathies, transverse myelitis, diphtheria, and acute intermittent porphyria.

Treatment

Even mildly affected patients should be hospitalized and closely observed for the insidious development of worsening respiratory status and bulbar weakness, which presents as difficulty handling secretions and maintaining the airway (see later). Once the diagnosis has been made, treatment should be initiated promptly in all patients who are nonambulatory or display signs of respiratory compromise or bulbar dysfunction. Both plasma exchange (PE) and IVIG have proven and equivalent efficacy in adults for shortening recovery time and improving long-term outcomes when given with four weeks of neurologic symptom onset. There is no additional benefit from combined therapy with PE and IVIG. Corticosteroids are of no benefit in GBS and should not be used. Both IVIG and PE are considered acceptable treatment options for GBS in children, despite the lack of large randomized-controlled trials in the pediatric population [24]. Because of its relative safety and ease of administration, IVIG therapy has become the preferred treatment for adults and children. Although no large randomized controlled trials of IVIG have been conducted with children, extensive positive experience has been published [25]. Plasma exchange is less suitable for children because of difficulty in obtaining large-bore double-lumen peripheral intravenous access, necessitating more invasive central line placement.

Psychological support is an important component of the compassionate care of the GBS patient. Patients are frequently terrified by the illness, a fear that may be exacerbated by their inability to communicate once ventilated. Caregivers should take the time to explain to the patients and their families the nature of the illness, the daily plan of care, and the generally favorable prognosis. A visit by a former GBS patient may be particularly helpful and may be arranged with the help of local or regional patient support groups.

Role of the Pediatric Intensive Care Unit Physician

Supportive critical care has dramatically decreased the mortality of GBS and is a cornerstone of therapy. Although one third of adult patients with GBS require admission to the intensive care unit, this number is likely lower for children [26]. The spectrum of PICU complications seen in GBS is summarized in Table 12.4.

The most common reason for PICU admission is neuromuscular *respiratory failure* caused by weakness of both the diaphragmatic and intercostal musculature. Neuromuscular respiratory failure is

TABLE 12.4. PICU Complications of Guillain-Barré syndrome.

Respiratory dysfunction
- Loss of airway control
- Weakness of inspiratory muscles
- Weakness of expiratory muscles

Autonomic dysfunction
- Cardiac arrhythmias (bradycardia, asystole, atrial fibrillation and flutter, sinus tachycardia, ventricular tachycardia, transient atrioventricular block)
- Sympathetic hyperfunction (hypertension)
- Sympathetic hypofunction (hypotension)
- Parasympathetic hyperfunction (excessive sweating, tearing and salivation)
- Parasympathetic hypofunction (gastroparesis, constipation, urinary retention)
- Syndrome of inappropriate antidiuretic hormone release
- Neurogenic pulmonary edema

Pain syndromes
- Neuropathic pain
- Deep muscular pain

Pressure palsies

Malnutrition caused by inadequate intake and catabolic state of illness
Complications related to plasma exchange therapy
- Pneumothorax (from central line placement)
- Line-related sepsis
- Symptomatic hypocalcemia
- Coagulation abnormalities
- Hypotension

Complications related to intravenous immunoglobulin therapy
- Anaphylaxis (immunoglobulin A deficiency)
- Aseptic meningitis
- Acute renal failure
- Transient hypercoagulability

characterized clinically by air hunger, staccato speech, accessory muscle use, paradoxical respirations, forehead sweating, and altered mentation. Vital capacity (VC) is the most commonly monitored paraclinical test of respiratory function, although maximum inspiratory and expiratory pressures are also useful. Continuous pulse oximetry and serial assessments (at least every 6–8hr) of these clinical and paraclinical indicators of respiratory function is crucial in order to anticipate the need for respiratory support. Elective tracheal intubation should be considered for patients who develop clinical signs of respiratory failure or whose VC falls below 15mL/kg or drops by more than 50% within 48hr [26]. In addition, patients with poor expiratory function (even in the presence of a normal VC) may require tracheal intubation because of poor cough effort, leading to atelectasis and the inability to clear secretions. Patients with marked bulbar weakness may require tracheal intubation for airway control, even in the presence of a normal VC and normal gas exchange [27].

Tracheostomy should generally be considered for patients requiring more than 3 weeks of continuous mechanical ventilatory support via a tracheal tube but can be performed earlier if rapid recovery is not anticipated (i.e., in axonal forms of GBS) or delayed if recovery of respiratory function appears imminent. Despite its invasive nature, patients often appreciate tracheostomy because it is more comfortable than oral or nasal intubations, facilitates oral hygiene, and may allow for oral communication. Tracheostomy also helps avoid complications of long-term intubation, such as tracheal stenosis and tracheomalacia [28].

Autonomic dysfunction is a frequent occurrence in hospitalized GBS patients, most commonly among patients with profound muscle weakness and respiratory failure. Paroxysmal hypertension, which occurs in 5%–10% of adults with GBS, seldom requires treatment unless there is evidence of end-organ damage (hypertensive encephalopathy, pulmonary edema, subarachnoid hemorrhage). Hypotension is equally common and is frequently orthostatic or triggered by gagging and tracheal suctioning. Hypotension seldom requires treatment, unless there is evidence of systemic hypoperfusion. Cardiac arrhythmias, although relatively uncommon, can be life threatening and therefore necessitate continuous cardiac monitoring of GBS patients. Abnormal excessive vagal activity may occasionally lead to profound bradycardia and asystole. In contrast, a sudden abnormal loss of vagal tone can lead to cardiac tachyarrhythmias, which may be benign (sinus tachycardia) but may also be life threatening (ventricular tachycardia, atrial fibrillation, and atrial flutter). Constipation and urinary retention should be anticipated and managed with stool softeners and bladder catheterization. Gastroparesis, caused by parasympathetic hypofunction and exacerbated by prolonged immobility and narcotic administration, may require adjustment of enteral nutrition and the use of prokinetic agents.

Pain syndromes occur in the majority of adults and children with GBS [23,29]. Two types of pain have been distinguished: neuropathic pain and deep aching muscular pain. Neuropathic pain is described as a burning or tingling in the affected extremities and is most common during the prodromal and recovery phases of GBS. Treatment options include gabapentin, carbamazepine, valproic acid, mexiletine and nortriptyline (which should be avoided in patients with severe autonomic dysfunction) [28]. Deep aching muscular pain in the lower back and legs is also commonly experienced by GBS patients. Treatment options include acetaminophen, nonsteroidal antiinflammatory drugs, and narcotics. This aching pain usually resolves within 8 weeks [29].

Guillain-Barré syndrome patients appear to be more vulnerable to *pressure palsies*, likely because of their coexistent inflammatory peripheral nerve injury. The ulnar and nerve should be protected by the use of hand and wrist splints and the peroneal nerve by the use of a trochanter roll and the avoidance of compression stockings that cover the proximal fibula [28].

Malnutrition can occur. Because of the systemic inflammatory autoimmune response, GBS patients are in a catabolic state that is comparable to acute trauma or sepsis. Furthermore, GBS patients who present with bulbar weakness may already be undernourished because of inadequate oral intake prior to hospitalization. Nutritional demands should be met promptly to prevent malnutrition and hypoalbuminemia. If gut motility is intact, then high-calorie and high-protein enteral feeding should be initiated promptly. Total parenteral nutrition is seldom required [28].

Complications of IVIG and PE therapy are summarized in Table 12.4. The rate of many complications during PE has been reduced by the use of modern, sophisticated apheresis equipment. In older children and adults, PE may be performed through a large-bore antecubital vein, which eliminates the risk of pneumothorax and may reduce the risk of line-related sepsis. Intravenous immunoglobulin therapy is generally well tolerated, and complications are uncommon. Anaphylaxis is a rare complication of IVIG therapy that occurs in some patients who are deficient in immunoglobulin A. Serum immunoglobulin levels may be measured prior to IVIG administration, and IVIG should be administered with particular caution to patients who are known to be immunoglobulin A deficient.

Outcome

Most patients with GBS have a favorable outcome. A recent prospective population-based Italian study of 120 adults and children reported that, at 2 years after diagnosis, 54% of patients had completely recovered and 80% of patients had a good recovery, defined as minor signs or symptoms of neuropathy but capable of manual work (Hughes grade <2) [30,31]. The remaining 20% of patients had a poor outcome at 2 years, defined as impairment of manual work or impairment of independent ambulation (Hughes grade ≥2). Seven patients died: six fatal cases were caused by pneumonia occurring during mechanical ventilation, and one patient died from a pulmonary embolus secondary to a deep vein thrombosis. Factors associated with a poor outcome at 2 years were more severe symptoms and signs at the nadir of illness and electromyographic evidence of axonal injury and history of gastroenteritis preceding GBS.

Limited data from case series indicate that the prognosis of GBS in children may be better than adults. Children with GBS typically have less severe weakness and less frequent bulbar involvement than adults. Children are less likely to require mechanical ventilation and typically recover more rapidly from paralysis than adults [23,32].

Disorders of the Neuromuscular Junction

Myasthenia Gravis

Classification

Autoimmune myasthenia gravis (MG) in children and adolescents (also termed *juvenile MG*) is a rare disorder. Myasthenia gravis in adults occurs with greater frequency. In North America, 10%–15% of MG cases begin before age 20 years, but onset before 1 year of age is exceptionally rare. The incidence in African-American children is greater than in Caucasian children. Among African-American children and adolescents, females are more commonly affected than males. Among Caucasian children, there is an equal sex ratio of MG incidence prior to puberty and a female predominance during and after puberty [33].

Neonatal myasthenia occurs transiently in about 10% of infants born to mothers with autoimmune MG. Maternal transmission of acetylcholine receptor antibodies can occur even if the mother is in clinical remission, and thus all women with a history of MG should be delivered in centers equipped to manage the neonatal complications. Newborn infants usually present on the first day of life with bulbar and respiratory difficulty, and some require mechanical ventilation. Neonatal symptoms can increase gradually over the first 24 hr after birth, and thus at-risk infants should be monitored closely for at least 48 hr. Affected infants improve with anticholinesterase therapy, and the condition resolves spontaneously over several days as maternally transmitted antibodies are cleared. Intravenous immunoglobulin infusion may improve respiratory function in severely affected neonates. Rarely, in utero transmission of acetylcholine antibodies leads to comprised fetal movements and associated development of limb contractures (arthrogryposis).

Congenital myasthenic syndromes (CMSs) are genetic disorders that result in defects of presynaptic, synaptic, or postsynaptic neuromuscular transmission. They are much rarer than autoimmune MG and usually present before age 2 years. More severe forms of CMS present at birth with respiratory failure, ocular muscle paralysis, facial and bulbar weakness, and profound hypotonia. Recognition of the CMSs is important, because many of them are treatable with medications that modulate pre- or postsynaptic neuromuscular transmission. Immunosuppressive therapies are of no benefit. The classification, diagnosis, and management of CMSs is beyond the scope of this chapter but have been recently reviewed [34].

Pathophysiology

Autoimmune MG is caused by antibody and T-cell mediated attack on elements of the postsynaptic neuromuscular junction. Approximately 75%–90% of patients are found to have antibodies to acetylcholine receptors (AChR). Of the remaining 10%–25% of patients, 30%–40% have antibodies to MuSK, a muscle-specific tyrosine kinase required for the proper clustering of AChR on the postsynaptic membrane [35,36]. Antibody and T-cell mediated attack on postsynaptic AChR and MuSK causes a reduction in the number of AChR and a simplification of postsynaptic membrane, which reduces the efficiency of neuromuscular transmission.

Neonatal myasthenia is caused by passive transfer to the fetus of AChR antibodies from a mother with autoimmune MG. There is no correlation between the risk for neonatal myasthenia and the current or past severity of MG in the mother or the length of time that the mother has been in clinical remission. Thus, all neonates born to women with active or remote MG should be delivered and monitored in centers equipped to manage neonatal respiratory failure. None of these infants should be discharged prior to 72 hr of life, as some affected infants may not present until day 3 of life.

Congenital myasthenic syndromes are not caused by an autoimmune process but rather by genetic abnormalities that affect presynaptic, synaptic, or postsynaptic neuromuscular transmission. Examples include congenital AChR deficiency, kinetic abnormalities of the AChR (slow-channel and fast-channel CMSs), congenital acetylcholinesterase deficiency, and congenital choline acetyltransferase deficiency [34].

Diagnosis

Clinical Presentation. The hallmark of MG is fluctuating muscle weakness. Weakness may be confined to the extraocular muscles (ocular myasthenia) or may extend to the facial and limb muscles (generalized myasthenia). Weakness may fluctuate from day to day and even from hour to hour and is typically worse late in the day. In ocular myasthenia, symptoms and signs are limited to diplopia, ptosis, and extraocular muscle weakness with preservation of pupillary function. In generalized myasthenia, weakness may involve any of the following: facial muscles, tongue and posterior pharyngeal muscles (causing slurred speech, dysphagia), vocal cords (causing stridor, which may require emergency intubation to maintain the airway), respiratory muscles (causing shallow respirations and inability to cough), and limb muscles. Proximal muscles (i.e., deltoids, quadriceps) are usually weaker than distal muscles. Muscle bulk, deep tendon reflexes, and sensation are preserved. Smooth muscle function (heart, gastrointestinal tract, bladder, uterus) is not affected.

Myasthenic crisis refers to a state of respiratory insufficiency or the inability to maintain a patent airway. A crisis may be caused by weakness of respiratory muscles (inability to maintain vital capacity, create adequate negative inspiratory force, or clear secretions by coughing) or by vocal cord paralysis leading to airway obstruction. Crisis may be precipitated by the use of drugs that exacerbate

TABLE 12.5. Drugs that exacerbate weakness in myasthenia gravis.

Corticosteroids
Thyroid preparations
Neuromuscular blocking agents (succinylcholine, botulinum toxin)
General anesthetic agents
Antiarrhythmics (procainamide, quinidine, verapamil)
Anticonvulsants (phenytoin, gabapentin)
Antibiotics (aminoglycosides, tetracyclines, clindamycin, erythromycin, ciprofloxacin)
Magnesium salts, Epsom salts

Source: Adapted from Keesey [37].

myasthenia (Table 12.5) and in numerous other clinical scenarios (Table 12.6). The incidence of crisis among patients with MG is 15%–20%, but the mortality rate has declined from 80% in the 1950s to 4% by the 1990s because of improved recognition of MG and advances in PICU management [37].

Confirmation. Confirmation of the diagnosis of MG may be made by pharmacologic, immunologic, and electrodiagnostic means. Pharmacologic confirmation of MG is made by assessing response to therapy with an intravenous injection of the short-acting anticholinesterase edrophonium chloride (Tensilon), administered in two to three incremental doses to a total of 0.15 mg/kg. A positive Tensilon test requires an objectively measurable improvement in a clinical sign (ptosis, gaze paresis, grip strength, respiratory function), which occurs within a few minutes of the injection. This may be compared with the response to a prior placebo injection. Atropine should be available in case bradycardia develops because of the muscarinic effects of Tensilon.

Immunologic confirmation of MG is performed using an assay for serum AChR binding antibodies, which are elevated in 85% of patients with generalized myasthenia. The sensitivity of the assay is lower for patients with ocular myasthenia. In the appropriate clinical context this is a highly specific test, with false-positive results reported in only a small percentage of patients with autoimmune thyroid disease or the Lambert-Eaton myasthenic syndrome. Patients without elevated levels of AChR antibodies should be tested for antibodies against MuSK, a muscle-specific tyrosine kinase (see earlier section on pathophysiology).

Electrodiagnostic testing is useful in documenting impaired neuromuscular transmission and can usually be performed urgently to confirm the diagnosis. For patients with MG, repetitive nerve stimulation at 2–3 Hz produces a characteristic decremental response in the compound muscle action potential (defined as a reduction in the size of the motor unit response with repetitive nerve stimulation). Single-fiber electromyography is a more sensitive technique that measures the instability in neuromuscular transmission that occurs in MG. Neuromuscular transmission defects are also demonstrable in the Lambert-Eaton myasthenic syndrome, the congenital myasthenic syndromes, and botulism.

TABLE 12.6. Precipitants of myasthenic crisis.

Upper and lower respiratory infections; aspiration
Sepsis
Surgical procedures
Initiation or rapid tapering of corticosteroid therapy
Exposure to drugs that exacerbate myasthenic weakness
Pregnancy

Treatment

Pharmacologic management of MG begins with an attempt to control symptoms using oral anticholinesterase medications such as pyridostigmine bromide (Mestinon) or neostigmine chloride (Prostigmin). These drugs block acetylcholinesterase, the enzyme that degrades the neurotransmitter acetylcholine in the neuro-muscular junction, allowing acetylcholine to remain longer in the synaptic cleft and thereby increasing the likelihood that the acetylcholine released by each nerve stimulation will have time to bind to AChRs not blocked by antibody. Pharmacologic blockade of ace-tylcholinesterase is short lived, peaking 1–2 hr after the ingestion of Mestinon and wearing off within 3–4 hr. These drugs cause mus-carinic cholinergic side effects such as hypersalivation and abdom-inal cramping, which may be reduced by the addition of oral anticholinergic drugs such as propantheline, if needed.

Plasma exchange is useful as a short-term treatment of MG in the setting of impending myasthenic crisis, prior to surgical proce-dures such as thymectomy, or to shorten the duration of mechani-cal ventilation. It is thought to work by removing pathogenic circulating AChR antibodies. The procedure is usually performed once daily for 5 days and requires a central line or large-bore double peripheral line, which may be difficult to obtain in young children.

Intravenous immunoglobulin therapy is an alternative to PE that in a small randomized controlled trial appeared to have equal effi-cacy in the management of myasthenic crisis [38]. However, a ret-rospective study indicated that PE is superior to IVIG in permitting extubation at 2 weeks [39], and it appears that some patients who fail to respond to IVIG subsequently respond to PE [40]. Although both PE and IVIG may cause considerable side effects, overall IVIG appears to cause fewer serious complications than PE therapy (see Table 12.4 and the discussion in the earlier section on Guillain-Barré syndrome).

Thymoma, a benign epithelioid tumor of the thymus gland asso-ciated with 15% of adult MG, is rare in childhood, present in only 2% of patients in a combination of two large pediatric series [33,41]. Thymectomy is indicated in all adult and pediatric MG patients who are found on chest computed tomography (CT) or MRI to have a thymoma. Children with nonthymomatous MG also appear to benefit from thymectomy, as symptoms improve in 57%–95% of patients, and a complete remission is achieved in 11%–75%. The greatest benefit is seen in peripubertal children and when thymec-tomy is performed within 12 months of symptom onset [33]. Thy-mectomy may be performed using a variety of operative techniques, ranging from more invasive transsternal approaches to less inva-sive video-assisted approaches [42]. The available evidence sug-gests that more complete resections produce better outcomes, although the optimal surgical technique continues to be a matter of debate [43].

Role of the Pediatric Intensive Care Unit Physician

Myasthenic crisis should be suspected in patients with nasal or staccato speech, shallow breathing with use of accessory muscles and paradoxical inward abdominal movement, weak cough, and nasal regurgitation of liquids. Patients should be admitted promptly to the PICU and their respiratory status closely monitored. Serial clinical assessments, including measurement of vital capacity and negative inspiratory force, should be conducted. A vital capacity of 15 mL/kg or less and a negative inspiratory force of 20 cm H_2O or less are signs of impending respiratory failure for which elective

TABLE 12.7. Distinguishing myasthenic from cholinergic crisis.

	Myasthenic crisis	Cholinergic crisis
Common precipitants	Infection, surgery, rapid taper of immunosuppressive medications	Recently increased dosage of anticholinesterase medications
Cholinergic symptoms	Absent	Present (miosis, sweating, lacrimation hypersalivation, gut hypermotility, etc.)
Muscle fasciculations	Uncommon	Common
Response to Tensilon (only if already intubated)	Improvement	Exacerbation or no change

tracheal intubation should be considered. Nasotracheal intubation is preferred over orotracheal intubation because of greater patient comfort and easier maintenance of oral hygiene. Prolonged ventila-tor requirement (>2 weeks) is less common in children than adult MG patients. Tracheostomy should be considered for patients requiring more than 2 weeks of mechanical ventilation but is seldom required in pediatric MG. Aggressive respiratory treatment including suctioning, chest physiotherapy, and bronchodilator treatments may prevent the development of atelectasis and pneu-monia and shorten the duration of mechanical ventilation and intensive care [44].

A myasthenic crisis may occasionally be precipitated by over-medication with anticholinesterase medications (Table 12.7). The resulting "cholinergic crisis" is characterized by respiratory insufficiency in the setting of symptoms of excessive cholinergic stimulation (miosis, hyperlacrimation, hypersalivation, excessive bronchial secretions, gut hypermotility, bradycardia). Muscle fas-ciculations are another sign that the patient is in a cholinergic crisis. The distinction of myasthenic crisis from cholinergic is not always straightforward. Upon endotracheal intubation of MG patients, anticholinesterase medications are generally discontin-ued and then gradually reinstated in order to minimize their mus-carinic side effects, particularly their production of excessive airway secretions.

Botulism

Botulism is a neuroparalytic illness caused by neurotoxins pro-duced by the organism *Clostridium botulinum*, which are among the most potent known toxins.

Classification

Three modes of acquisition of botulism are recognized: food borne, wound, and intestinal colonization in adults and infants. Food-borne botulism is caused by ingestion of preformed neurotoxin from improperly canned foods. Wound botulism occurs when a traumatic wound is contaminated by spores of *C. botulinum*, which produce toxin that is systemically absorbed. Intestinal colonization occurs in the setting of alterations in endogenous gut flora. In adults, this is most commonly caused by abdominal surgery, gas-trointestinal tract abnormalities, and antibiotic use. In infants, there appears to be a window of susceptibility to intestinal coloni-zation by *C. botulinum* between ages 2 weeks and 1 year, which may be related to the establishment of normal gut flora and withdrawal from breast milk. Infants may also be at greater risk because of their small size, which renders them more vulnerable to small doses of botulinum toxin. Because infant botulism is the most frequent type, it is the focus of this section.

Epidemiology

Infant botulism usually occurs in infants between the ages of 2 weeks and 1 year (median age 10 weeks). The incidence has remained stable at 75–100 cases per year in the United States, with the most cases occurring in California, Utah, and Pennsylvania [45,46]. Exposure to contaminated dust or soil is responsible for the majority of cases of infant botulism. *Clostridium botulinum* spores are found in 20% of soil samples in the United States. Infants born into rural homes or areas of new home construction appear to be at greater risk [45,46]. Consumption of contaminated honey has become a less frequent cause of infant botulism in the United States since the institution of widespread public awareness campaigns. Although 6%–10% of commercial honey samples may contain spores of *C. botulinum*, honey consumption is now linked to only 20% of infant botulism cases in the United States compared with 59% of cases in Europe [47].

Pathophysiology

Exposure to a neurotoxin produced by the anaerobic spore-forming Gram-positive bacilli *C. botulinum* causes the great majority of cases of botulism. A handful of cases of infant botulism have been linked to *Clostridium baratii* and *Clostridium butyricum*, species closely related to *Clostridium botulinum* that produce similar neurotoxins [46]. *Clostridium botulinum* produces eight neurotoxins (types A–F), of which type A and type B cause the vast majority of disease. Botulinum toxin inhibits the presynaptic release of the neurotransmitter acetylcholine by cleaving the proteins SNAP-25 and synaptobrevin, which are required for the active exocytosis of vesicles containing acetylcholine into the synaptic cleft. Botulinum toxin is thought to irreversibly bind to presynaptic nerve terminals, and recovery is thought to require collateral sprouting of new nerve terminals to form new motor endplates, a process that takes weeks to months. Both autonomic and neuromuscular cholinergic synapses are affected, and autonomic synapses appear to recover more slowly than neuromuscular synapses [48].

Diagnosis

Infants with botulism classically present with hypotonia, a weak cry, feeding difficulty, constipation, and flaccid paralysis that begins in the cranial nerve distribution and descends symmetrically to involve the truncal and extremity muscles and finally the diaphragm. Common findings include ptosis and absence of cranial nerve reflexes (absent pupillary responses, corneal reflexes, oculocephalic reflexes). The paralysis progresses over hours to a few days. Approximately 50% of infants will require mechanical ventilation [45]. Deep tendon reflexes are usually diminished or absent. Infants typically remain afebrile. Routine laboratory investigations and serum and CSF cultures, electroencephalography, and neuroimaging are typically within normal limits.

Electrophysiologic testing provides sensitive and relatively specific evidence to support the diagnosis of infantile botulism. Nerve conduction studies reveal normal conduction velocities but may show reduced CMAPs. Rapid repetitive nerve stimulation at 20–30 Hz produces a characteristic incremental response (facilitation), whereas slow repetitive nerve stimulation at 2–3 Hz produces a decremental response. Single-fiber EMG may show increased *jitter* in incompletely paralyzed muscles, reflecting the instability in neuromuscular transmission.

In patients with botulism, there is no response to edrophonium (Tensilon), which inhibits acetylcholinesterase and prolongs the presence of acetylcholine in the region of postsynaptic AChRs, because presynaptic terminals affected by botulinum toxin are not able to release acetylcholine. Thus, a lack of improvement following administration of edrophonium is helpful in distinguishing presynaptic defects from myasthenia gravis.

Microbiologic testing provides the most sensitive and specific confirmation of the diagnosis; however, such testing may take several weeks. Isolation of *C. botulinum* spores from stool samples supports the diagnosis, whereas detection of botulinum toxin in stool or CSF samples using a mouse bioassay remains the gold standard for confirming the diagnosis. Stool samples should be collected serially until the diagnosis has been confirmed. Although naturally passed stool samples are optimal for diagnostic testing, in the frequent setting of constipation, a sterile water enema is an acceptable alternative.

The differential diagnosis of infant botulism includes sepsis, myasthenia gravis, GBS, SMA, poliomyelitis-like syndromes, tick paralysis, and organophosphate poisoning.

Treatment

Until recently, the treatment of botulism consisted of supportive care during the weeks required for natural recovery from the neuromuscular paralysis. In 2003, human botulism immune globulin (BIG) was approved in the United Stated for the treatment of infant botulism. Human BIG is manufactured from the pooled plasma of adults who have been immunized with the pentavalent botulinum vaccine, selected for samples with high titers of neutralizing antibodies against type A and B botulinum toxin. Human BIG was approved based on evidence that it significantly shortened the length of hospital stay (2.6 vs. 5.7 weeks), length of mechanical ventilation (0.7 vs. 2.4 weeks), and duration of tube feeding (3.6 vs. 10 weeks) [46]. The most common side effect of BIG was an erythematous rash occurring in 14% of infants. In the United States, BIG is available from the Centers for Disease Control and Prevention in Atlanta, Georgia. In adults, trivalent equine immunoglobulin against types A, B, and E toxins is an additional therapeutic option. The equine antitoxin is not recommended in infants because of both the 9% incidence of hypersensitivity reactions and its short half-life, which renders it less effective in infants who experience ongoing absorption of toxin from their colonized intestine.

Role of the Pediatric Intensive Care Unit Physician

Supportive care remains the mainstay of therapy. Recognition of impending respiratory insufficiency because of bulbar dysfunction or diaphragmatic and intercostal muscle weakness is essential for timely endotracheal intubation and mechanical ventilation. Medications that interfere with neuromuscular transmission should be avoided (see Table 12.5), particularly aminoglycoside antibiotics, which have been demonstrated to increase the need for ventilatory assistance in this population [49]. Nutritional support via enteral feeding should be initiated promptly. Stool samples should be monitored for *C. difficile* colitis, which may occur as a complication of colonic stasis.

Outcome

The overall prognosis of infant botulism is excellent. Infants can be expected to make a full recovery, and mortality rates for hospitalized patients are as low as 3%–5%. Infants requiring mechanical ventilation have longer hospital stays (median 38.5 days vs. 27 days for nonventilated infants) [45]. Infants should remain in the hospital until they demonstrate strong gag and cough reflexes and are able to maintain adequate oral intake to meet their nutritional requirements without enteral supplementation.

Tetanus

Epidemiology

Tetanus remains a major public health problem, causing an estimated 800,000–1,000,000 deaths per year worldwide, the great majority of which occur in the developing world [50]. Because of incomplete immunization programs, tetanus remains endemic in 90 countries worldwide [51]. Fortunately, tetanus has been largely eliminated in the developed world by active childhood immunization programs, with only 40–60 cases reported per year in the United States [52].

Tetanus is commonly classified by age of infection into neonatal and non-neonatal forms. Neonatal tetanus is most common worldwide, responsible for a nearly 500,000 infant deaths annually [50]. Neonatal tetanus is caused by contamination of the umbilical cord with *Clostridium tetani* spores during delivery because of unsanitary birth practices. It can be prevented by routine antepartum administration to expectant mothers of at least two doses of tetanus toxoid. Non-neonatal tetanus is caused by contamination of deep penetrating wounds with *C. tetani* spores. It can be prevented by active childhood immunization with at least three doses of tetanus toxoid between 2 and 6 months of age, followed by boosters at ages 15 months, 4 years, and again every 10 years.

Pathophysiology

Clostridium tetani spores are ubiquitous in the environment and in human and animal gastrointestinal flora but only become pathogenic when they germinate in a wound and produce the toxin tetanospasmin. In nonimmune individuals, tetanospasmin binds to peripheral nerves at the site of infection and undergoes retrograde axonal transport to anterior horn cells in the spinal cord. The toxin then spreads up and down the spinal cord transsynaptically. Tetanospasmin acts by cleaving synaptobrevin, which is required for neurotransmitter vesicle release at the presynaptic membrane. The primary targets of tetanospasmin are GABAergic inhibitory interneurons, resulting in a lack of inhibitory input to anterior horn cells, which leads to the characteristic clinical presentation of tetany (sustained muscular contraction). The binding of tetanospasmin is thought to be irreversible, and recovery of synaptic function is thought to require collateral sprouting of new presynaptic nerve terminals.

Diagnosis

The diagnosis is made based on the characteristic clinical presentation and a history of potential *C. tetani* exposure; however, the wound may be trivial, and in up to 30% of patients no portal of entry is found [53]. The incubation period following exposure ranges from 24 hr to several months, depending on the quantity of toxin produced and the distance of the wound from the central nervous system. Tetanus may remain localized, in which case the symptoms of muscle spasm and pain remain restricted to site of injury, and the mortality rate is low. Cephalic tetanus refers to localized tetanus caused by injury in the head and facial regions and carries a higher mortality rate.

Generalized tetanus, the most common form, presents with pain, headache, and the characteristic symptom of trismus (lockjaw), which is caused by the inability to open the mouth because of masseter spasm. In newborns, trismus may present simply as feeding difficulty and excessive drooling. The muscle rigidity and spasms subsequently generalize and become excruciatingly painful. Involvement of the paraspinal muscles results in opisthotonus, which can be so severe as to cause vertebral fractures and rhabdomyolysis. Spasms may be provoked by the mildest of stimuli, including touch, noise, and even light. It is important to remember that patients' levels of consciousness often remain normal throughout the illness, although their ability to communicate may be severely limited by the muscular rigidity. Respiratory compromise is common and may be secondary to laryngospasm or rigidity of the diaphragm and intercostal muscles. Autonomic disturbance frequently accompanies the spasms, leading to cardiac arrhythmia and blood pressure lability.

The differential diagnosis of tetanus includes rabies meningoencephalitis, strychnine poisoning, hypocalcemic tetany, and acute dystonic reactions to phenothiazines.

Treatment

The goals of therapy are to neutralize any unbound tetanus toxin and to provide supportive care until the muscular rigidity and spasms improve. Unbound tetanus toxin is eliminated by a combination of passive immunization with tetanus immunoglobulin, appropriate antibiotic therapy, and thorough debridement of the causative wound. Tetanus immunoglobulin shortens the course and may reduce the severity of the disease and thus should be administered as early as possible. The human form of immunoglobulin is preferred because of its longer half-life and lower incidence of anaphylactic reactions than the equine form. The antibiotic of choice is metronidazole, although penicillin remains the standard therapy in many parts of the world (however, penicillin can act as a competitive GABA antagonist, causing CNS hyperexcitability at high doses, potentially exacerbating tetany). Pyridoxine (vitamin B_6), a co-factor for glutamate decarboxylase, the enzyme that produces GABA, reduced the duration of spasms and mortality in an unblinded trial of 20 neonates [54].

Role of the Pediatric Intensive Care Unit Physician

Patients with generalized tetanus require sedation or paralysis for the treatment of the spasms. Curare-based neuromuscular blocking agents (pancuronium, vecuronium) are commonly used, in addition to benzodiazepines. When the control of spasms is attempted with benzodiazepines alone, the doses required invariably cause coma and respiratory depression, necessitating tracheal intubation and mechanical ventilation. Poor compliance because of muscle rigidity and spasms can be overcome using positive end-expiratory pressure (PEEP) and pressure-controlled ventilation. Tracheostomy may be required in the case of laryngospasm and should be considered electively to increase patient comfort and to facilitate oral hygiene.

Complications of tetanus include sympathetic overactivity (causing tachyarrhythmias and blood pressure lability), which may be managed with β-adrenergic blockers, and renal failure secondary to rhabdomyolysis. Because patients with tetanus are in are in a catabolic state, prompt initiation of enteral or parenteral nutrition is essential.

Outcome

Poor outcome is predicted by an interval of less than 7 days between injury and the onset of trismus and by progression to spasms within 3 days or less. The worldwide mortality rate for generalized non-neonatal tetanus is 45%–55%, and for neonatal tetanus it is greater than 60% [55]. In industrialized countries, the availability of modern intensive care has considerably reduced mortality [56]. Although muscle rigidity may persist for several months, survivors of the acute illness generally experience few long-term neurologic sequelae.

Tick Paralysis

Commonly mistaken for Guillain-Barré syndrome, the syndrome of tick paralysis should always be considered in the differential diagnosis of the child presenting with acute flaccid paralysis. Failure to consider this diagnosis and conduct a thorough search for ticks can have severe consequences, because paralysis will progress until the tick is removed or detaches spontaneously.

Epidemiology

Young children between ages 2 and 5 years are the most common victims of tick paralysis, possibly because of their relatively small body mass, which may make them more vulnerable to a given dose of toxin. Tick paralysis is also reportedly more common among girls, possibly because the tick is more difficult to find in children with long hair. Three species of ticks are responsible for the majority of disease: the Australian marsupial tick *Ixodes holocyclus*, the North American wood tick *Dermacentor andersoni*, and the common dog tick *Dermacentor variabilis*.

Pathophysiology

The causative toxin is secreted into the host by the salivary gland of the engorged tick. Neither the *Dermacentor* nor the *Ixodes* toxin has been well characterized, and the mechanism by which they cause paralysis remains unknown, with varying lines of evidence implicating both a peripheral and central nervous system site of action.

Diagnosis

Symptoms begin 2 to 6 days following attachment of the tick and may be indistinguishable from those of Guillain-Barré syndrome [57,58]. A prodromal phase consisting of fatigue, malaise, and gait instability is followed by a symmetric ascending flaccid paralysis. Early cranial nerve involvement is common, characterized by ptosis, oculomotor paresis, dilated nonreactive pupils, and bulbar weakness resulting in dysarthria and dysphagia. Respiratory insufficiency may occur as a result of bulbar dysfunction and weakness of respiratory muscles, necessitating intubation and mechanical ventilation. Deep tendon reflexes are diminished or absent. Although patients may complain of limb paresthesias, objective sensory testing remains normal. The Australian *Ixodes* tick causes a particularly severe and long-lasting paralysis that may transiently worsen for 24–28 hr following tick removal [59].

Results of complete blood counts and electrolytes are typically normal. Cerebrospinal fluid analysis is also within normal limits, in contrast to the elevated protein levels characteristic of GBS. Mild transient elevations in serum creatine kinase levels may be seen, indicating some degree of myositis or myocarditis. Electrophysiologic studies typically demonstrate a nonspecific pattern of low-amplitude CMAPs, with preservation of sensory responses and a normal response to slow and fast repetitive nerve stimulation.

Treatment

Any child presenting with acute flaccid paralysis should be carefully inspected for the presence of a tick (Figure 12.1). Ticks are usually found on the scalp, typically behind the ear. They may be well hidden, particularly in patients with long hair, and detection may literally require careful combing through the hair. Removal of the tick in its entirety should be performed using forceps, and any remaining parts should be excised and the wound disinfected. An antitoxin prepared from exposed dogs is available but has unproven efficacy in humans and carries a high risk of hypersensitivity reactions. The need for respiratory support because of bulbar or respiratory muscle weakness should be anticipated. The duration of mechanical ventilation seldom exceeds 2 weeks, and thus a tracheostomy is not usually required.

Outcome

Provided children receive adequate supportive care, they can be expected to make a full recovery. The severity of paralysis and speed of recovery depend on the causative tick species. Following removal of the North American *Dermacentor* species, complete recovery typically occurs within 24 hr. Following removal of the Australian *Ixodes* species, symptoms may transiently worsen in the 24–28 hr, and recovery may require days to several weeks. Myositis and myocarditis are occasional complications of tick paralysis but resolve spontaneously and seldom require treatment.

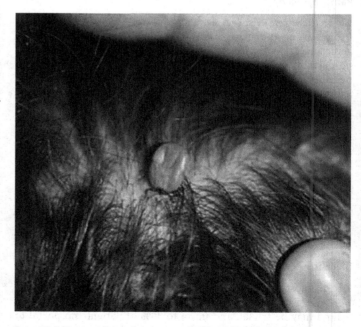

FIGURE 12.1. Engorged female *Dermacentor variabilis* tick in the scalp of a 6-year-old girl. (Felz et al. [58]. © 2000 Massachusetts Medical Society. All rights reserved. Reprinted with permission.)

Disorders of Muscle

Rhabdomyolysis

Epidemiology

Rhabdomyolysis is characterized by acute skeletal muscle fiber destruction, with release of intracellular muscle proteins, including creatine kinase (CK) (hyperCKemia) into the blood and myoglobin into the urine (myoglobinuria) [60,61]. Renal excretion of myoglobin carries the risk of renal failure. There are numerous etiologies for rhabdomyolysis (Table 12.8). Of particular relevance to the PICU population are postanesthetic crises associated with malignant hyperthermia, acute metabolic crises in patients with inborn errors of metabolism, and trauma-induced fulminant muscle necrosis. Less commonly, acute endocrinopathy can lead to metabolic decompensation (discussed later), and occasional patients will present with rhabdomyolysis as a component of neuroleptic malignant syndrome (NMS).

Elevated serum CK values alone are not necessarily sufficient for the diagnosis of rhabdomyolysis [60]. Patients with muscular dystrophy, particularly boys with mutations in the dystrophin gene, have chronically elevated serum CK values. Only during intercurrent crises, such as extreme overexertion or as an adverse reaction to anesthetic, do patients with dystrophy develop fulminant muscle necrosis. Rhabdomyolysis accounts for %–25% of all cases of acute renal failure [60]. The incidence of rhabdomyolysis in the PICU is not clearly reported.

The etiology of rhabdomyolysis relates to direct injury to the muscle fiber surface membrane or to intracellular failure of muscle energy metabolism. Induction of rhabdomyolysis can occur as a consequence of medication exposure. A careful medication exposure history must be obtained. Neuroleptic malignant syndrome, in which patients develop rhabdomyolysis and severe muscle rigidity, is classically associated with the older neuroleptics, such as haloperidol. However, NMS has been reported rarely in children treated with newer, atypical neuroleptic agents [62]. These agents are becoming more frequently prescribed in the pediatric population, and clinicians must be aware of the risk of NMS. Adults exposed to lipid-lowering agents, and to some of the medications used in the treatment of HIV disease can lead to acute rhabdomyolysis. To the best of our knowledge, this has not been reported in pediatric HIV patients or in children treated with lipid-lowering agents.

Diagnosis

Clinical diagnosis of rhabdomyolysis requires appreciation of the signs and symptoms. Children who are well-enough to articulate symptoms often complain of muscle pain, as rhabdomyolysis is typically associated with severe myalgia. Many but not all patients will manifest with clinical muscle weakness. Urinary dipstick testing may show a false-positive result for hemoglobin. Microscopic assessment of urine will be negative for red blood cells. Biochemical analyses of urine can detect very small amounts of myoglobin, and, if the serum CK and myoglobin levels reach values of more than 20,000 U/L, myoglobin becomes visible in the urine. The change in urine color is best described as resembling the color of coca-cola or tea, to be distinguished from the faintly reddish hue typically seen with hematuria.

Delineation of the etiology of acute rhabdomyolysis requires a careful review of precipitating illness or trauma. Acute viral illness can be directly causal or can be a sufficient metabolic stress to precipitate metabolic decompensation in patients with inborn errors of metabolism. Viral myositis may be best diagnosed by serum serologic measurements, such as for influenza. Parasitic infection should be considered in individuals from endemic regions. Viral-induced metabolic failure is particularly relevant in patients with defects of fatty acid metabolism (such as carnitine palmitoyltransferase deficiency), who are unable to mobilize fatty acids required for energy metabolism during viremia. Many children with fatty acid oxidation defects were otherwise completely healthy children in the past, and only after an acute triggering event is their metabolic disease identified. Other children with metabolic myopathies may report a history of limited exercise tolerance, muscle cramps, or past episodes of myoglobinuria or may have clinical features of myopathy. In patients with trauma-induced myonecrosis, it is critical to exclude compartment syndrome or localized ischemic injury. Patients with generalized burns may require fasciotomy if intramuscular pressure recordings indicate that tissue edema is impeding vascular flow to the injured muscle.

Muscle biopsy is generally of little value in the acute illness. Widespread muscle necrosis generally precludes the ability to delineate the presence or absence of any underlying myopathy or metabolic disease. In patients with suspected metabolic myopathies, diagnostic muscle biopsies should be performed after recovery from the acute illness. Investigation of metabolic muscle diseases requires specialized laboratory studies, and thus consideration should be given to patient referral to specialized centers. Paraffin-embedded muscle alone does not enable enzyme histochemistry, and thus routine muscle biopsies in centers in which histochemical analyses are not available will not be diagnostic. The

TABLE 12.8. Diagnoses to consider in the etiology of acute rhabdomyolysis.

Type of disorder	Specific disorders
Trauma	Compartment syndrome
	Crush Injury
	Burns
	Vascular compression or occlusion
	Heat stroke
Inborn error of metabolism	Defects of fatty acid oxidation
	Mitochondrial myopathies
	Glycogenoses
	Myoadenylate deaminase deficiency
Acute viral, bacterial, or parasitic infection	Influenza A or B
	Infectious mononucleosis
	Human immunodeficiency virus (HIV)
	Coxsackie virus
	Mycoplasma
	Escherichia coli sepsis
Muscular dystrophy	Dystrophinopathies (Duchenne's or Becker's muscular dystrophy)
	Calpainopathies
	Rarely other forms of muscular dystrophy
Medication induced	Neuroleptics
	Lipid-lowering agents
	HIV-associated medications
Endocrine	Diabetic ketoacidosis
	Hyperosmolar coma
	Severe hypothyroidism
	Hyokalemia
	Hypophosphatemia

laboratory techniques required to diagnose specific inborn errors of metabolism in muscle, or in cultured skin fibroblasts, are described elsewhere [60].

Treatment

The most important aspects of care for patients with rhabdomyolysis are to optimize renal perfusion and to ensure adequate hydration. Electrolyte imbalance, such as hypocalcemia, hypokalemia, or hypophosphatemia, must be corrected. Mannitol or osmotic diuretics and bicarbonate can reduce the risk of renal failure [61]. Recently, however, the value of bicarbonate and mannitol as a means of reducing the risk of renal failure in patients with acute rhabdomyolysis has been questioned [63]. In patients with renal failure and marked elevation of the serum and urine myoglobin, dialysis can be considered. Myoglobin is poorly dialyzable. Continuous venovenous hemofiltration using conventional methods or with a super high-flux membrane can lead to rapid reduction in circulating myoglobin levels [64].

Role of the Pediatric Intensive Care Unit Physician

The most important roles of the ICU physician are awareness and prompt action. Initiation of diuresis may reduce the risk of subsequent renal failure. Recognition of compression syndromes or vascular occlusion is particularly critical in comatose or sedated patients who are otherwise unable to communicate pain.

Outcome

Rhabdomyolysis is associated with a low, but still appreciable mortality. Survivors typically recover renal function over time and generally recover muscle strength. Patients with metabolic myopathies are at risk of further episodes and require detailed counseling on prevention of metabolic crises. Patients with defined metabolic disorders are encouraged to carry a detailed management care plan, generally devised in consultation with an expert in metabolic disease.

Neuromuscular Manifestations of Endocrinopathy in the Pediatric Intensive Care Unit

Epidemiology and Clinical Features

Endocrinologic dysfunction can be the precipitant of, or consequence of, critical illness. Muscle weakness can be one of the presenting features of thyrotoxic crises, diabetes insipidus, hyperosmolar coma, and adrenal insufficiency. Children with fulminant sepsis or multiorgan failure or who require multiple medications can develop hyperglycemia, adrenal suppression, and sick euthyroid syndromes, all of which may contribute to acquired muscle weakness in the critical care setting. Secondary endocrinopathic dysfunction in critically ill children not further discussed in this section, as the major clinical manifestations are discussed in the section on critical illness–acquired myopathies.

The neuromuscular effects of thyroid dysfunction include thyrotoxic myopathy, thyrotoxic hypokalemic periodic paralysis, and inhibition of neuromuscular transmission (MG) [65]. Approximately 50% of patients with hyperthyroidism experience at least some muscle weakness. Severely affected patients may experience bulbar weakness or respiratory failure. Thyrotoxic periodic paralysis is relatively rare. Patients present with recurrent attacks of weakness lasting from 30 min to several days [65]. Fluctuating weakness also occurs in patients with concomitant thyrotoxicosis and MG. A new fatal syndrome has been recently reported, largely in adolescent males, as the initial presentation of diabetes mellitus. Clinical features include hyperglycemic hyperosmolar coma complicated by a malignant hyperthermia-like picture with fever, rhabdomyolysis, and severe cardiovascular instability [66]. The increasing rate of obesity in North American children may lead to an increasing incidence of the fulminant presentation.

Pathophysiology

Thyroid dysfunction leads to an overall reduction in skeletal muscle contractility and in extreme cases can lead to muscle necrosis [65]. Thyrotoxicosis leads to a marked increase in basal metabolic rate, which in turn leads to mitochondrial energy depletion, accelerated gluconeogenesis, and lipid oxidation. The muscle weakness experienced in patients with acute diabetic ketoacidosis may relate to derangement in electrolytes. Hyperkalemia, hyperosmolality, and acidosis impair cellular metabolism in multiple tissues, including skeletal muscle.

Diagnosis

Endocrinologic crises associated with muscle weakness are diagnosed by laboratory measures of glucose, electrolytes, thyroid stimulating hormone, and thyrotoxin levels.

Treatment

Correction of acid–base balance and normalization of glucose, electrolyte, and thyroid function are the mainstay of therapy. Overall management of thyroid storm and of diabetic ketoacidosis are described in further detail elsewhere [67].

Outcome

Most children will recover from acute endocrinologic emergencies and will gradually recover muscle strength. However, a considerable mortality still exists. In particular, children with the hyperglycemic hyperosmolar syndrome have a high mortality rate and may experience multiple complications such as rhabdomyolysis and hypovolemic shock [68].

Myopathies

Epidemiology

Children with congenital myopathy or muscular dystrophy may present to the intensive care unit because of acute respiratory infection or compromise, postoperatively because of difficulty weaning from mechanical ventilation, or with progressive respiratory failure that occurs as part of their underlying disease. Acute rhabdomyolysis (discussed earlier) may occur in children with muscular dystrophy, typically in the context of excessive exertion.

Diagnosis

The diagnosis of congenital structural myopathies and muscular dystrophies is beyond the scope of this chapter. However, it is important that the PICU staff appreciate that many children with congenital myopathies can improve with age, even if they are profoundly hypotonic at birth [69]. Discussions regarding long-term prognosis should involve an experienced neuromuscular clinician and geneticist. For the intensive care staff, the key issue relates to the correct diagnosis of the acute crisis that has precipitated admission to the PICU. Acute respiratory infection must be excluded. Respiratory compromise in patients with muscular dystrophy may be associated with intercurrent chest infection or may develop as a chronic component of the underlying muscle disease [70–75]. Factors that may contribute to an apparent acute deterioration include chronic poor nutrition caused by bulbar weakness and acute or chronic hypoventilation.

A careful history may reveal symptoms of impending respiratory failure such as exertional dyspnea [75] or symptoms related to nocturnal hypoventilation [76]. Poor sleep, frequent nocturnal awakenings, night terrors or nightmares, nocturnal seizures, morning headaches, reduced school performance, and daytime hypersomnolence are symptoms of nocturnal hypoventilation [70,71,77]. For children well enough to perform pulmonary function tests, results may be useful in predicting respiratory reserve and the likelihood that the child with require mechanical ventilation. Weakness of the respiratory muscles results in a restrictive ventilatory defect and eventual hypercapnia [77]. Reduction of the vital capacity (VC) closely reflects the degree of general disability [78] and predicts the need for artificial ventilation [79]. A VC < 1.5 L, especially if combined with hypercarbia ($PaCO_2$ > 45 mm Hg) or hypoxemia (PaO_2 < 75 mm Hg), indicates that ventilatory support is needed [77]. During the period of intercostal and accessory muscle atonia associated with rapid eye movement (REM) sleep, ventilation is supported by movements of the diaphragm muscle. Diaphragmatic weakness, particularly prominent in Duchenne dystrophy, results in orthopnea and REM-sleep associated hypoventilation [70].

Admission to the PICU may also be precipitated by atelectasis or aspiration pneumonia. Many children with severe congenital myopathies or progressive muscular dystrophies have an ineffective cough, leading to mucous plugging and microatelectasis, which will eventually decrease O_2-diffusing capacity and lead to hypoxemia.

Treatment

Antibiotics, chest physiotherapy, and pulmonary toilet are the major therapies required for children with myopathies who are admitted to the PICU. Mechanical ventilation is often required but raises numerous concerns about many children regarding the likelihood of successful tracheal extubation. Children with static congenital myopathies typically wean from mechanical ventilation successfully but may still require some measure of ventilatory support. For these patients, long-term nocturnal ventilation at home can dramatically improve the quality of life [75]. Biphasic positive airway pressure (BiPAP) delivered via nasal mask is well tolerated provided the mask is fitted well and the child and family are well educated and supported in its use. It rapidly improves the nocturnal hypoxemia, restores normal sleep patterns, eliminates morning headaches, reduces daytime somnolence, and prevents cor pulmonale [76]. In a study of children with neuromuscular disease, initiation of nocturnal BiPAP led to an 85% reduction in the number of hospital admission days and a 68% reduction in the number of days of intensive care admission [80].

Patients with progressive muscular dystrophies, particularly boys with Duchenne's muscular dystrophy, may have significantly greater difficulty weaning from ventilation. Mechanical ventilation of patients with a progressive disability raises numerous ethical, financial, emotional, and practical issues for affected patients and their families. These issues must be discussed openly and ideally would have been discussed prior to an acute crisis leading to a PICU admission. In Japan, nearly all boys with Duchenne's muscular dystrophy offered assisted ventilation chose to pursue this option [79]. It has been shown that health care providers underestimate the quality of life of ventilated patients [81]. The use of assisted ventilation can prolong life by as much as 10 years [82].

Cardiac muscle involvement can be prominent in patients and manifesting carriers of dystrophinopathies and in patients with Emery Dreifuss muscular dystrophy or myotonic dystrophy [83–86]. Rarely, patients with fascioscapulohumeral [85], congenital muscular dystrophy associated with merosin deficiency (87), or sarcoglycanopathies [88,89] develop cardiac disease. Holter monitoring, His bundle electrocardiograms, or echocardiography may help define the extent of cardiac involvement and will direct cardiac management [84].

Role of the Pediatric Intensive Care Unit Physician

Correct delineation of the mechanism for acute decompensation in children with congenital muscle disease is the cornerstone of effective PICU care. A multidisciplinary approach is also essential, particularly for children facing end-of-life decisions. A dedicated respiratory care team with expertise in the management of children requiring home ventilation is invaluable, as they can provide a *real life* view of the pros and cons of invasive mechanical ventilation or noninvasive ventilation.

Peripheral Nervous System Complications of Critical Illness

Acute respiratory distress syndrome, acquired cardiac failure, renal failure, anemia of chronic illness, and acquired infection are medical issues familiar to all involved in the care of critically ill children. Muscle and nerve are also organs affected by critical illness. Failure of the PNS leads to weakness of limb, intercostals, and diaphragm muscles, which can result in respiratory compromise and the requirement of ventilatory support.

Neuromuscular complications of critical illness are associated with significant short- and long-term morbidity and prolonged PICU stays. Awareness of the impact of critical illness on nerve and muscle health is of the utmost importance if preventative strategies are to be employed and patient management optimized. Most patients who survive their underlying illness will ultimately recover their muscle strength. Failure to appreciate PNS causes of PICU-acquired weakness or paralysis may lead to false assumptions of brain damage or to other assumptions of a dismal prognosis for a child for whom potential recovery is possible. The impact of critical illness on the PNS is now reviewed as it pertains to the anterior horn cell, peripheral nerve, neuromuscular junction, and muscle. Each disease is discussed in terms of its epidemiology, clinical features, diagnostic evaluation, treatment, the role of the PICU physician, and outcome.

Pediatric Intensive Care Unit–Related Anterior Horn Cell Disorder: Hopkins Syndrome (Acute Postasthmatic Amyotrophy)

Hopkins syndrome, first reported by Hopkins and Shield in 1974, consists of a poliomyelitis-like paralysis typically occurring within

1 week of an acute asthma exacerbation [90,91]. This syndrome appears to occur only in childhood, with onset of paralysis reported between ages 13 months and 12 years (mean 5.7 years) [92].

Pathophysiology

The paralysis of Hopkins syndrome is clinically very similar to poliomyelitis and appears to be caused by the destruction of anterior horn cells. The etiology is unknown, but the most accepted theory is that of an autoimmune process. An adverse reaction to corticosteroids or other medications is unlikely, because no consistent medication was administered to all reported patients. Poliovirus infection is an unlikely cause, because nearly all reported patients had received poliovirus vaccination, and a postparalysis elevation in poliovirus titers has not been observed. Various other organisms (coxsackieviruses A and B, enterovirus, echovirus, varicella, and *Mycoplasma*) have been identified in affected patients; however, no consistent organism has been identified, and a role in the pathogenesis remains unproven.

Diagnosis

Within 1 week of an acute exacerbation of asthma, the affected patient presents with acute weakness and loss of deep tendon reflexes, developing over hours to days. Monoplegia of an arm or leg is the most common symptom, but involvement of multiple limbs and even respiratory compromise may occur. Paralysis of the affected limb is frequently total or near total. Myalgia frequently accompanies the onset of weakness, and meningismus has occasionally been reported. Sensory function is uniformly preserved.

Cerebrospinal fluid examination may be normal or may show pleocytosis or elevated protein. The findings on electromyography and nerve conduction studies are identical to those of the poliomyelitis-like syndrome, with diminution or loss of CMAPs, and preservation of nerve conduction velocities and sensory nerve action potentials. Spinal MRI may be normal or may show high signal on T2 and FLAIR sequences in the cord, which may be localized to the anterior horn cells [93].

Treatment

As with poliomyelitis-like syndromes, treatment is supportive. There is no proven therapy to slow the progression of the paralysis or to facilitate recovery. There is one case report of a 15-year-old boy who experienced nearly complete recovery following treatment with IVIG [94].

Role of the Pediatric Intensive Care Unit Physician

Although Hopkins syndrome is rare, awareness on the part of the PICU physician is important. The diagnosis of acute postasthmatic amyotrophy should be considered for any child who experiences recurrent respiratory compromise following an asthma exacerbation, particularly in the setting of limb weakness. Patients and family members should be advised before hospital discharge of the potential for this syndrome and instructed to seek medical attention at the earliest signs of myalgia, weakness, or worsening respiratory status.

Outcome

The paralysis of untreated Hopkins syndrome is usually permanent, with little or no recovery of function in affected muscle groups. The affected muscles become atrophic over several weeks. Electromyography usually fails to demonstrate any evidence of muscle reinnervation. Physiotherapy may allow patients to partially compensate for their weakness by training adjacent unaffected muscle groups.

Pediatric Intensive Care Unit–Acquired Focal Neuropathies

The impact of critical illness on the peripheral nerve can manifest as a focal dysfunction, typically associated with nerve compression or traumatic injury, or as a more general polyneuropathy. Acquired generalized dysfunction of peripheral nerves, often associated with sepsis, is discussed later in the section on muscle, as the two conditions are often co-existent.

The incidence of development of compressive neuropathy in pediatric ICU patients is not well documented. In a prospective study of 830 children cared for in our PICU over a 12-month period, 2 children were identified with focal neuropathy [95]. However, mild focal weakness is likely underappreciated during PICU admission and may be fully appreciated only as a child approaches more active stages of recovery.

Compressive and traumatic neuropathies result from damage to focal regions of the peripheral nerve. Compression typically leads to focal demyelination, often with preservation of the underlying axon. The region of peripheral nerve myelin under compression is displaced from the areas of high pressure to adjacent regions, leading to exposure and subsequent demyelination of myelin internodes [96]. Surgical or external trauma to the phrenic nerve may be complete, with transection of the entire nerve, or partial in which the nerve may be stretched leading to injury to the axon with preservation of the overlying myelin sheath. Compression neuropathy can occur in the absence of external force when local tissue edema or hematoma leads to compression of the nerve in an enclosed space. As an example, focal or generalized edema of the distal upper extremity can lead to compression of the median nerve as it passes under the flexor retinaculum at the wrist. Compartment syndromes can also be associated with nerve compression, although the mechanism in these cases may relate more to pressure-induced ischemia.

The nerve fibers most sensitive to compression are the large, myelinated fibers, and thus vibration and position sense may be the first clinical manifestations. Continued compression leads to axonal damage, termed neurapraxia. Depending on the extent of nerve injury, recovery typically proceeds over 6–8 weeks.

Diagnosis requires recognition that muscle weakness corresponds to the innervation pattern of a specific nerve. Patients with rapid weight loss, constitutively thin body habitus, and patients exposed to prolong bed rest, prolonged care in a fixed position, or immobilization with fixed restraints are a particular risk for compressive neuropathies. The typical sites of compressive neuropathy include the common peroneal, femoral, and ulnar nerves. Injury to the phrenic nerve because of chest surgery for trauma is also a well-recognized issue in PICU patients. Peroneal neuropathy is caused by compression of the common peroneal nerve as it cross medially over the fibula and occurs in patients who require prolonged positioning in the lateral decubitus position or whose lower limb was held in a fixed position by a pressure restraint. Damage to the common peroneal nerve leads to weakness of dorsiflexion of the ankle (foot drop), inability to evert at the ankle, and numbness over the lateral aspect of the lower leg. Femoral neuropathy is caused by compression of the femoral nerve and typically occurs in patients who require prolonged care in the prone position. Femoral neuropathy manifests as inability to extend at the knee because of weakness of the quadriceps muscle, numbness over the anterior aspect of the thigh and medial aspect of the lower leg, and it is associated with loss of the knee jerk reflex. Ulnar neuropathy is mediated by compressive injury to the ulnar nerve at the elbow and occurs relatively infrequently. Ulnar neuropathy presents as weakness of wrist flexion and small muscles of the hand and numbness of the last three digits and palm. Phrenic nerve dysfunction is demonstrated by ultrasound evidence of paradoxical diaphragm movement and absence of diaphragm contraction.

Nerve conduction studies demonstrate reduced nerve transmission, or complete conduction block, above the site of compression. Needle examination of weak muscles will demonstrate denervation characterized by polyphasic motor units and fibrillations.

Treatment is largely supportive. Nursing care should be optimized to remove ongoing compression. Frequent changes in patient positioning and use of an air mattress are helpful. Physiotherapy should be instituted promptly to maintain range of motion, to increase muscle activation, and to avoid contractures. Surgical fixation of the diaphragm muscle (plication) can improve respiratory function in patients with phrenic nerve injury. Patients who do not recover from compression neuropathies would be considered for tendon transfers or other surgical strategies. These procedures are not part of the PICU care.

The most important role of the PICU physician is to reduce the risk of compression neuropathies. Education of PICU staff on the importance of patient positioning and embracing a philosophy of early mobilization of critically ill patients will reduce the risk of compression neuropathies. Most patients will ultimately recover functional strength in the affected region of compression neuropathies. Loss of muscle bulk is not always regained. Phrenic nerve injury, especially surgical transaction of the phrenic nerve, typically does not recover spontaneously, but plication of the diaphragm is associated with improvement in respiratory function.

Pediatric Intensive Care Unit–Related Disorders of the Neuromuscular Junction

Approximately 20% of patients will develop limb and occasionally ocular weakness if treated for more than 6 days with neuromuscular blocking agents [97]. Neonates treated for several weeks with neuromuscular blockage developed muscle atrophy and fixed muscle contractures [98]. Prolonged paralysis following neuromuscular blockade has also been reported in children [99].

The metabolism of nondepolarizing neuromuscular blocking agents varies depending on the agent used. Vecuronium is metabolized by the liver and is primarily eliminated in bile, with only 10%–25% of the drug undergoing renal excretion [100]. Pancuronium and tubocurarine are predominantly excreted by the kidney. Reduced hepatic metabolism of neuromuscular blocking agents has been well documented in patients with liver failure, sepsis, and critical illness [97,101], leading to impaired neuromuscular junction transmission that far exceeds the normal duration of pharmacologic blockade. Markedly elevated serum levels of vecuronium and its metabolite 3-desacetylvecuronium have been documented in a patient with profound muscle paralysis and hepatic dysfunction more than 14 days following cessation of vecuronium therapy [101].

Autopsy studies of adults exposed to prolonged neuromuscular blockade who subsequently succumbed from their underlying illness demonstrated upregulation of nicotinic acetylcholine receptors at the postsynaptic junction [102]. These findings are similar to the response of the postsynaptic region of muscle to denervation and suggest that pharmacologically mediated neuromuscular blockade may have similar pathobiology to that of polyneuropathy.

In addition to neuromuscular blocking agents, exposures to aminoglycoside antibiotics, acidosis, and hypermagnesemia have also been found to impair neuromuscular transmission [103]. Treatment with aminoglycoside antibiotics has been shown to reduce presynaptic release of acetylcholine. Aminoglycoside antibiotic therapy alone rarely reduces neuromuscular transmission sufficiently to lead to clinical muscle weakness but may contribute to prolonged weakness in children exposed to depolarizing or nondepolarizing agents.

A history of exposure to medications that impair neuromuscular transmission in a patient with acquired muscle weakness should prompt an evaluation to exclude persistent neuromuscular blockade. Bedside examination using the "train of four" repetitive stimulation test can be used to determine whether neuromuscular transmission is impaired [103]. Supportive therapy is required until the putative pharmacologic agent is metabolized. If the child is receiving medications, such as aminoglycoside antibiotics, that impair neuromuscular transmission, use of alternative therapies should be considered if possible.

In children for whom muscle weakness is solely on the basis of neuromuscular blockade, full recovery of muscle strength is expected. Prolonged exposure to neuromuscular blocking agents increases the risk of disuse atrophy and muscle contractures and has been implicated as a risk factor for acute quadriplegic myopathy (discussed below).

Pediatric Intensive Care Unit–Related Disorders of Muscle

The development of muscle weakness is a well-recognized, serious sequela of critical illness in adults [104–107] and more rarely in critically ill children [95]. In adults with sepsis and multiorgan failure, the incidence of muscle weakness often manifesting as failure to wean from mechanical ventilation approaches 70% [108]. In a prospective study of patients with status asthmaticus requiring mechanical ventilation, high-dose corticosteroids, and neuromuscular blockade, 76% were documented to have elevated serum CK levels, and 36% developed muscle weakness of a severity that necessitated prolonged ventilatory support [109].

Several forms of critical illness–associated muscle weakness have been described: critical illness myopathy (CIM) or acute quadriplegic myopathy (AQM), necrotizing myopathy, and critical illness polyneuropathy (CIP). Persistence of neuromuscular blockade was discussed earlier. In a prospective study performed in the PICU at our institution, 14 of 830 children (1.7%) developed muscle weakness [95]. Muscle biopsies specimens from three children confirmed AQM. Eight of the 14 children (50%) had received solid organ or bone marrow transplantation, suggesting that this subgroup of the PICU population may be at particular risk for PICU-acquired muscle weakness.

Multiorgan failure, organ transplantation, status asthmaticus, sepsis, and prolonged exposure to neuromuscular blocking agents or corticosteroids are putative risk factors for the development of muscle weakness [104,105,110–114]. Prolonged immobility alone likely contributes significantly to muscle weakness [115]. Antigravity muscle movements are important signals for muscle growth and for maintenance of muscle health, as evidenced by the negative effects of space travel on muscle integrity [116,117].

Critical illness is associated with profound catabolic stress, immobilization, and elevated circulating levels of proinflammatory and antiinflammatory cytokines [118]. Breakdown of muscle proteins provides amino acids essential for hepatic gluconeogenesis and for oxidation directly for cellular energy [119]. Muscle proteolysis is increased in critical illness, mediated through the ubiquitin-proteasomal, calcium-dependent calpain and the ATP-independent, lysosomal cathepsin B pathways [119,120]. The availability of myofibrillar proteins for degradation to amino acids is controlled in part through the activity of m-calpain, a calcium-dependent protease situated at the z-disc of skeletal muscle that functions to release myosin thick filaments from the sarcomere [121]. Myosin thick filament loss is prominent in atrophic fibers in AQM. Electrophoretic studies of muscle from patients with AQM reveal a markedly reduced ration of myosin relative to actin [122]. Activation of the transforming growth factor (TGF)-β/MAPK pathway has been recently demonstrated, implicating proapoptotic mechanisms in the etiology of AQM [123]. The presence of DNA fragmentation and abnormalities of nuclear morphology in atrophic fibers further supports a role for apoptosis in AQM [124].

The presence of one or more of muscle weakness, loss of muscle bulk, reduced or absent tendon reflexes, elevated serum CK values, or failure to wean from mechanical ventilation should prompt consideration of critical illness–acquired muscle weakness. Laboratory investigations should include serum CK; and electrolyte imbalance, profound hypothyroidism, or marked deficiency of carnitine should be excluded. With the exception of necrotizing myopathy, serum CK values are normal or reduced in most patients with critical illness–associated weakness.

Electromyographic studies are helpful in distinguishing CIP from CIM/AQM. In patients with CIM or AQM, nerve conduction velocities of motor and sensory nerves are normal, but needle examination reveals small-amplitude motor unit potentials and fibrillations [114]. In patients with severe weakness, muscle may be electrically inexcitable [125]. Electromyographic studies in patients with CIP demonstrate slowing of motor and/or sensory nerve conduction [126].

Clinical and electrodiagnostic studies are often sufficient for the diagnosis of critical illness–acquired muscle weakness. However, confirmation of the diagnosis is aided by pathologic study of muscle. Muscle biopsy tissue features of AQM include muscle fiber atrophy and basophilia, selective loss of myosin thick filaments in atrophic fibers, and increased immunoreactivity of affected fibers for proteolytic enzymes [111,127–129]. Muscle fiber necrosis is rare in AQM but is the pathologic hallmark of toxic/necrotizing myopathy [130]. Biopsy findings of atrophy of type I and type II fibers are characteristic of CIP, although recent electron microscopy studies have shown myosin thick filament loss even in patients in whom the clinical phenotype and routine histochemistry studies in muscle suggest CIP [131].

Various strategies have been proposed to reduce the incidence of muscle weakness during critical illness. Passive stretching [132], electrical stimulation [133], and early mobilization [118] have all been advocated. These strategies can be implemented at the bedside and in most patients can be initiated almost immediately after admission to the PICU. Hemodynamic instability and placement of indwelling catheters are limitation in many PICU patients but often do not preclude passive range of motion exercises.

Protein hyperalimentation was shown to reduce myofibrillar proteolysis [134]. Provision of protein nutrition as a means to reduce catabolism of muscle proteins is biologically plausible [135], and it has been shown that malnutrition leads to increased fatigability and impaired muscle contractility [136]. However, aggressive nutritional support does not prevent protein loss in critically ill adults [137,138], suggesting that provision of amino acids through the gut may not be sufficient to reduce mobilization of myofibrillar proteins during catabolic crises. Further study of nutritional intervention in critical illness is required [139]. Future therapeutic strategies may include interruption of the proteolytic and proapoptotic components of the MAPK cascade implicated in AQM [123].

Appropriate diagnosis of acquired muscle weakness is of the utmost importance to avoid falsely attributing lack of purposeful limb movement to impairment of the central nervous system. In a series of comatose adults with quadriparesis caused by AQM rather than to brain injury, six of seven patients recovered fully despite the fatal outcome predicted by their attending physicians [104]. Critical illness–associated muscle weakness is associated with significant morbidity both during the acute illness and in the months that follow [118]. Reduced exercise tolerance has been documented up to 2 years after lung transplantation [140,141] and up to 12 months after acute respiratory distress syndrome [142]. Ultimately, many patients, even those with profound weakness, can recover fully. This point must be recognized by the PICU staff involved in the counseling of families of critically ill children.

Conclusion

Multiorgan failure in critical illness can include muscle and nerve, and more research is needed to reduce neuromuscular complications of critical illness. Strategies might include nutritional support and specifically designed physiotherapy techniques. Future interventions may utilize medications that can impede the pathobiologic cascade leading to loss of muscle proteins, reduce the release of harmful cytokines, or decrease oxidative stress. Patient care strategies to avoid preventable complications of critical illness, such as compression neuropathies, should be optimized in all intensive care units.

References

1. Pearn JH. The gene frequency of acute Werdnig-Hoffmann disease (SMA type 1). A total population survey in North-East England. J Med Genet 1973;10(3):260–265.
2. Pearn J. Incidence, prevalence, and gene frequency studies of chronic childhood spinal muscular atrophy. J Med Genet 1978;15(6):409–4013.
3. Zerres K, Rudnik-Schoneborn S, Forrest E, Lusakowska A, Borkowska J, Hausmanowa-Petrusewicz I. A collaborative study on the natural history of childhood and juvenile onset proximal spinal muscular atrophy (type II and III SMA): 569 patients. J Neurol Sci 1997;146(1):67–72.
4. Lefebvre S, Burlet P, Liu Q, Bertrandy S, Clermont O, Munnich A, et al. Correlation between severity and SMN protein level in spinal muscular atrophy. Nat Genet 1997;16(3):265–269.
5. Ben Hamida M, Hentati F, Ben Hamida C. Hereditary motor system diseases (chronic juvenile amyotrophic lateral sclerosis). Conditions combining a bilateral pyramidal syndrome with limb and bulbar amyotrophy. Brain 1990;113(Pt 2):347–363.

6. Rabin BA, Griffin JW, Crain BJ, Scavina M, Chance PF, Cornblath DR. Autosomal dominant juvenile amyotrophic lateral sclerosis. Brain 1999;122(Pt 8):1539–1550.

7. Rosen DR, Sapp P, O'Regan J, McKenna-Yasek D, Schlumpf KS, Haines JL, et al. Genetic linkage analysis of familial amyotrophic lateral sclerosis using human chromosome 21 microsatellite DNA markers. Am J Med Genet 1994;51(1):61–69.

8. Bensimon G, Lacomblez L, Meininger V. A controlled trial of riluzole in amyotrophic lateral sclerosis. ALS/Riluzole Study Group. N Engl J Med 1994;330(9):585–591.

9. Borasio GD, Miller RG. Clinical characteristics and management of ALS. Semin Neurol 2001;21(2):155–166.

10. Mostashari F, Bunning ML, Kitsutani PT, Singer DA, Nash D, Cooper MJ, et al. Epidemic West Nile encephalitis, New York, 1999: results of a household-based seroepidemiological survey. Lancet 2001;358(9278):261–264.

11. Petersen LR, Marfin AA, Gubler DJ. West Nile virus. JAMA 2003;290(4):524–528.

12. West Nile Virus Surveillance and Control: An Update for Health-Care Providers in New York City. New York: New York City Department of Health; 2001.

13. Madden K. West Nile virus infection and its neurological manifestations. Clin Med Res 2003;1(2):145–150.

14. Leis AA, Stokic DS. Neuromuscular manifestations of human West Nile virus infection. Curr Treat Options Neurol 2005;7(1):15–22.

15. Watson NK, Bartt RE, Houff SA, Leurgans SE, Schneck MJ. Focal neurological deficits and West Nile virus infection. Clin Infect Dis 2005;40(7):e59–e62.

16. CDC. Progress toward global eradication of poliomyelitis, 2002. MMWR 2003;52:366–369.

17. Jeha LE, Sila CA, Lederman RJ, Prayson RA, Isada CM, Gordon SM. West Nile virus infection: a new acute paralytic illness. Neurology 2003;61(1):55–59.

18. Sejvar JJ, Leis AA, Stokic DS, Van Gerpen JA, Marfin AA, Webb R, et al. Acute flaccid paralysis and West Nile virus infection. Emerg Infect Dis 2003;9(7):788–793.

19. Al-Shekhlee A, Katirji B. Electrodiagnostic features of acute paralytic poliomyelitis associated with West Nile virus infection. Muscle Nerve 2004;29(3):376–380.

20. Hahn AF. Guillain-Barré syndrome. Lancet 1998;352(9128):635–641.

21. Morris AM, Elliott EJ, D'Souza RM, Antony J, Kennett M, Longbottom H. Acute flaccid paralysis in Australian children. J Paediatr Child Health 2003;39(1):22–26.

22. Yuki N. Infectious origins of, and molecular mimicry in, Guillain-Barré and Fisher syndromes. Lancet Infect Dis 2001;1(1):29–37.

23. Jones HR. Childhood Guillain-Barre syndrome: clinical presentation, diagnosis, and therapy. J Child Neurol 1996;11(1):4–12.

24. Hughes RA, Wijdicks EF, Barohn R, Benson E, Cornblath DR, Hahn AF, et al. Practice parameter: immunotherapy for Guillain-Barre syndrome: report of the Quality Standards Subcommittee of the American Academy of Neurology. Neurology 2003;61(6):736–740.

25. Abd-Allah SA, Jansen PW, Ashwal S, Perkin RM. Intravenous immunoglobulin as therapy for pediatric Guillain-Barre syndrome. J Child Neurol 1997;12(6):376–380.

26. Chalela JA. Pearls and pitfalls in the intensive care management of Guillain-Barre syndrome. Semin Neurol 2001;21(4):399–405.

27. Lawn ND, Fletcher DD, Henderson RD, Wolter TD, Wijdicks EF. Anticipating mechanical ventilation in Guillain-Barre syndrome. Arch Neurol 2001;58(6):893–898.

28. Tripathi M, Kaushik S. Carbamazepine for pain management in Guillain-Barre syndrome patients in the intensive care unit. Crit Care Med 2000;28(3):655–658.

29. Moulin DE, Hagen N, Feasby TE, Amireh R, Hahn A. Pain in Guillain-Barre syndrome. Neurology 1997;48(2):328–331.

30. Hughes RA, Newsom-Davis JM, Perkin GD, Pierce JM. Controlled trial prednisolone in acute polyneuropathy. Lancet 1978;2(8093):750–753.

31. Chio A, Cocito D, Leone M, Giordana MT, Mora G, Mutani R. Guillain-Barre syndrome: a prospective, population-based incidence and outcome survey. Neurology 2003;60(7):1146–1150.

32. Bos AP, van der Meche FG, Witsenburg M, van der Voort E. Experiences with Guillain-Barre syndrome in a pediatric intensive care unit. Intensive Care Med 1987;13(5):328–331.

33. Andrews PI. Autoimmune myasthenia gravis in childhood. Semin Neurol 2004;24(1):101110.

34. Harper CM. Congenital myasthenic syndromes. Semin Neurol 2004;24(1):111–123.

35. Hoch W, McConville J, Helms S, Newsom-Davis J, Melms A, Vincent A. Auto-antibodies to the receptor tyrosine kinase MuSK in patients with myasthenia gravis without acetylcholine receptor antibodies. Nat Med 2001;7(3):365–368.

36. Vincent A, Bowen J, Newsom-Davis J, McConville J. Seronegative generalised myasthenia gravis: clinical features, antibodies, and their targets. Lancet Neurol 2003;2(2):99–106.

37. Keesey JC. Clinical evaluation and management of myasthenia gravis. Muscle Nerve 2004;29(4):484–505.

38. Gajdos P, Chevret S, Clair B, Tranchant C, Chastang C. Clinical trial of plasma exchange and high-dose intravenous immunoglobulin in myasthenia gravis. Myasthenia Gravis Clinical Study Group. Ann Neurol 1997;41(6):789–796.

39. Qureshi AI, Choudhry MA, Akbar MS, Mohammad Y, Chua HC, Yahia AM, et al. Plasma exchange versus intravenous immunoglobulin treatment in myasthenic crisis. Neurology 1999;52(3):629–632.

40. Stricker RB, Kwiatkowska BJ, Habis JA, Kiprov DD. Myasthenic crisis. Response to plasmapheresis following failure of intravenous gammaglobulin. Arch Neurol 1993;50(8):837–840.

41. Evoli A, Batocchi AP, Bartoccioni E, Lino MM, Minisci C, Tonali P. Juvenile myasthenia gravis with prepubertal onset. Neuromuscul Disord 1998;8(8):561–567.

42. Kolski HK, Kim PC, Vajsar J. Video-assisted thoracoscopic thymectomy in juvenile myasthenia gravis. J Child Neurol 2001;16(8):569–573.

43. Jaretzki A, Steinglass KM, Sonett JR. Thymectomy in the management of myasthenia gravis. Semin Neurol 2004;24(1):49–62.

44. Juel VC. Myasthenia gravis: management of myasthenic crisis and perioperative care. Semin Neurol 2004;24(1):75–81.

45. Thompson JA, Filloux FM, Van Orman CB, Swoboda K, Peterson P, Firth SD, et al. Infant botulism in the age of botulism immune globulin. Neurology 2005;64(12):2029–2032.

46. Fox CK, Keet CA, Strober JB. Recent advances in infant botulism. Pediatr Neurol 2005;32(3):149–154.

47. Aureli P, Franciosa G, Fenicia L. Infant botulism and honey in Europe: a commentary. Pediatr Infect Dis J 2002;21(9):866–868.

48. Vita G, Girlanda P, Puglisi RM, Marabello L, Messina C. Cardiovascular-reflex testing and single-fiber electromyography in botulism. A longitudinal study. Arch Neurol 1987;44(2):202–206.

49. Wilson R, Morris JG, Jr., Snyder JD, Feldman RA. Clinical characteristics of infant botulism in the United States: a study of the non-California cases. Pediatr Infect Dis J 1982;1(3):148–150.

50. Dietz V, Milstien JB, van Loon F, Cochi S, Bennett J. Performance and potency of tetanus toxoid: implications for eliminating neonatal tetanus. Bull WHO 1996;74(6):619–628.

51. Whitman C, Belgharbi L, Gasse F, Torel C, Mattei V, Zoffmann H. Progress towards the global elimination of neonatal tetanus. World Health Stat Q 1992;45(2–3):248–256.

52. Leads from the MMWR. Tetanus—United States, 1982–1984. JAMA 1985;254(20):2873, 2877–2878.

53. Farrar JJ, Yen LM, Cook T, Fairweather N, Binh N, Parry J, et al. Tetanus. J Neurol Neurosurg Psychiatry 2000;69(3):292–301.

54. Godel JC. Trial of pyridoxine therapy for tetanus neonatorum. J Infect Dis 1982;145(4):547–549.

55. Brook I. Tetanus in children. Pediatr Emerg Care 2004;20(1):48–51.

56. Khoo BH, Lee EL, Lam KL. Neonatal tetanus treated with high dosage diazepam. Arch Dis Child 1978;53(9):737–739.

57. Vedanarayanan V, Sorey WH, Subramony SH. Tick paralysis. Semin Neurol 2004;24(2):181–184.

58. Felz MW, Smith CD, Swift TR. A six-year-old girl with tick paralysis. N Engl J Med 2000;342(2):90–94.

59. Grattan-Smith PJ, Morris JG, Johnston HM, Yiannikas C, Malik R, Russell R, et al. Clinical and neurophysiological features of tick paralysis. Brain 1997;120 (Pt 11):1975–1987.

60. Lofberg M, Jankala H, Paetau A, Harkonen M, Somer H. Metabolic causes of recurrent rhabdomyolysis. Acta Neurol Scand 1998;98(4):268–275.

61. Tein I, DiMauro S, Rowland L. Myoglobinuria. In: Rowland L, DiMauro S, eds. Handbook of Clinical Neurology. New York: Elsevier Science; 1992:553–593.

62. Hanft A, Eggleston CF, Bourgeois JA. Neuroleptic malignant syndrome in an adolescent after brief exposure to olanzapine. J Child Adolesc Psychopharmacol 2004;14(3):481–487.

63. Brown CV, Rhee P, Evans K, Demetriades D, Velmahos G. Rhabdomyolysis after penetrating trauma. Am Surg 2004;70(10):890–892.

64. Naka T, Jones D, Baldwin I, Fealy N, Bates S, Goehl H, et al. Myoglobin clearance by super high-flux hemofiltration in a case of severe rhabdomyolysis: a case report. Crit Care 2005;9(2):R90–R95.

65. Doherty C. The neurological manifestations of thyroid disease. In: Noseworthy J, ed. Neurological Therapeutics: Principles and Practice. London: Martin Dunitz; 2003:1455–1463.

66. Hollander AS, Olney RC, Blackett PR, Marshall BA. Fatal malignant hyperthermia-like syndrome with rhabdomyolysis complicating the presentation of diabetes mellitus in adolescent males. Pediatrics 2003;111(6 Pt 1):1447–1452.

67. Goldberg PA, Inzucchi SE. Critical issues in endocrinology. Clin Chest Med 2003;24(4):583–606.

68. Carchman RM, Dechert-Zeger M, Calikoglu AS, Harris BD. A new challenge in pediatric obesity: pediatric hyperglycemic hyperosmolar syndrome. Pediatr Crit Care Med 2005;6(1):20–24.

69. Wallgren-Pettersson C, Thomas N. 45th ENMC Workshop: Myotubular Myopathy. September13–15, 1996, Naarden, the Netherlands. Neuromuscul Disord 1997;7(4):268–271.

70. Barbe F, Quera-Salva MA, McCann C, Gajdos P, Raphael JC, de Lattre J, et al. Sleep-related respiratory disturbances in patients with Duchenne muscular dystrophy. Eur Respir J 1994;7(8):1403–1408.

71. Barthlen GM. Nocturnal respiratory failure as an indication of non-invasive ventilation in the patient with neuromuscular disease. Respiration 1997;64(Suppl 1):35–38.

72. Birnkrant DJ, Pope JF, Eiben RM. Management of the respiratory complications of neuromuscular diseases in the pediatric intensive care unit. J Child Neurol 1999;14(3):139–143.

73. Howard RS, Wiles CM, Hirsch NP, Spencer GT. Respiratory involvement in primary muscle disorders: assessment and management. Q J Med 1993;86(3):175–189.

74. Kelly BJ, Luce JM. The diagnosis and management of neuromuscular diseases causing respiratory failure. Chest 1991;99(6):1485–1494.

75. Polkey MI, Lyall RA, Moxham J, Leigh PN. Respiratory aspects of neurological disease. J Neurol Neurosurg Psychiatry 1999;66(1):5–15.

76. Heckmatt JZ, Loh L, Dubowitz V. Nocturnal hypoventilation in children with nonprogressive neuromuscular disease. Pediatrics 1989;83(2):250–255.

77. Scheuerbrandt G. First meeting of the Duchenne Parent Project in Europe: Treatment of Duchenne Muscular Dystrophy. November 7–8, 1997, Rotterdam, the Netherlands. Neuromuscul Disord 1998;8(3–4):213–219.

78. Smith PE, Calverley PM, Edwards RH, Evans GA, Campbell EJ. Practical problems in the respiratory care of patients with muscular dystrophy. N Engl J Med 1987;316(19):1197–1205.

79. Fukunaga H, Okubo R, Moritoyo T, Kawashima N, Osame M. Long-term follow-up of patients with Duchenne muscular dystrophy receiving ventilatory support. Muscle Nerve 1993;16(5):554–558.

80. Katz S, Selvadurai H, Keilty K, Mitchell M, MacLusky I. Outcome of non-invasive positive pressure ventilation in paediatric neuromuscular disease. Arch Dis Child 2004;89(2):121–124.

81. Bach JR, Campagnolo DI, Hoeman S. Life satisfaction of individuals with Duchenne muscular dystrophy using long-term mechanical ventilatory support. Am J Phys Med Rehabil 1991;70(3):129–135.

82. Yasuma F, Sakai M, Matsuoka Y. Effects of noninvasive ventilation on survival in patients with Duchenne's muscular dystrophy. Chest 1996;109(2):590.

83. Ortiz-Lopez R, Li H, Su J, Goytia V, Towbin JA. Evidence for a dystrophin missense mutation as a cause of X-linked dilated cardiomyopathy. Circulation 1997;95(10):2434–2440.

84. Stollberger C, Finsterer J, Keller H, Mamoli B, Slany J. Progression of cardiac involvement in patients with myotonic dystrophy, Becker's muscular dystrophy and mitochondrial myopathy during a 2-year follow-up. Cardiology 1998;90(3):173–179.

85. de Visser M, de Voogt WG, la Riviere GV. The heart in Becker muscular dystrophy, fascioscapulohumeral dystrophy, and Bethlem myopathy. Muscle Nerve 1992;15(5):591–596.

86. Harper PS, Rudel R, Faole R, Camici PG, Muntoni F. Myotonic dystrophy. In: Engel AG, Franzini-Armstrong C, ed. Myology. New York: McGraw-Hill; 1994:1192–1219.

87. Spyrou N, Philpot J, Foale R, Camici PG, Muntoni F. Evidence of left ventricular dysfunction in children with merosin-deficient congenital muscular dystrophy. Am Heart J 1998;136(3):474–476.

88. Melacini P, Fanin M, Duggan DJ, Freda MP, Berardinelli A, Danieli GA, et al. Heart involvement in muscular dystrophies due to sarcoglycan gene mutations. Muscle Nerve 1999;22(4):473–479.

89. Mascarenhas DA, Spodick DH, Chad DA, Gilchrist J, Townes PL, DeGirolami U, et al. Cardiomyopathy of limb-girdle muscular dystrophy. J Am Coll Cardiol 1994;24(5):1328–1333.

90. Hopkins IJ. A new syndrome: poliomyelitis-like illness associated with acute asthma in childhood. Aust Paediatr J 1974;10(5):273–276.

91. Hopkins IJ, Shield LK. Letter: poliomyelitis-like illness associated with asthma in childhood. Lancet 1974;1(7860):760.

92. Liedholm LJ, Eeg-Olofsson O, Ekenberg BE, Nicolaysen RB, Torbergsen T. Acute postasthmatic amyotrophy (Hopkins' syndrome). Muscle Nerve 1994;17(7):769–772.

93. Arita J, Nakae Y, Matsushima H, Maekawa K. Hopkins syndrome: T2-weighted high intensity of anterior horn on spinal MR imaging. Pediatr Neurol 1995;13(3):263–265.

94. Cohen HA, Ashkenasi A, Ring H, Weiss R, Wolach B, Paret G, et al. Poliomyelitis-like syndrome following asthmatic attack (Hopkins' syndrome)—recovery associated with i.v. gamma globulin treatment. Infection 1998;26(4):247–249.

95. Banwell BL, Mildner RJ, Hassall AC, Becker LE, Vajsar J, Shemie SD. Muscle weakness in critically ill children. Neurology 2003;61(12):1779–1782.

96. Ochoa J, Fowler TJ, Gilliatt RW. Anatomical changes in peripheral nerves compressed by a pneumatic tourniquet. J Anat 1972;113(3):433–455.

97. Op de Coul AA, Lambregts PC, Koeman J, van Puyenbroek MJ, Ter Laak HJ, Gabreels-Festen AA. Neuromuscular complications in patients given Pavulon (pancuronium bromide) during artificial ventilation. Clin Neurol Neurosurg 1985;87(1):17–22.

98. Rutledge ML, Hawkins EP, Langston C. Skeletal muscle growth failure induced in premature newborn infants by prolonged pancuronium treatment. J Pediatr 1986;109(5):883–886.

99. Benzing G, 3rd, Iannaccone ST, Bove KE, Keebler PJ, Shockley LL. Prolonged myasthenic syndrome after one week of muscle relaxants. Pediatr Neurol 1990;6(3):190–196.

100. Bencini AF, Scaf AH, Sohn YJ, Meistelman C, Lienhart A, Kersten UW, et al. Disposition and urinary excretion of vecuronium bromide in anesthetized patients with normal renal function or renal failure. Anesth Analg 1986;65(3):245–251.

101. Barohn RJ, Jackson CE, Rogers SJ, Ridings LW, McVey AL. Prolonged paralysis due to nondepolarizing neuromuscular blocking agents and corticosteroids. Muscle Nerve 1994;17(6):647–654.

102. Dodson BA, Kelly BJ, Braswell LM, Cohen NH. Changes in acetylcholine receptor number in muscle from critically ill patients receiving muscle relaxants: an investigation of the molecular mechanism of prolonged paralysis. Crit Care Med 1995;23(5):815–821.

103. Segredo V, Caldwell JE, Matthay MA, Sharma ML, Gruenke LD, Miller RD. Persistent paralysis in critically ill patients after long-term administration of vecuronium. N Engl J Med 1992;327(8):524–528.

104. Latronico N, Fenzi F, Recupero D, Guarneri B, Tomelleri G, Tonin P, et al. Critical illness myopathy and neuropathy. Lancet 1996;347(9015): 1579–1582.

105. Lacomis D, Petrella JT, Giuliani MJ. Causes of neuromuscular weakness in the intensive care unit: a study of ninety-two patients. Muscle Nerve 1998;21(5):610–617.

106. Deconinck N, Van Parijs V, Beckers-Bleukx G, Van den Bergh P. Critical illness myopathy unrelated to corticosteroids or neuromuscular blocking agents. Neuromuscul Disord 1998;8(3-4):186–192.

107. Wijdicks EF. Neurologic complications in critically ill patients. Anesth Analg 1996;83(2):411–419.

108. Bolton CF, Young GB, Zochodne DW. The neurological complications of sepsis. Ann Neurol 1993;33(1):94–100.

109. Douglass JA, Tuxen DV, Horne M, Scheinkestel CD, Weinmann M, Czarny D, et al. Myopathy in severe asthma. Am Rev Respir Dis 1992;146(2):517–519.

110. Gooch JL. AAEM case report #29: Prolonged paralysis after neuromuscular blockade. Muscle Nerve 1995;18(9):937–942.

111. Waclawik AJ, Sufit RL, Beinlich BR, Schutta HS. Acute myopathy with selective degeneration of myosin filaments following status asthmaticus treated with methylprednisolone and vecuronium. Neuromuscul Disord 1992;2(1):19–26.

112. Hirano M, Ott BR, Raps EC, Minetti C, Lennihan L, Libbey NP, et al. Acute quadriplegic myopathy: a complication of treatment with steroids, nondepolarizing blocking agents, or both. Neurology 1992;42(11):2082–2087.

113. Perea M, Picon M, Miro O, Orus J, Roig E, Grau JM. Acute quadriplegic myopathy with loss of thick (myosin) filaments following heart transplantation. J Heart Lung Transplant 2001;20(10):1136–1141.

114. Gorson KC, Ropper AH. Generalized paralysis in the intensive care unit: emphasis on the complications of neuromuscular blocking agents and corticosteroids. J Intensive Care Med 1996:219–231.

115. Kauhanen S, Leivo I, Michelsson JE. Early muscle changes after immobilization. An experimental study on muscle damage. Clin Orthop Rel Res 1993(297):44–50.

116. Riley DA, Ilyina-Kakueva EI, Ellis S, Bain JL, Slocum GR, Sedlak FR. Skeletal muscle fiber, nerve, and blood vessel breakdown in space-flown rats. FASEB J 1990;4(1):84–91.

117. Baldwin KM, Herrick RE, Ilyina-Kakueva E, Oganov VS. Effects of zero gravity on myofibril content and isomyosin distribution in rodent skeletal muscle. FASEB J 1990;4(1):79–83.

118. Winkelman C. Inactivity and inflammation: selected cytokines as biologic mediators in muscle dysfunction during critical illness. AACN Clin Issues 2004;15(1):74–82.

119. Tawa N, Goldberg AL. Protein and amino acid metabolism in muscle. In: Engel AG, ed. Myology. New York: McGraw-Hill; 1994:683–707.

120. Mansoor O, Beaufrere B, Boirie Y, Ralliere C, Taillandier D, Aurousseau E, et al. Increased mRNA levels for components of the lysosomal, Ca^{2+}-activated, and ATP-ubiquitin–dependent proteolytic pathways in skeletal muscle from head trauma patients. Proc Natl Acad Sci USA 1996;93(7):2714–2718.

121. Goll DE, Thompson VF, Taylor RG, Christiansen JA. Role of the calpain system in muscle growth. Biochimie 1992;74(3):225–237.

122. Stibler H, Edstrom L, Ahlbeck K, Remahl S, Ansved T. Electrophoretic determination of the myosin/actin ratio in the diagnosis of critical illness myopathy. Intensive Care Med 2003;29(9):1515–1527.

123. Di Giovanni S, Molon A, Broccolini A, Melcon G, Mirabella M, Hoffman EP, et al. Constitutive activation of MAPK cascade in acute quadriplegic myopathy. Ann Neurol 2004;55(2):195–206.

124. Di Giovanni S, Mirabella M, D'Amico A, Tonali P, Servidei S. Apoptotic features accompany acute quadriplegic myopathy. Neurology 2000;55(6):854–858.

125. Rich MM, Teener JW, Raps EC, Schotland DL, Bird SJ. Muscle is electrically inexcitable in acute quadriplegic myopathy. Neurology 1996;46(3):731–736.

126. Bolton CF. Electrophysiologic studies of critically ill patients. Muscle Nerve 1987;10(2):129–135.

127. al-Lozi MT, Pestronk A, Yee WC, Flaris N, Cooper J. Rapidly evolving myopathy with myosin-deficient muscle fibers. Ann Neurol 1994;35(3): 273–29.

128. Danon MJ, Carpenter S. Myopathy with thick filament (myosin) loss following prolonged paralysis with vecuronium during steroid treatment. Muscle Nerve 1991;14(11):1131–1139.

129. Showalter CJ, Engel AG. Acute quadriplegic myopathy: analysis of myosin isoforms and evidence for calpain-mediated proteolysis. Muscle Nerve 1997;20(3):316–322.

130. Zochodne DW, Ramsay DA, Saly V, Shelley S, Moffatt S. Acute necrotizing myopathy of intensive care: electrophysiological studies. Muscle Nerve 1994;17(3):285–292.

131. Sander HW, Golden M, Danon MJ. Quadriplegic areflexic ICU illness: selective thick filament loss and normal nerve histology. Muscle Nerve 2002;26(4):499–505.

132. Griffiths RD, Palmer TE, Helliwell T, MacLennan P, MacMillan RR. Effect of passive stretching on the wasting of muscle in the critically ill. Nutrition 1995;11(5):428–432.

133. Gibson JN, Smith K, Rennie MJ. Prevention of disuse muscle atrophy by means of electrical stimulation: maintenance of protein synthesis. Lancet 1988;2(8614):767–770.

134. Goodman MN, del Pilar Gomez M. Decreased myofibrillar proteolysis after refeeding requires dietary protein or amino acids. Am J Physiol 1987;253(1 Pt 1):E52–E58.

135. Wilmore DW. Catabolic illness. Strategies for enhancing recovery. N Engl J Med 1991;325(10):695–702.

136. Lopes J, Russell DM, Whitwell J, Jeejeebhoy KN. Skeletal muscle function in malnutrition. Am J Clin Nutr 1982;36(4):602–610.

137. Streat SJ, Beddoe AH, Hill GL. Aggressive nutritional support does not prevent protein loss despite fat gain in septic intensive care patients. J Trauma 1987;27(3):262–266.

138. Wernerman J, von der Decken A, Vinnars E. Protein synthesis in skeletal muscle in relation to nitrogen balance after abdominal surgery: the effect of total parenteral nutrition. JPEN J Parenter Enteral Nutr 1986;10(6):578–582.

139. Griffiths RD, Jones C, Palmer TE. Outcome of nutrition therapies in the intensive care unit. Nutrition 1995;11(2 Suppl):224–228.

140. Evans AB, Al-Himyary AJ, Hrovat MI, Pappagianopoulos P, Wain JC, Ginns LC, et al. Abnormal skeletal muscle oxidative capacity after lung transplantation by 31P-MRS. Am J Respir Crit Care Med 1997; 155(2):615–621.

141. Wang XN, Williams TJ, McKenna MJ, Li JL, Fraser SF, Side EA, et al. Skeletal muscle oxidative capacity, fiber type, and metabolites after lung transplantation. Am J Respir Crit Care Med 1999;160(1):57–63.

142. Herridge MS, Cheung AM, Tansey CM, Matte-Martyn A, Diaz-Granados N, Al-Saidi F, et al. One-year outcomes in survivors of the acute respiratory distress syndrome. N Engl J Med 2003;348(8):683–693.

143. Munsat TL. International SMA Collaboration. Neuromuscul Disord 1991;1(2):81.

Index